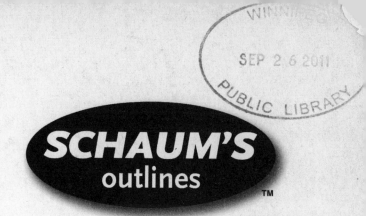

SCHAUM'S
outlines
™

Psychiatric Nursing

SCHAUM'S
outlines

Psychiatric Nursing

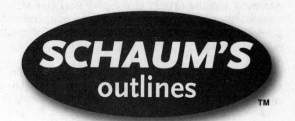

Psychiatric Nursing

Daminga Bynum-Grant

Psychiatric and Mental Health Nurse
Adjunct Professor, Pace University,
Dorothea Hopfer School of Nursing, and
Westchester Community College

Margaret M. Travis-Dinkins

Psychiatric and Mental Health Nurse
Adjunct Professor, Pace University and
Westchester Community College

Schaum's Outline Series

New York   Chicago   San Francisco   Lisbon   London   Madrid
Mexico City   Milan   New Delhi   San Juan   Seoul
Singapore   Sydney   Toronto

DAMINGA BYNUM-GRANT received her BSN from Molloy College in 1982 and her MS in Nursing Education from Mercy College in 2006. She is currently an adjunct nursing professor and clinical nurse educator at Pace University, Dorothea Hopfer School of Nursing, and Westchester Community College, and is a practicing psychiatric and mental health nurse at a large teaching hospital.

MARGARET M. TRAVIS-DINKINS received her BSN from Mount Saint Mary College in 1982 and her MSN in Nursing Education from Walden University in 2007. She is currently an adjunct professor and clinical nurse educator at Pace University and Westchester Community College, and is a practicing psychiatric and mental health nurse at a large teaching hospital.

Schaum's Outline of
PSYCHIATRIC NURSING

1 2 3 4 5 6 7 8 9 10 ROV/ROV 1 9 8 7 6 5 4 3 2 1 0

ISBN: 978-0-07-162364-3
MHID: 0-07-162364-7

Library of Congress Cataloging-in-Publication Data

Bynum-Grant, Daminga.
Schaum's outline of psychiatric nursing / Daminga Bynum-Grant, Margaret Travis-Dinkins.
    p. ; cm. – (Schaum's outlines)
  Other title: Outline of psychiatric nursing
  ISBN 0-07-162364-7 (alk. paper)
  1. Psychiatric nursing—Outlines, syllabi, etc. I. Travis-Dinkins, Margaret. II. Title. III. Title: Outline of psychiatric nursing.
IV. Series: Schaum's outline series.
  [DNLM: 1. Psychiatric Nursing—Examination Questions. 2. Psychiatric Nursing—Outlines. 3. Mental Disorders—nursing—Examination Questions. 4. Mental Disorders—nursing—Outlines. WY 18.2 B994s 2011]

  RC440.B96 2011
  616.89'0231—dc22   2010022228

Contents

Acknowledgments

This text would not have been possible if not for the unconditional love of my parents, Gertrude and Roosevelt Bynum. They instilled in me from the time I entered kindergarten, the importance of education. I'd also like to thank my very supportive siblings, Katina, Carmena, and Darryl Bynum, who provided me with much needed support throughout this endeavor, and my very understanding and tolerant sons, Brandon and Harrison. Lastly, thank you Margie for your belief and confidence in our abilities.

DAMINGA BYNUM-GRANT

Though this certainly was a labor of love, I do need to extend my appreciation and gratitude to my wonderful parents (Peg and Larry Travis), my sons (Willie and Travis), and a special thanks to my rock, voice of reason, and forever supporter, my dear husband Willie.

MARGARET TRAVIS-DINKINS

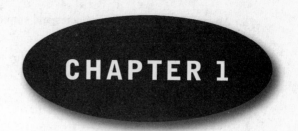

Foundations of Psychiatric Nursing

1.1 The Mental Illness–Mental Health Continuum

The study of the nursing profession, in general, is an exciting and challenging experience. Entering the realm of psychiatric nursing typically results in even more excitement, dubiety, apprehension, and self-doubt. The concepts of mental health and illness are difficult to define specifically. In general, we identify that those individuals who are able to function and fulfill their roles in the community while exhibiting appropriate and adaptive behaviors as mentally healthy. In contrast, those who have failed to effectively and efficiently perform in society or who demonstrate indecorous behaviors are described as mentally ill. Cultural awareness and embracing concepts of ethnic diversity are important considerations in assessing where on the continuum a person may fall. Many cultures conflict in their definition of acceptable behavior. Therefore, it is essential that the nurse be proficient in acknowledging cultural differences.

Mental Health

There are various reports defining mental health. We will refer to the perception of mental health being psychical well-being with acceptable adjustment to society and the customary demands of life. In consideration of the spectrum of mental health and mental illness, it is apparent that mental health encompasses more than the absence of illness. Individuals that are mentally healthy are able to engage in positive interpersonal relationships; communicate effectively and efficiently; demonstrate reality-based thinking; and exhibit self-awareness, an accepting self-image, and self esteem. Overall, they hold the ability to cope adaptively to everyday stress and issues, have the ability to find joy in life, employ resiliency, experience life harmony, embrace flexibility, and enjoy self-actualization. When their ability to deal effectively falters, persons who are mentally healthy are able to identify this vulnerability and seek appropriate assistance. The National Mental Health Association cites 10 characteristics of people who are mentally healthy (see Figure 1-1). They are as follows:

1. Exhibits a positive self-image
2. Are able to maintain control of their emotional responses (fear, anger, love, jealousy, guilt, or anxiety)
3. Are able to enter and maintain positive, fulfilling, and lasting interpersonal relationships
4. Are able to relate to and experience feelings of comfort in dealing with others
5. Are equipped to find humor in self and with others
6. Experience positive self-regard and respect of others, even in diversity
7. Are able to effectively manage life disappointments

8. Are able to meet life's exigencies and employ effective coping skills in addressing problems
9. Demonstrate self-determination
10. Influence environment as able and display adjustability when needed

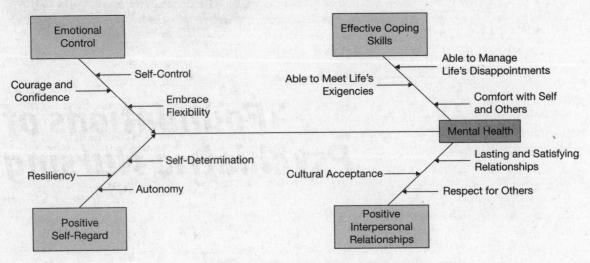

Figure 1-1 Mental health diagram.

The determination of mental health for a child or adolescent includes the attainment of scheduled developmental, cognitive, social, and emotional milestones and the ability to develop secure attachments, satisfying social relationships, and effective coping skills.

Mental Illness

In the United States, mental disorders are diagnosed based on the *Diagnostic and Statistical Manual of Mental Disorders, Fourth Edition (DSM-IV)*. The concept of mental illness is beleaguered with many myths and false impressions. Historically, the presence of a mental illness was attributed to those who exhibited behaviors that were perceived as "weird," "strange," or "odd." Hindsight demonstrates that this characterization of a person demonstrating behaviors not conducive to society's norms cannot, and should not, be used in determining the presence of a psychiatric disorder. Using these criteria would significantly impact the works of innovative and progressive individuals. Instead, mental illness is considered a condition in which a person with emotional or behavioral impairments experiences difficulty in activities of:

- Daily living
- Acceptable social demeanor
- Alteration in cognition

Any of the above may be caused by:

- Social factors
- Psychological factors
- Biochemical factors
- Genetic factors
- Health-related factors such as infection or head trauma

Mental illnesses are medical disorders that result in disruptions in an individual's cognition, emotions, interpersonal skills, and activities of daily living. The American Psychiatric Association defines a mental disorder as "a clinically significant behavioral or psychological syndrome or pattern that occurs in an individual and that is associated with present distress, disability, or with a significantly increased risk of suffering death, pain, disability, or an important loss of freedom." Comparable to the impact of a medical condition on the physical functioning of the human body, mental disorders negatively influence the ability to cope effectively with the demands of every-day living. Psychiatric conditions occur across the life span regardless of gender, ethnicity, religious preference, or financial position. The profession's definition of mental illness has changed over time as well. Prior to 1973, homosexuality was a diagnosis in the *Diagnostic and Statistical Manual of Mental Disorder.*

1.2 Epidemiology of Mental Health Disorders

Epidemiology of mental health disorders is the study of the incidence and prevalence of mental illness in the population to provide important indications related to the cause of the disorders. That allows for the identification of high-risk individual and factors, ranging from demographic factors to biological risks. There are two measures of prevalence:

1. *Clinical prevalence*—Identifies how many people who seek out mental health services actually suffer from mental illness.
2. *Actual prevalence*—Measures the percentage of people who suffer from mental illness in all of society.

This information can enable appropriate assessments and interventions to decrease the possible impact of the disease. *The DSM-IV-TR* includes the results of epidemiological studies to provide occurrence consequences. This information is helpful in dissecting the frequency of concurrent symptoms. More specifically, clinical epidemiology is a field that studies the natural history of an illness, diagnostic screening assessments, and observational and experimental examination of actions employed in the treatment of individuals experiencing symptoms or the disease. It is much simpler to study clinical than actual prevalence, but the actual prevalence is the area in which epidemiologists are most interested.

Psychiatric illness occurs in an estimated 26.2 percent of Americans ages 18 and older. About one in four adults suffer from a diagnosable mental disorder in a given year. In respect to the 2004 United States Census of residential population of individuals aged 18 and over, this calculates to 57.7 million people. Though mental disorders are widespread in the population, the main burden of illness is concentrated in a much smaller proportion—about 6 percent, or 1 in 17—who suffer from a serious mental illness, and many people suffer from more than one mental disorder at a given time. Nearly half (45 percent) of those with any mental disorder meet criteria for two or more disorders, with severity strongly related to comorbidity. The leading cause of disability in the United States, Canada, and other developed countries for ages 15 to 44 are mental disorders. The prevalence of selected psychiatric disorders occurring in the United States is shown in Table 1-1.

PSYCHIATRIC DISORDER	PREVALENCE	MEDIAN AGE OF ONSET	SPECIAL NOTATIONS
Mood disorders	20.9 million American adults (9.5%)	30 years	Women are affected twice as often as men.
Major depressive disorder (MDD)	14.8 million American adults (6.7%)	32 years	Often occurs with individuals diagnosed with anxiety disorders and substance abuse issues.
Dysthymic disorder	3.3 million American adults (1.5%)	31 years	
Bipolar disorder	5.7 million American adults (2.6%)	25 years	
Schizophrenia	2.4 million American adults (1.1%)	Males—late teens to early 20s Females—20s to early 30s	Affects men and women with equal frequency.

(Continued...)

PSYCHIATRIC DISORDER	PREVALENCE	MEDIAN AGE OF ONSET	SPECIAL NOTATIONS
Anxiety disorders	40 million American adults (18.1%) Anxiety disorders occur co-morbidly with depressive disorders, and substance abuse, and most often individuals have another anxiety disorder.	21.5 years	Anxiety disorders frequently occur with depressive disorders, eating disorders, and substance abuse.
Panic disorder	6 million American adults (2.7%)	Early adulthood but can extend throughout adulthood.	Generally occurs in adolescence or early adulthood. Approximately 1 in 3 individuals with panic disorder develop agoraphobia.
Obsessive-compulsive disorder (OCD)	2.2 million American adults (1.0%)	19 years	First symptoms typically occur in childhood or early adolescence.
Post-traumatic stress disorder (PTSD)	7.7 million American adults (3.5%) 19% of Vietnam Veterans experienced PTSD	Can develop at any age; median is 23 years.	Can develop at any age. About 30% of Vietnam veterans experienced PTSD postwar. High percentage of first responders to 9/11/01 terrorist attack in the United States experienced PTSD.
Generalized anxiety disorder (GAD)	6.8 million American adults (3.1%)	31 years	Can begin throughout the life span.
Social phobia	15 million American adults (6.8%)	13 years	Typically begins in childhood or adolescence.
Attention deficit hyperactivity disorder (ADHD)	(4.1%)	7 years	Usually becomes evident in preschool or early elementary years. One of the most common mental disorders in children and adolescents.
Autism	3.4 cases per 1000 children	Develops in childhood and generally diagnosed by age three.	Four times more common in males than females, although females diagnosed tend to have more severe symptoms with greater cognitive impairment.
Alzheimer's disease	4.5 million American adults	Most exhibit symptoms after age 65; however, it can occur as early as the 30s (rare).	The number of Americans diagnosed has doubled since 1980. Increasing age is the greatest risk factor. From the time of diagnosis, survival rate is half.

Data from National Institute of Mental Health. (2001; updated June 2008). *The numbers count: Mental disorders in America* (NIH Publication no.01–4584). Retrieved January 24, 2009 from the Web site www.nimh.nih.gov/health/publications/the-numbers-count-mental-disorders-in-america.shtml.

1.3 Cultural Considerations

The greatest influence of an individual's health-care beliefs and practices is culture. While Western medicine generally relies on a biochemical explanation of disease and illness, non-Western cultures have two prevalent types of beliefs regarding the etiology of illness:

- *Personalistic belief*—Identifies the cause to the intervention of an outside agent (spirit, deity, force, etc.).
- *Naturalistic belief*—Considers the illness is a result of elements such as cold, heat, wind, wetness, and so on.

Awareness of this difference in etiological belief is essential for the nurse to consider in relation to compliance with treatment modalities. Cultural competence is essential in ensuring that our approach in mental health treatment is aligned with the patient's beliefs. The nurse is charged with investigating cultural values, beliefs, and practices in the population served. While such information can be found in texts and journals, to ensure accuracy and individual care, it is recommended that the nurse obtain this information directly from the patient/family. The inclusion of a cultural assessment is paramount in the assessment phase.

Understanding the lived experiences of patients will allow health-care staff to remember that experiences of racism can be a major factor influencing the perception and use of health services for many people from ethnic minorities. An open and objective approach to patients is essential in the development and maintenance of the therapeutic relationship. There are several basic tenets that should be adhered to regarding the provision of culturally competent care:

Patients and Family

- To be treated with respect
- To be interviewed by staff with relevant language skills, or accompanied by an interpreter
- To be encouraged to explain their views, and to have the views of the doctor explained to them

Clinicians

- To understand issues of racism and stigma in relation to the mental health of ethnic minority groups
- To be aware of, and be instructed in, the cultural norms and religious beliefs of the main ethnic groups consulting them
- To elicit and attempt to understand the explanatory models of illness used by their patients, and to consider the value of traditional healing methods

Ethnic Minority Groups

- To be provided with information about Western concepts of mental illness and its treatments
- To be consulted and involved in developing services
- To be encouraged to join patient support and advocacy groups

Given the multicultural nature of many communities, it is critical that nurses understand how culture can influence diagnosis and treatment and affects how an individual defines health and illness, including the meanings of specific physical and psychological sensations. Nurses should strive to surpass the designated illness and address the patient's individual needs. To accomplish this aspect of care, the nurse must ensure cultural competence. With the high number of ethno-cultural groups, it is impossible to address each individually. This chapter will identify some considerations of importance, but individual research is encouraged to increase familiarity with the characteristics and customs aligned with specific geographical areas.

Each culture provides ways of explaining mental illness, answering questions about why, and under what circumstances, someone becomes mentally ill. Western cultures place emphasis on psychological factors, life events, and the effects of stress; while in many parts of the Third World, explanations of mental illness take into account wider social and religious factors, such as:

- Spirit possession
- Witchcraft
- Breaking of religious taboos
- Divine retribution
- Capture of the soul by a spirit

These factors need to be considered to improve the goal of patient/family compliance. For example, taking prescribed medication may not make sense to a patient who feels that the behaviors are a result of a nonbiological etiology.

Culture-bound syndrome has been included in the current *Diagnostic and Statistical Manual of Mental Disorders* to define a combination of psychiatric and somatic symptoms recognized only within specific societies or cultures. Western medicine focuses on the etiology of mental disorders as biological; however, this approach does not allow for the impact of the social environment on psychiatric problems. Although these disorders are not recognized in other cultures, it is essential that mental health clinicians at least consider how such clinical situations may influence assessment and treatment.

The following lists are examples of culture-bound syndromes adapted from lists provided in the *DSM-IV-TR*:

- *Amok* (origin is Malaysia)—A spree of sudden violent attacks on people, animals, or property affecting men in Malaysia. The common saying of "running amok" stems from this syndrome.
- *Koro* (origins are China, Malaysia, and Indonesia)— Also referred to as genital retraction syndrome, a belief that the penis is shrinking into the abdomen. Though this can occur in females, it is much rarer.
- *Evil eye*—A belief among Latin Americans that illness is caused by the stare of a jealous person.
- *Susto*—A belief in Latin America in the loss of the soul.
- *Latah*—Syndrome of increased suggestibility and imitative behavior found in Southeast Asia. Typically occurring in middle-aged females, this phenomenon evidences itself subsequent to the person being startled. The individual, instead of regaining composure after a couple seconds, experiences a lengthened response of screaming, increased psychomotor activity, and the mimicking of others' behaviors.

1.4 Theoretical Models of Personality Development

To increase one's understanding of maladaptive behaviors exhibited in psychiatric disorders, one must have a basic understanding of the human personality development. There are various developmental theories which assign behaviors to life span stages. Recognizing these expected behaviors allows for determination of appropriateness for the specific developmental level. Many child development specialists hold the belief that the origin and occurrence of developmental change happen within infancy and early childhood. The developmental stages are defined by age, allowing for the ability to determine if one's behaviors are age-appropriate.

Psychoanalytic Theory

Sigmund Freud, recognized as the father of psychiatry, was the first to identify an individual's development in stages, believing that a person's basic character is formed by the age of five (see Figure 1-2). He revolutionized approaches to mental health disorders by introducing his ideas about the development of the personality, awareness levels, anxiety, ego defense mechanisms, and stages of psychosexual development.

He believed that the basic structure of the personality is composed of three parts:

- *The id*—The center of instinctual drives that is present from birth. Referred to as the "pleasure principle," behaviors driven by the id are impulsive and can be irrational.

- *The ego*—The rational self, or the "reality principle." Beginning development from ages four to six, it experiences the reality of the external world, adapts to it, and responds in kind. The ego's primary function is to mediate the external world, the id, and the superego.
- *The superego*—The "perfection principle." Developing between the ages three and six, there is an internalization of values and morals learned from caregivers.

AGE	STAGE	MAJOR DEVELOPMENTAL TASK
Birth-18 months	ORAL	Relief from anxiety through oral gratification of needs
18 months-3 years	ANAL	Learning independence and control with a focus on the excretory function
3-6 years	PHALLIC	Identification with the parent of same sex; the development of sexual identity; focus on genitial organs
6-12 years	LATENCY	Sexuality is repressed; focus on relationships with same-sex peers
13-20 years	GENITAL	The libido is reawakened as the genital organs mature; opposite-sex relationships get focus

Figure 1-2 Freud's stages of psychosexual development.

Interpersonal Theory

Harry Stack Sullivan, the first American theorist to develop a comprehensive personality theory which believed that development of the personality occurred within the context of the social group, initially followed Freud's theory. His perception of the development of the personality only began gaining popularity since his death in 1949 (see Figure 1-3 for the main concepts).

ANXIETY	A contagious entity that we learn from our caregivers. The main motive force of personality is the avoidance and reduction of anxiety. Sullivan believed that anxiety is the "chief disruptive force in interpersonal relationships and a main factor in the development of serious difficulties in living"
SATISFACTION OF NEEDS	Attainment of all physical, psychosocial requirements of an individual - anything that when not fulfilled will cause discomfort
INTERPERSONAL SECURITY	Feelings experienced with relief from anxiety; sense of whole well-being
SELF-SYSTEM	The collection of lived or security measures embraced by an individual as protection against anxiety. Comprised of 3 components: 1. "good me" - personality developed in response to positive feedback from primary caregiver 2. "bad me" - part of the personality developed in response to negative feedback elicited from the primary careprovider 3. "not me"- part of the personality developed in response to events that resulted in intense anxiety in the child

Figure 1-3 Sullivan's interpersonal theory of main concepts.

Stack embraced the belief that the goal of all human behavior is to achieve needs through interpersonal interactions, and to decrease or avoid anxiety. Consideration and understanding of this theory has a particular influence on psychiatric and mental health nursing. Sullivan's theory is the building block for Hildegard Peplau's nursing theory of interpersonal relationships. Core elements of both theories include the following:

- Mutuality
- Respect
- Acceptance
- Empathy
- Presence

The establishment of this therapeutic and positive relationship with patients (individual, family, or community) is a primary intervention for the behavioral health nurse. The goal is for the patient to develop skills needed to interact successfully with others. Gaining an understanding of behaviors resulting from anxiety experiences, as well as appropriate nursing actions for relieving the discomfort associated with anxiety, allows the nurse to assist his or her clients to achieve more independence and be higher functioning interpersonally. (See Figure 1-4 for Sullivan's stages of personality development.)

INFANCY: BIRTH-18 MONTHS	Major developmental task is gratification of needs. Accomplished by oral activities (crying, sucking, etc.)
CHILDHOOD: 18 MONTHS-6 YEARS	Learning that interference with wishes/goals may result in delayed gratification. Parental approval may be associated with managing delayed gratification appropriately, making this acceptable and bringing comfort. Tools used: mouth, anus, language, experimentation, manipulation, and identificaton
JUVENILE: 6-9 YEARS	Major task is establishing positive relationships within the peer group. Tools used: competition, cooperation, compromise.
PREADOLESCENCE: 9-12 YEARS	Task is developing same-sex relationships. Tools used: ability to collaborate, demonstrate love and affection for another.
EARLY ADOLESCENCE: 12-14 YEARS	Development of individuality from parents. Major task is establishing opposite-sex relationships. Major focus: emergence of lust in response to biological changes
LATE ADOLESCENCE: 14-21 YEARS	Characterized by tasks related to achieving interdependence in society and the ability to form a lasting, intimate relationship with a member of the opposite-sex. Major focus are the genital organs.

Figure 1-4 Sullivan's stages of personality development.

Erikson's Ego Theory

Although Erik Erikson, a psychoanalyst, also accepted Freud's theory, he focused on the role of the ego, emphasizing that a person's progression as self has more contributing to it than merely the parent-child relationship. He believed that society had a significant impact on the development of the personality. His model addresses the entire life span and, differing from Freud, does not preclude corrective measures past the age of five (see Figure 1-5).

AGE	STAGE	DEVELOPMENTAL TASK
INFANCY: BIRTH-18 MONTHS	TRUST vs MISTRUST	Establish trust in mothering figure, develops trust in others as result
EARLY CHILDHOOD: 18 MONTHS-3 YEARS	AUTONOMY vs SHAME and DOUBT	Gain self-control and environmental independence
LATE CHILDHOOD: 3-6 YEARS	INITIATIVE vs GUILT	Develop purposefulness, directiveness
SCHOOL AGE: 6-12 YEARS	INDUSTRY vs INFERIORITY	Gain self-confidence through development of social, physical, and school-based skills
ADOLESCENCE: 12-20 YEARS	IDENTITY vs ROLE CONFUSION	Develop a sense of individuality and identity, transition from child to adult
EARLY/YOUNG ADULTHOOD: 20-30 YEARS	INTIMACY vs ISOLATION	Establish intimate relationships, enable commitment to persons, ideals, causes
MIDDLE ADULTHOOD: 30-65 YEARS	GENERATIVITY vs STAGNATION	Achievement of family, career, societal life goals, focus on the future generation
OLD AGE: 65-DEATH	EGO INTEGRITY vs DESPAIR	Evaluation of life's paths chosen with acceptance, resulting in a positive self-assessment

Figure 1-5 Erikson's developmental model.

Erikson's developmental model is applied in the assessments of the nurse. Analysis of behavior patterns using this theory assists in identifying the individual's development of interpersonal skills and allows determination of appropriateness in response. It is common that persons with mental illness experience difficulty mastering developmental tasks.

Humanistic Theories

Humanistic theories differ from the psychoanalytical perspective in that the focus is on freedom to choose your own behavior, rather than reacting to environmental stimuli and reinforcements. Issues dealing with self-esteem, self-fulfillment, and needs are dominant, the goal being self-actualization. The major focus is to facilitate personal development. Carl Rogers and Abraham Maslow are the most recognized humanistic theorists.

Abraham Maslow developed the theory of human motivation, known as Maslow's Hierarchy of Needs. A psychologist, Maslow noted that some human needs were more powerful than others. He divided those needs into five general categories, from most urgent to most enlightened:

- Physiological
- Safety
- Belonging/love
- Esteem
- Self-actualization

The nursing profession embraces this theory both for its reflection on the importance of an individual's strengths in the establishment of the therapeutic relationship and for its driving force in determining the prioritization of care (see Figure 1-6). Paramount is the provision of basic physiologic needs (air, food, water, oxygen, rest, elimination) and then safety (limits, security, protection, structure, and stability). Once these have been met, work can begin on higher-functioning needs.

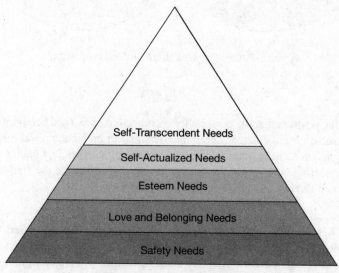

Maslow's Hierachy of Needs

(adapted from Maslow, A.H. (1972). *The farther reaches of human nature.* NY: Viking.)

Figure 1-6

Carl Rogers

Carl Rogers expressed a similar belief to that of Maslow, except that he expanded his focus past human beings, applying his theoretical ideals to all living creatures, even the ecosystem. His theory is built on a single concept he calls "the actualizing tendency." This concept embraces the consideration that innate to every life-form is the provocation to develop its potentials to the fullest extent possible. As opposed to the survival instinct, Rogers believes that more than just to live, all creatures strive to make the very best of their existence.

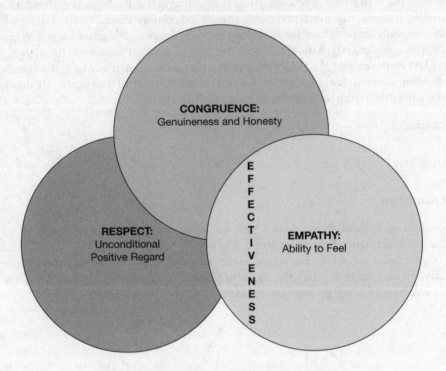

Carl Rogers is best known for his contributions to therapy. His experiences as a therapist led him to the use of the term "client-centered," which encompasses his belief that individuals are not looking for solutions from others, rather for a guide to determine the solutions inside of themselves. Rogers believed that to be effective, a therapist need only ensure three components in the relationship: congruence, respect, and empathy (see Figure 1-7). These same components are identified as essential in the establishment of the therapeutic relationship, and will be discussed at greater length in the second chapter.

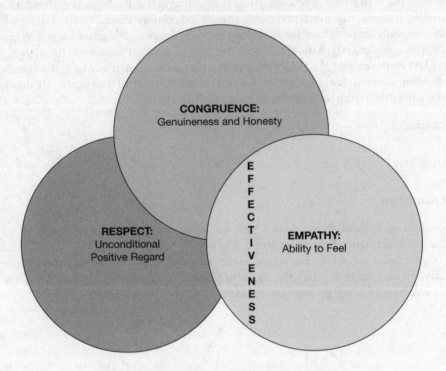

Figure 1-7 Carl Rogers: Therapist requirements.

Behavioral Theories

Behavioral models hold the position that the personality is composed of learned behaviors. The premise: change the behavior and the personality will change. These theories inspect how behavioral responses are learned and how to effect modifications on these learned behaviors. The three theorists that center on use of the intervention of conditioning (connecting behavior with a situation that will influence the frequency of its occurrence) we will review include Ivan Pavlov, John Watson, and B. F. Skinner.

Ivan Pavlov

Ivan Pavlov initialized behavioral models in the nineteenth century. As he studied the functioning of the salivary glands on canines, his interest grew to the causation of the salivation. He assigned the results of his study to a theory known as classic conditioning. He discovered that when a benign stimulus (bell) was associated with another stimulus (food), it resulted in his desired response from the dogs (salivation). Though his work was fixed on physiologic responses, it did lay the foundation for further research related to psychological responses.

John Watson

John Watson is considered to have developed behaviorism. He applied Pavlov's concepts to humans. He is most recognized for what is referred to as "The Little Albert Experience." Albert, the son of a wet nurse employed at the hospital, participated in this experiment at nine months. Watson and his assistant exposed Albert to a variety of situations, none which elicited fear. At 11 months, Watson began making a loud noise (unconditioned stimulus) when he was in sight of one previously neutral stimulus, eliciting a fear response (unconditioned response).

Ultimately, merely the loud noise (unconditioned stimulus) produced the fear (unconditioned response). (Make note of this event for the future discussions regarding ethics.)

B. F. Skinner

B. F. Skinner's theory focuses on operant conditioning, the collusion of chosen reinforcers to elicit and strengthen desired behavioral responses. As the individual "operates" in his or her environment, the individual happens upon certain special stimuli or "reinforcers," which results in an increased chance of the behavior that occurred just before the stimulus. Positive reinforcement will encourage the operant behavior; negative reinforcement will deter the behavior.

How does this influence nursing practice? Behavioral modification is effective in children, adolescents, and adults with various mental illness diagnoses. This approach enables nurses to address maladaptive coping skills and assist individuals in the development and utilization of effective management capabilities.

1.5   Biological Theories

Biological causes of mental illness, like those of other diseases, must also be considered. The advent of psychotropic medication, specifically Chlorpromazine in 1950, provided a different path from psychodynamic approaches. Many other medications have been developed and recognized for their positive effect on the symptoms of psychiatric illnesses. The effectiveness of chemical interventions suggests that perhaps these behaviors are biological in occurrence. The biological model of psychiatric illness attempts to address the mind-body connection, and centers on the neurological, biological, chemical, and familial impact on an individual. The unusual behavioral responses to mental illness are viewed as symptoms, just as atypical findings are present in illnesses such as cardiac disease and endocrine disorders. These symptoms can be treated with medications. Most treatment providers encourage the use of both therapy and prescription medication for the best prognosis.

As the perspective of a biological influence progresses in the treatment of mental health issues, it is important to consider the implications for nursing. Basic interventions will remain unchanged: meeting the physical and psychosocial needs of patients. The concern arises if one allows the concept of a biological causation to negate one's personal responsibility and accountability for behavior and events. While nurses certainly need to convey unconditional acceptance, they must also strive to motivate treatment participation. A biological approach can also influence the perception of environmental, societal, cultural, spiritual, and interpersonal influence on the mental health–mental illness continuum. It would be a disservice for patients and their families if nursing staff did not consider all possible factors.

1.6   Historical Influences of Psychiatric Nursing

The first training for psychiatric nursing encompassed primarily custodial care. Strategies centered on nutrition, hygiene, and activity; however, as somatic therapies were introduced, the role of the psychiatric nurse broadened. Nurses adapted their knowledge of medical-surgical nursing techniques in conjunction with compassionate care to address the needs of the psychiatric patient.

Johns Hopkins was the first nursing school to include a course in psychiatric nursing in 1913, and the educational inclusion for experience in psychiatric nursing was formally included in school curriculum by the National League for Nursing in 1950. Harriet Bailey wrote the first psychiatric nursing textbook, *Nursing Mental Diseases*, which was published in 1920. (See Figure 1-8.)

The progression of psychiatric nursing practice continued with the development of standards of care by the American Nurses Association in 1973. These standards of care describe nursing practice responsibilities clinicians are accountable to follow. These professional standards are essential for the formalization of nursing approaches and considerations. Adherence ensures safe practice, and may offer protection in legal circumstances by demonstrating safe techniques. To be considered legal requirements of practice, the standards must be introduced in the state's Nurse Practice Act or adopted by the state's Board of Nursing (BON). These standards depict the nursing process in psychiatric and mental health nursing.

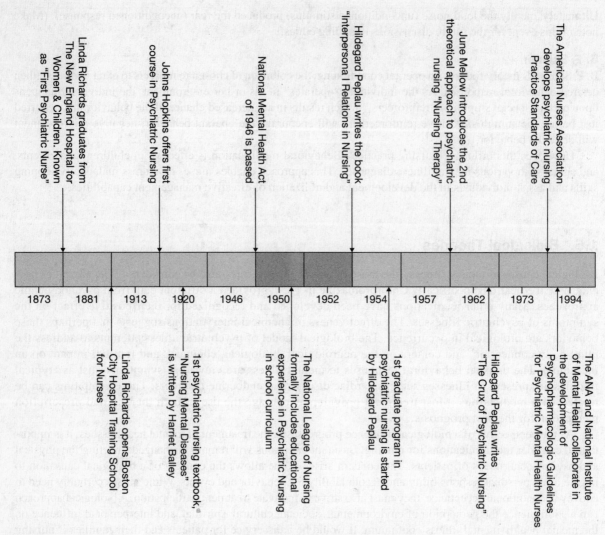

Figure 1-8 History of psychiatric nursing.

Nursing Theories

Many nursing theorists influenced the practice of nursing and of the psychiatric and mental health nurse. Jean Watson, Madeleine Leininger, Betty Neuman, and Martha Rogers all discussed the concept of caring as an essential component of nursing practice and how individuals relate within themselves and with their environment. Caring is an essential component in the establishment of the therapeutic relationship.

Mentioned earlier in the chapter, Hildegard Peplau is a pioneer of psychiatric and mental health nursing. She was influenced by the studies of Sullivan, developing the primary theoretical theory for psychiatric nursing in her publications *Interpersonal Relations in Nursing* (1952) and *The Crux of Psychiatric Nursing* (1962). She provided a foundation of the recognition of the importance in the care of psychiatrically ill individuals by focusing on the importance of the relationship between the care provider and the patient. Peplau coined the term "psychodynamic nursing," which means the nurse must understand his or her own attitudes and behaviors in order to guide the patient to identify and address his or her own problems.

The nurse assumes multiple roles in these interpersonal relationships with patients:

- *Counselor*—Working with the patient on current problems
- *Leader*—Working with the patient democratically
- *Surrogate*—Figuratively standing in for a person in the patient's life
- *Stranger*—Accepting the patient objectively
- *Resource person*—Interpreting the medical plan for the patient and explaining it to him or her
- *Teacher*—Offering information and helping the patient learn

STANDARDS OF PSYCHIATRIC MENTAL HEALTH CLINICAL NURSING PRACTICE

Standards of Care

Standard I. Assessment
The psychiatric-mental health nurse collects client health data

Standard II. Diagnosis
The psychiatric-mental health nurse analyzes the data in determining diagnoses

Standard III. Outcome Identification
The psychiatric-mental health nurse identifies expected outcomes individualized to the patient

Standard IV. Planning
The psychiatric-mental health nurse develops a plan of care that prescribes interventions to attain expected outcomes

Standard V. Implementation
The psychiatric-mental health nurse implements the interventions identified in the plan of care

Standard Va. Counseling
The psychiatric-mental health nurse uses counseling interventions to assist clients in improving or regaining their previous coping abilities, fostering mental health, and preventing mental illness and disability

Standard Vb. Milieu Therapy
The psychiatric-mental health nurse provides, structures, and maintains a therapeutic environment in collaboration with the client and other health care providers

Standard Vc. Self-Care Activities
The psychiatric-mental health nurse structures interventions around the client's activities of daily living to foster self-care and mental and physical well-being

Standard Vd. Psychobiologic Interventions
The psychiatric-mental health nurse uses knowledge of psychobiologic interventions and applies clinical skills to restore the client's health and prevent further disabilities

Standard Ve. Health Teaching
The psychiatric-mental health nurse, through health teaching, assists the clients in achieving satisfying, productive, and healthy patterns of living

Standard Vf. Case Management
The psychiatric-mental health nurse provides case management to coordinate comprehensive health services and ensure continuity of care

Standard Vg. Health Promotion and Maintenance
The psychiatric-mental health nurse employs strategies and interventions to promote and maintain mental health and prevent mental illness. (Interventions Vh-Vj are advanced practice interventions and may only be performed by clinical nurse specialist or psychiatric nurse practitioner (prescriptive authority and treatment)

Standard VI. Evaluation
The psychiatric-mental health nurse evaluates the client's progress in attaining expected outcomes

STANDARDS OF PROFESSIONAL PERFORMANCE

Standard I. Quality of Care
The psychiatric-mental health nurse systematically evaluates the quality of care and effectiveness of psychiatric-mental health nursing practice

Standard II. Performance Appraisal
The psychiatric-mental health nurse evaluates his/her own nursing practice in relation to professional practice standards and relevant statutes and regulations

Standard III. Education
The psychiatric-mental health nurse acquires and maintains current knowledge in nursing practice

Standard IV. Collegiality
The psychiatric-mental health nurse contributes to the professional development of peers, colleagues, and others

Standard V. Ethics
The psychiatric-mental health nurse's decisions and actions on behalf of others are determined in an ethical manner

Standard VI. Collaboration
The psychiatric-mental health nurse collaborates with the client, significant others, and health-care providers in providing care

Standard VII. Research
The psychiatric-mental health nurse contributes to nursing and mental health through the use of research

Standard VIII. Resource Utilization
The psychiatric-mental health nurse considers factors related to safety, effectiveness, and cost in planning and delivering client care

Hildegard Peplau also established a four-staged concept of the relationship development (see Figure 1-9). The main achievement in this concept is the idea that nurses should embrace caring in nursing through envisioning the patient as an individual, not a diagnosis or illness. Certainly a common consideration today, this principle was not well received in 1952 when first introduced.

ORIENTATION	Occurring during the **assessment phases** of the nursing process, it is during this stage the nurse and patient (individual, family, or community) identity, verify, and give meaning to the problem.
IDENTIFICATION	During the **planning phase** of the nursing process, this is the stage where the patient identifies who can assist in reaching the agreed upon goals. The nurse should help strengthen positive attributes of the personality. The patient may respond by working dependently, independently, or interdependently.
EXPLOITATION	During the **implementation phase** of the nursing process, this is the stage where the patient actively seeks and employs knowledge and expertise of caregivers in their quest towards wellness. The patient becomes an active participant in their care.
RESOLUTION	During the **evaluation phase** of the nursing process, this stage occurs when the patient is no longer reliant on the care of others. Having the strength and independence to provide self-care, resolution is the successful completion of the previous 3 stages. Termination of the nurse–patient relationship occurs at this point.

Figure 1-9 Phases of the nursing–patient relationship.

Another important nursing theory specific to psychiatric and mental health nursing is Roy's Adaptation Theory (after Sister Callista Roy). This model is based on consideration of the internal and external environmental stimuli affecting the development and behavior of the person. In applying this theory to practice, one assesses the individual's response to a stimulus and works with him or her to remove, improve, or maintain the cause.

Chapter 1 Questions

Matching

1. Birth to 18 months.

2. Failure to resolve developmental crisis; results in dissatisfaction with self and others; suspiciousness.

3. Successful resolution of a developmental crisis, which results in mastery of reliable work habits and the development of behaviors of trustworthiness.

4. Age 65 to death.

5. Failure to resolve crisis results in self-consciousness, doubt, and confusion over one's role.

6. A sense of personal and professional satisfaction, and concern for future generations.

7. Task is to achieve self-confidence by learning, competing, performing, and receiving recognition by others.

8. Sense of self-disappointment with life events. Presence of the emotions of anger, depression, and loneliness, resulting from perceived failures.

9. Ages 20 to 30.

A. Intimacy versus isolation

B. Industry

C. Generativity

D. Intimacy

E. Trust versus mistrust

F. Despair

G. Mistrust

H. Autonomy

I. Role confusion

10. Development of a sense of control and the ability to delay gratification.

11. Task is to inform a meaningful, intense, and lasting intimate relationships.

J. Ego integrity versus despair

K. Industry versus inferiority

Chapter 1 Answers

1. E
2. G
3. B
4. J
5. I
6. C

7. K
8. F
9. A
10. H
11. D

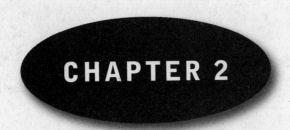

CHAPTER 2

Core Competencies in Psychiatric Nursing Practice

2.1 The Therapeutic Relationship

The therapeutic relationship is at the very core of nursing and is established using knowledge and skills, as well as by applying caring attitudes and behaviors. The nurse-client relationship differs from the social encounter in that unsuccessful or uncomfortable conversations do not come with an option to discontinue the relationship. Therapeutic relationships are goal oriented, directed toward learning and growth promotion to facilitate a change in the client's life. The therapeutic intention is to enter into a nurse-client relationship that encourages the client to use what the nurse has to offer for reparative and adaptive purposes. To accomplish this relationship, it is important to understand and embrace the behaviors that will assist in developing therapeutic relationships. Characteristics that will help to promote this growth and change in patients and that are valued for establishing a therapeutic relationship are as follows:

- *Genuineness*—A self-awareness of feelings experienced within the relationship and the ability to express these feelings when appropriate. It is the ability to use communication techniques in a relaxed and spontaneous manner rather than rigidly or parrotlike.
- *Empathy*—When one understands the ideas expressed by and the feelings that are present in the other person. It includes the following attributes:
  - Accurately perceiving the client's situation, perspectives, and feelings
  - Communicating one's understanding to the client and checking for accuracy
  - Acting on this understanding in a therapeutic way toward the client
- *Positive regard*—The ability to see another individual as worthy of being cared about and as someone who has strengths and achievement potential. Demonstrating respect to another typically is exhibited nonverbally.
  - Attitudes—Showing that this is "not just a job"
  - Actions—Being with the client, not being judgmental, facilitating the client's self-resolution

Nursing involves the formation of a meaningful relationship accomplished through the development of an effective interpersonal process. The clinician may take on various roles during the care of their client (teacher, counselor, socializing agent, liaison, etc.), but in a therapeutic relationship the focus is consistently on the client. Key to the development of this therapeutic relationship is effective communication techniques and understanding of the nurse-patient therapeutic relationship.

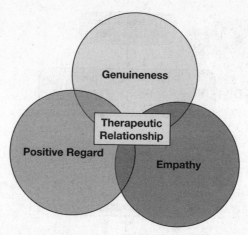

Figure 2-1 Phases of the therapeutic relationship.

Phases of the Therapeutic Relationship

Orientation Phase

1. A major emphasis during this phase is establishing trust. Trust is facilitated by the use of:
   A. Genuineness, empathy, positive regard
   B. Consistency, offering assistance in alleviating the clients problems or pain
2. Four essential issues are as follows:
   A. Parameters of the relationship—Who you are, what your role is, the purpose of the relationship.
   B. Formal or informal contract—Use of a contract demonstrates working with, not for, the client.
   C. Confidentiality—The client has the right to know what information will be shared, what information will not be shared, and with whom the information will be shared.
   D. Termination—Begins in the orientation phase and can be renegotiated as needed.

Working Phase

1. Specific tasks of this phase are as follows:
   A. Maintain the relationship.
   B. Gather further information.
   C. Promote the client's problem-solving skills, self-esteem, and use of language.
   D. Facilitate behavioral changes.
   E. Overcome resistance behaviors.
   F. Evaluate problems and goals; redefine as needed.
   G. Promote practice and expression of alternative adaptive behaviors.

Termination Phase

1. Reasons to terminate the therapeutic relationship
   A. Symptom relief
   B. Improved social functioning
   C. Increased sense of identity
   D. Development of adaptive behavior
   E. Achievement of goals
   F. Impasse in therapy—The nurse is unable to help the client further resolve issues.
   G. Forced termination—Completion of course, completion of employment, change in staff, client discharged due to financial issues (see Figure 2-2).

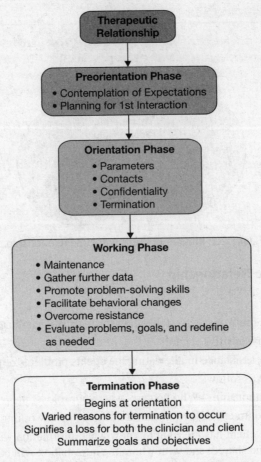

Figure 2-2 Phases of the therapeutic relationship.

Not all therapeutic relationships follow the guidelines in the textbooks. Sometimes they never progress past the orientation phase. Behaviors that facilitate the formation of a therapeutic relationship and those behaviors that function as debilitations are important to understand in order that health-care staff focus on the positive influences in fostering therapeutic relationships.

- Facilitators:
  1. Consistency
  2. Pacing
  3. Listening
  4. Initial impressions
  5. Comfort and control
  6. Client factors
- Debilitations:
  1. Inconsistency and unavailability
  2. The nurse's feelings and awareness

The development of the therapeutic relationship is necessary to allow the setting for the nurse to provide care for their clients. To facilitate the delivery of that care, the nurse needs to understand the interpersonal communication techniques and their role and its relationship in the care of that client. Verbal and nonverbal communication are tools used by caring professionals to assist the client in achieving his or her goals. To use this technique effectively, the nurse must be knowledgeable of therapeutic and nontherapeutic communication techniques, and skilled in their use.

Though generally focused on in the psychiatric setting, these skills are relevant to all practice areas.

2.2 Therapeutic Communication

The use of therapeutic communication techniques is a core requirement in the establishment of the therapeutic relationship. Our interactions must be clear, concise, and comprehensible. To accomplish these effects, we must understand the intricacy of communication. While there are many theories and recommendations focusing on communication, this review will include a basic theory of communication, *the transactional theory*, and common facilitations and barriers in interactions. It will also investigate the impact of nonverbal and paralanguage and discuss the importance of self-awareness in communication.

Transactional Model of Communication

Individuals communicate in many ways, as every word spoken and every action taken or not taken conveys a message to others. Communication is a process where a message is sent to one or more individuals. There are many models of communication. The transactional model involves face-to-face communication where verbal and nonverbal messages are sent and received simultaneously. Each participant mutually perceiving the other, and the participants are simultaneously engaged in the process of creating meaning in a relationship. In the analysis of the influences on communication, consideration is given to preexisting conditions, environment in which the communication occurs, and nonverbal communication, as follows:

Box 2-1: Influences on Communication

- **Preexisting conditions**
  1. Values
  2. Attitudes/beliefs
  3. Culture
  4. Knowledge
  5. Religion
  6. Gender
  7. Age/developmental level
  8. Social status

- **Environment**
  1. Territoriality
  2. Density
  3. Distance

- **Nonverbal communication**
  1. Dress and appearance
  2. Physical characteristics
  3. Kinesics and posture
  4. Touch
     A. Functional—Professionalism
     B. Social—Politeness
     C. Friendship—Warmth
     D. Love—Intimacy
     E. Sexual—Arousal
  5. Facial expression
  6. Eye behavior
  7. Paralanguage

The importance of socially skilled communication can never be undermined in the caring profession, and it is imperative that nursing education begin with and continue to advance the art of communication for effective practice. Ineffective communication continues to be a major issue in health care, with patients tending to be more dissatisfied with poor communication than with any other aspect of care. Studies have demonstrated that the use of effective communication and the establishment of therapeutic relationships produce greater satisfaction in perceived care by the patient, as well as in work conditions by the nurse.

Communication is both one of the most demanding and difficult aspects of a nurse's job and one which, although central to the quality of patient care, is frequently avoided or done badly. There are intervening variables that will influence communication in the therapeutic relationship. Knowledge of the principles of communication, ability to identify therapeutic and nontherapeutic techniques, and ability to perform these techniques is necessary in establishing positive rapport with the patients and enabling quality patient care. For example, the use of open-ended questions, rather than "yes" or "no," can help the clinician determine how well the patient understands the information given, facilitates the drawing out of additional information, and provides the clinician with relevant data.

It is important to recognize that communication with clients occurs at different levels. Nurses interact with patients using both phatic and therapeutic communication. All nurses use communication other than purely therapeutic techniques with their clients. This decreases the impersonal nature of therapeutic communication; however, if the interaction remains at that perceived social level, little if no formal communication can take place. Therefore, it is important to recognize that though nurses strive to use therapeutic techniques to facilitate information seeking/retrieving from patients, it is necessary to interject some "social talk."

Nurses use a variety of effective communication techniques and interpersonal strategies to appropriately establish, maintain, reestablish, and terminate the nurse-client relationship. Following are expected behaviors that the nurse demonstrates using therapeutic communication techniques:

- Introduces self to the client using name and title.
- Addresses the client by the name and title he or she prefers.
- Allows time, opportunity, and ability of the client to express him- or herself, and listens with the intent to understand and without diminishing the client's feelings or immediately giving advice.
- Informs the client that information will be shared with the health-care team, identifying who constitutes the team members.
- Is aware of verbal and nonverbal communication and the possible perception of the client.
- Modifies communication to meet the needs of the client.
- Assists the client in determining the best care solution by assessing the level of knowledge and discussing the client's beliefs and wishes.
- Considers the preference of the client, encourages his or her advocacy, and, if needed, becomes his or her advocate.
- Offers information to facilitate the client's ability to make an informed decision.
- Listens to, understands, and respects the client's values, options, needs, and ethno-cultural beliefs. Integrates these into the client's plan of care.
- Recognizes that behavior has meaning, and seeks to understand the cause of an unusual comment, attitude, or behavior.
- Listens to concerns of the family and significant others, and acts upon them when appropriate and consistent with the client's wishes.
- Refrains from self-disclosure unless it meets a specific, identified client need.
- Reflects on interactions with the client and the health-care team, investing time and effort to continually improve communication skills.
- Discusses throughout the therapeutic relationship ongoing needs after termination of this therapeutic relationship (discharge planning).

Therapeutic Communication Techniques

Following are techniques that foster communication between nurse and patient:

TECHNIQUE	RATIONALE/EXPLANATION	EXAMPLE
Formulating a plan of action	When a plan is identified in a stressful situation, it may prevent anger/anxiety from escalating.	"The next time this comes up, what can you do to manage it?"
Using silence	Allows the patient to gather thoughts, think through a point, or consider introducing a different topic.	Encourage talking by waiting for an answer.
Accepting	Conveys an attitude of reception and regard, that the patient has been understood.	"I follow what you are saying." "Uh huh."
Giving recognition	Acknowledges and demonstrates awareness; more positive than complimenting (nurse's judgment).	"Good morning, Ms. Smith." "I see that you have styled your hair today."
Offering self	Availability on an unconditional basis, facilitates increased self-esteem with the patient.	"I would like to speak with you for a few minutes." "I'll stay with you for a while."
Giving broad openings	Allows the patient to take the initiative in introducing the topic; emphasizes the importance of the patient's role in the interaction.	"Is there something you would like to talk about?" "Where would you like to start?"
Offering general leads	Offers the patient encouragement to continue.	"Tell me more about that." "Please continue."
Placing the event in time or sequence	Clarifies the relationship of events in time so that the nurse and patient can view them in perspective.	"When did this happen?" "What was going on before that occurred?"
Making observations	Verbalizing what is observed. Encourages the patient to recognize certain behaviors and compare the perceptions with the nurse.	"I noticed you are tapping your foot, are you feeling anxious?" "You hesitated before you answered."
Encouraging description of perceptions	Asking the patient to state what is being perceived; often used with patients experiencing hallucinations.	"What does the voice say to you?" "Describe for me how you feel when you are anxious." "What does that word mean to you?"
Encouraging comparison	Asks the patient to compare similarities and differences in ideas, experiences, or interpersonal relationships. Encourages the patient to recognize life experiences that tend to recur as well as those aspects that are changeable.	"Have you felt like this before?" "What was effective when this happened before?"
Restating	The main idea of what the patient said is repeated; allows the patient to make sure that what he or she said is perceived correctly, letting the patient either clarify or continue.	Patient: "I was awake all last night. I can't sleep." Nurse: "You have trouble sleeping?"

(Continued...)

TECHNIQUE	RATIONALE/EXPLANATION	EXAMPLE
Reflecting	Questions and feelings are referred back to the patient to allow recognition and acceptance, lets the patient know that his or her views are valued. Most appropriate when the nurse is asked for advice.	Patient: "What should I do about my child's acting out behavior?" Nurse: "What do you think you should do?"
Focusing	Taking notice of a single idea or even word; most effective with patients exhibiting flight of ideas/tangentially. Ineffective with anxious patients.	"You've mentioned many things. Let's go back to talking about limit setting." "That is a good point you made. Perhaps we can discuss that a little more together."
Exploring	Going further into a subject, idea, experience, or relationship. Most effective with patients that tend to remain superficial in communication.	"Can you tell me a little more about that?" "How did you feel when you heard that voice?"
Seeking clarification and validation	Addressing a vague or incomprehensible concept. Allows for mutual understanding. Facilitates and increases understanding for both the nurse and patient.	"Let me make sure I understand what you said." "I don't understand what you mean. Can you explain further?"
Presenting reality	The nurse defines reality or indicates his or her perception of the situation for the patient.	"I am not your sister. I am your nurse." "That was a car backfire."
Voicing doubt	Expressing uncertainty of the reality of the patient's perception. Often used with patients experiencing delusional thoughts.	"Isn't that unusual?" "I find that difficult to believe."
Verbalizing the implied	Putting into words what the patient has only implied or said indirectly. Effective with patients experiencing mutism or other impaired verbal communication.	Patient: "This is a waste of my time. I can't talk to you." Nurse: "Do you think that I don't understand you?"
Attempting to translate words into feelings	When feelings are expressed indirectly, the nurse can try to "desymbolize" what is said and translate the words into true feelings.	Patient: "I am floating on a cloud." Nurse: "Are you saying that you feel happy?"
Suggesting collaboration	Emphasizes working with the patient, not doing things for the patient. Encourages the idea that change is possible by working together.	"Perhaps together we can develop a plan to manage your anger the next time."
Summarizing	Brings together important points of the interaction and allows the chance to clarify.	"During the past hour, you and I discussed …" "During our last interaction …"

Adapted from Hayes & Larson (1963). *Interacting with patients*. New York: MacMillan.

Barriers to Communication and Nontherapeutic Communication Techniques

Barriers to communication include language issues and expressive/receptive impairments. It is important to recognize these techniques and strive to eradicate their use during interaction with patients. Avoiding these communication barriers will maximize communication effectiveness and will enhance the nurse-patient relationship.

TECHNIQUE	RATIONALE/EXPLANATION	EXAMPLE
Reassurance	Indicates to the patient that there is no cause for their response, thereby devaluing the patient's feelings. May cause the patient not to interact, as he or she may feel ridiculed or devalued.	"I wouldn't worry about that." "Everything will be fine."
Rejecting	Not accepting, or showing contempt for, the patient's ideas or behaviors. Will stop interaction due to fear of further rejection.	"Let's not think about that." "I don't want to hear that."
Approval or disapproval	Sanctioning or denouncing the patient's ideas or behaviors. Implies that the nurse can pass judgment on what is "good" or "bad" for the patient.	"That's good. I'm glad that you did that" "That's bad. I'd prefer it if you wouldn't do that." "You really should have come to that medication group."
Agreeing/disagreeing	Indicate congruence with or opposition to the patient's ideas or opinions. Implies that the nurse has the ability to judge what is "right" or "wrong."	"I agree with your decision." "I'm proud of you for applying for that job." "I don't think you should do that."
Giving advice	Directing the patient's actions. Implies that the nurse determines appropriate responses for the patient, negates self-determination. Nurtures dependent role for the patient.	"I think you should take your medication." "Why don't you just hang up the phone?"
Probing	Persistent questioning, pushing for responses to matters the patient does not wish to discuss at that time. Can result in the patient experiencing feelings of being used and only valued for what he or she is willing to share with the nurse.	"Tell me about how your mother abused you when you were young." "Tell me about how you feel about her now that she is dead" "Tell me about …"
Defending	Protecting someone or something from a verbal attack. To defend what the patient criticizes is to imply that the patient has no right to express his or her views, ideas, opinions, or feelings. This technique will not change the patient's perception but will result in feeling the nurse is "taking sides" against the patient.	"Your doctor is great. I'm sure he cares about you." "No one here would lie to you." "This is a great hospital."
Asking "why"	Asking the patient to provide the reason for his or her thoughts, feelings, behaviors, and events. Can be intimidating for the patient and implies that the patient must defend him- or herself.	"Why do you feel that way? "Why did you do that?" "Why did you stop taking your medication?"

(Continued...)

TECHNIQUE	RATIONALE/EXPLANATION	EXAMPLE
Indicating the existence of an external power	Attributes the source of the patient's feelings, thoughts, and behavior to others or an outside source. This encourages projection for the patient.	"What makes you say that?" "What made you so angry the last time we spoke?"
Minimizing	Indicates that the nurse is unable to understand or empathize with the patient. The patient's feelings or experiences are belittled, which results in the devaluing of the patient.	Patient: "I have nothing to live for. I wish I were dead." Nurse: "Everybody feels down at times. I feel that way myself sometimes." "I know what you mean."
Making value judgments	Prevents problem-solving and can result in the patient feeling guilty, angry, misunderstood, not supported, and/or anxious to leave.	"How come you requested dessert when you are on a diet?" "How come you are still smoking when your husband has lung cancer?"
Using denial	When the nurse denies that a problem exists, this blocks interaction with the patient and avoids assisting the patient in identifying and exploring the areas of difficulty.	Patient: "I'm nothing." Nurse: "Of course you're something. Everybody has worth."
Interpreting	Attempt to make conscious what is unconscious, assist to give the patient meaning of experience.	"What you really mean to say is … "
Showing nonverbal signs of boredom or resentment	Decreases the patient's self-esteem, resulting in patient feeling demeaned and blocking interaction.	The nurse looks at watch, rustles papers, avoids eye contact, does not respond to the patient's concerns, and reflects annoyance or disapproval nonverbally.
Introducing a new subject	Changing the subject allows the nurse to take over the direction of the interaction. This may occur because the nurse has a specific topic to discuss or does not want to get involved in the discussion the patient introduces.	Patient: "I feel like I'd like to die." Nurse: "Did you go to Recreation Therapy today?"
Making stereotyped comments	Clichés and trite expressions are meaningless in the nurse-patient relationship. Use of empty conversation by the nurse encourages the same of the patient.	"I'm good. How are you?" "Keep your chin up"
Excessive questioning	Overwhelms the patient and results in his or her inability to respond timely and can lead to confusion.	Nurse: "How's your appetite? Have you recently lost weight? Are you eating enough?" Patient: "No."

2.3   Facilitating Active Listening Attending Behaviors

Most people want more than just physical presence in human communication. They want the other person to be there psychologically, socially, and emotionally. Listening well requires an active mind and increased energy, and is most probably the most important factor in effective communication. To listen actively is to be attentive to the words a patient is speaking as well as the message he or she is conveying nonverbally. Attentive listening will create an environment conducive to communication by demonstrating respect and acceptance by the nurse for the patient and enhancing trust. Active listening includes the following:

- Observing the patient's nonverbal communications
- Listening to and understanding the person in the context of the social setting of their life
- Listening for inconsistencies or things the patient says that need clarifying
- Providing the patient with feedback information about him- or herself about which the patient may not be aware

Principles that are important in active listening include the following:

- The answer is always inside the patient.
- Objective truth is never as simple as it appears.
- Everything that the clinician hears has been modified by the patient's filter.
- Everything the clinician hears has been modified by his or her own filters.
- It is "normal" to feel confused and uncertain.
- Listen to yourself.

Nonverbal behaviors are significant in conveying interest, regard, respect, and attentiveness during interactions and are conducive in facilitating the interactions. Important considerations to bear in mind when conducting a one-on-one is your positioning toward the patient, maintaining openness in body language, conveying interest through strategic positioning, maintaining appropriate eye contact, and, most importantly, presenting yourself in a relaxed manner.

2.4 Evaluating Communication

Once the basics are understood and integrated into practice, the learning does not end. The establishment of a therapeutic relationship relies upon the use of effective communication techniques and behaviors by the clinician and avoidance of nontherapeutic methods and behaviors. These skills must be learned, practiced, and reviewed with regularity.

Process recordings are frequently used learning tools in clinician-patient communication. These recordings are not considered official documentation, but rather are intended to be used as a learning tool for students and practicing clinicians. A major disadvantage of this method is the reliance on memory and potential distortion. The practice is to document, verbatim, the interactions and behaviors of the nurse and patient. During review, the nurse analyzes therapeutic/nontherapeutic techniques and behaviors/emotions during the interaction. (See Figure 2-3.)

Nurse's Response (verbal and nonverbal)	Client's Response (verbal and nonverbal) Defense Mechanisms	Therapeutic or Nontherapeutic Technique Used	Nurse's Thoughts and Feelings about the Interaction

Figure 2-3 Process recording.

2.5   Communicating with Special Needs Patients

Impaired communication can result from various circumstances and conditions. It is a state in which an individual experiences or is at risk of experiencing difficulty in exchanging thoughts, ideas, desires, wants, or needs to others, either as sender or receiver of the message. The characteristics of a patient experiencing impaired communication include the following:

- Difficulty with speech or hearing
- Inappropriate, absent speech or response
- Aphasia, stuttering, dysarthria
- Incongruence between spoken word and nonverbal message
- Impaired volume
- Reported inability to understand or of being misunderstood

There are various causes for impairment in communication, as well as identified actions to improve effectiveness of communication.

Interventions for Specific Impairments in Communication

IMPAIRMENT	INTERVENTION
Sensory impairments	Use factors that will promote hearing and understanding.
Language barriers	Provide alternative methods of communication.
Emotionally responsive	Provide a non-rushed environment.
Cognitive impairments	Make an effort to understand when the patient is speaking.
Psychosis	Teach techniques to improve speech.

2.6   Language Barriers

According to the Office of Civil Rights, the 1964 Civil Rights Act affords patients with limited English proficiency the right, at no cost, to have an interpreter when obtaining care from any service provider who receives federal funding (Medicare or Medicaid). The clinician has special considerations when communicating due to language barriers. The use of a translator is imperative; however, the translation may be compromised by the person who serves the role. Family members' support of the patient may be enhanced by participating in the communication process. They may, however, have separate issues and mask relevant symptoms in the translation. Therefore, it is not recommended that family members be used as translators unless the situation is emergent and no other immediately available resource is available. Additionally, the clinician needs to ensure cultural sensitivity and awareness when interpreting nonverbal communication patterns.

Health-care providers under the Americans with Disabilities Act (ADA) must ensure that disabled patients have access to health-care services and be able to adequately communicate with their providers.

Psychotic Disorders

Therapeutic strategies for communicating with clients experiencing alterations in sensory and thought perceptions address lowering the patient's anxiety, decreasing defensive patterns, encouraging participation in the therapeutic milieu, and raising the level of self-worth.

Depressive Disorders

Communicating with a severely depressed patient can be difficult and frustrating without awareness and knowledge of communication techniques and their effectiveness. This is an opportunity to employ the technique of silence. In addition, making observations can help the patient maintain reality orientation.

Dementia/Cognitive Disorders

A considerable number of patients experiencing cognitive disorders have secondary behavioral disturbances, including depression, hallucinations and delusions, agitation, insomnia, and wandering. Communication with these patients influences their maintenance of self-esteem and ability/willingness to participate in their care. Basic verbal interventions for patients with cognitive disturbances include the following:

- Identify self and patient by name during each contact.
- Speak slowly and clearly.
- Use uncomplicated communication (short, simple words).
- Ensure visual connection.
- Consider distance.
- Address one topic at a time.
- Ensure any prescribed sensory equipment is in proper use.

2.7 Cultural Competence

Chapter 1 reviewed the importance of cultural awareness in the application of the nursing process. Interactions with a patient (individual, family, or community) allow opportunities to observe cultural aspects that may influence care. This cultural assessment is considered imperative and represents another core competency. Note that if and when you do assess data that may be useful in addressing medical, spiritual, social, physical, or other types of needs for the patient, it is your responsibility to share this information within the multidisciplinary approach.

The communication abilities of the client are a primary consideration (verbal and nonverbal). Psychiatric nursing's primary intervention involves communication skills and techniques; therefore, it is essential that the patient and family have a full understanding of information provided and be able to communicate effectively with the care provider.

The assessment phase of the nursing process enables collection of relevant data to help determine not only the problems that patients are experiencing but also their strengths. Success in analysis of the data requires that cultural questions are included.

There are many examples that demonstrate the importance of gathering the information specified in Figure 2-4. For instance, in some American Indian tribes the decision regarding seeking treatment for an illness is determined through a family council meeting. In this circumstance, it is generally the eldest family member that bears the greatest decision-making weight.

Gathering information about your client's race, ethnicity, use of language, length of time in the country, and community affords considerations that may impact the patient's perception and engagement in treatment procedures and indicate specific needs of the patient. This essential information helps determine those that may require extra time, support, and financial implications on care decisions. Continuing treatment, especially for the psychiatric patient, can be affected by financial insecurity. Noncompliance, a significant issue, has many causes. A major barrier is inability to afford treatment and/or medications. The presence of a good social support can be pivotal in the success of treatment. Knowledge of the role of the patient's significant other (SO) can give added insight into prediction of success. It is important that the presence of the SO is respected, even if the relationship is not considered "traditional." The level of independence acknowledged by a culture can offer insight into the expectations of patients. This is an important consideration when you are developing the patient-centered goal. Some cultures value independence in the elderly, while in others an elderly individual is not expected to be physically active.

Cultural competency allows one to recognize and embrace the knowledge that each individual has a distinctive background and history. The person's lived cultural experience will affect how the world is viewed and what the person considers as appropriate care. It also encourages the clinician to consider known group beliefs yet have the flexibility to allow each individual to express his or her own positions. The patient (individual, family, community) has an expectation that their care provider will see him or her as unique individuals. Remember that everyone wants to be acknowledged and respected regardless of illness, belief, race, creed, or color.

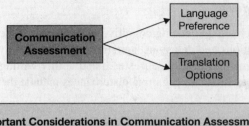

Important Considerations in Communication Assessment

1. Is there a preferred language?
2. Is there a secondary language?
3. In what language do you read?

Considerations for Translation

1. Offer the use of language assistance services promptly when needed.
2. Although convenient, it is not recommended to use a family member/friend for translation purposes:
   - Person may be unable to interpret crucial health information.
   - Person may feel uncomfortable sharing certain information.
   - Person may try to have the patient's responses "make sense".

Figure 2-4 Communication assessment.

2.8   Legal and Ethical Considerations in Psychiatric Nursing Practice

Psychiatric and mental health nursing is wrought with legal and ethical issues. Knowledge of ethical and legal considerations in nursing care will facilitate enhanced quality in patient care, while providing nurses with information and guidance that can protect them legally. A basic understanding of the definition of ethics and bioethics is required.

Box 2-2

Ethics: Branch of philosophy dealing with values relating to human conduct, with respect to the rightness and wrongness of certain actions and to the goodness and badness of the motives and ends of such actions.

Bioethics: Field of study concerned with the ethics and philosophical implications of certain biological and medical procedures, technologies, and treatments, such as organ transplants, genetic engineering, and care of the terminally ill.

The American Nurses Association has formulated a specific code of ethics for nurses to use as a guide in practice for ethical choices and decision making.

Box 2-3: American Nurses Association Code of Ethics for Nurses

1. The nurse, in all professional relationships, practices with compassion and respect for the inherent dignity, worth, and uniqueness of every individual, unrestricted by consideration of social or economic status, personal attributes, or the nature of health problems.
2. The nurse's primary commitment is to the patient, whether an individual, family, group, or community.

3. The nurse promotes, advocates for, and strives to protect the health, safety, and rights of the patient.

4. The nurse is responsible and accountable for individual nursing practice and determines the appropriate delegation of tasks consistent with the nurse's obligation to provide optimum patient care.

5. The nurse owes the same duties to self as to others, including the responsibility to preserve integrity and safety, to maintain competence, and to continue personal and professional growth.

6. The nurse participates in establishing, maintaining, and improving health-care environments and conditions of employment conducive to the provision of quality health care and consistent with the values of the profession through individual and collective action.

7. The nurse participates in the advancement of the profession through contributions to practice, education, administration, and knowledge development.

8. The nurse collaborates with other health professionals and the public in promoting community, national, and international efforts to meet health needs.

9. The profession of nursing, as represented by associations and their members, is responsible for articulating nursing values, for maintaining the integrity of the profession and its practice and for shaping social policy.

Reprinted with permission from the American Nurses Association Code of Ethics for Nurses with Interpretative Statements, © 2001. American Nurses Publishing, American Nurses Foundation/American Nurses Association, Washington, D.C.

There are five key ethical principles used by health-care professionals to guide resolution of an ethical dilemma.

Box 2-4: Key Ethical Principles

1. *Beneficence*—The duty to act to benefit or promote the good of others.
2. *Autonomy*—The right to make one's own decisions and the respect for the right of others to make their own decisions.
3. *Justice*—The treating of others fairly and equally.
4. *Nonmaleficence (fidelity)*—The maintenance of loyalty and commitment to the patient, doing no harm/wrong to the patient.
5. *Veracity*—Responsibility to always be truthful to the patient.

An ethical dilemma occurs when an individual is required to make a choice between equally unfavorable alternatives. During these situations, there is evidence that would support something right and wrong in each choice selection. The individual in charge of the decision making experiences a conflict in selection. Typically, ethical dilemmas are emotionally charged occurrences (right to life, abortion, end-of-life decisions, etc.). The principles that help guide the decision include autonomy, beneficence, nonmaleficence, justice, and veracity. There is a Model for Making Ethical Decisions (see Figure 2-5) that resembles the phases of the nursing process and may serve as a guide in resolving ethical decisions. When faced with making an ethical decision, you should review and consider the following resources:

- Legal advice
- Nurse practice acts
- Facility policies and procedures
- Patient's Bill of Rights
- Input from colleagues

- Input from clergy
- Consideration of individual ideals and morals
- Code of Ethics for Nurses (Box 2-3)
- Standards of Care from the Scope and Standards of Psychiatric Mental Health Nursing Practice (Refer back to Chapter 1.)

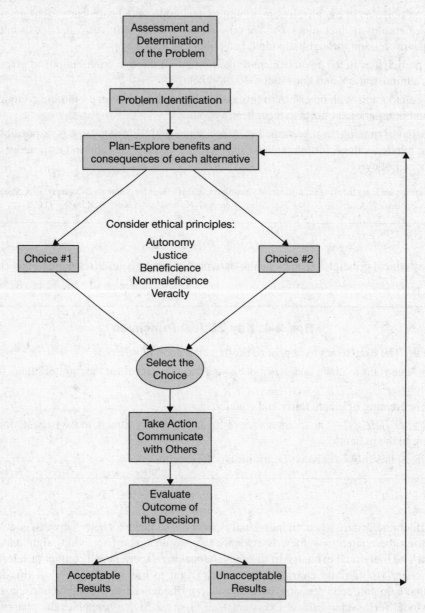

Figure 2-5 Model for making ethical decisions.

    While ethical issues require a review of individual beliefs and values, legal considerations are dictated by state and federal laws. The psychiatric patient population can be vulnerable for mistreatment and abuse; therefore, laws have been enacted to afford them with legal protection. A Patient's Bill of Rights, first adopted by the American Hospital Association in 1973, specifies the basic rights afforded. Additionally, in 1980, the 96th Congress of the United States passed the Mental Health Systems Act, which includes a Patient's Bill of Rights. See Box 2-5 for a review of these rights.

Box 2-5: Bill of Rights for Psychiatric Patients

1. The right to appropriate treatment and related services in the setting that is most supportive and least restrictive to personal freedom.

2. The right to an individualized, written treatment or service plan; the right to treatment based on such a plan; and the right to a periodic review and revision of the plan based upon treatment needs.

3. The right, consistent with one's capabilities, to participate in and receive a reasonable explanation of the care and treatment process.

4. The right to refuse treatment, except in an emergency situation or as permitted by law.

5. The right not to participate in experimentation in the absence of informed, voluntary, written consent.

6. The right to freedom from restraint or seclusion, except in an emergency situation.

7. The right to a humane treatment environment that affords reasonable protection from harm and appropriate privacy.

8. The right to confidentiality of medical records (also applicable following a patient's discharge).

9. The right of access to medical records except information received from third parties under promise of confidentiality, and when access would be detrimental to the patient's health (also applicable following a patient's discharge).

10. The right of access to use a telephone, personal mail, and visitors, unless deemed inappropriate for treatment purposes.

11. The right to be informed of these rights in a comprehensible language at the time of admission.

12. The right to assert grievances if rights are infringed.

13. The right to exercise these rights without reprisal.

14. The right to referral, as appropriate, to other providers of mental health services upon discharge.

Title II, Public Law 99–319, *Restatement of Bill of Rights of Mental Health Patients*, Title II – Restatement of Bill of Rights for Mental Health Patients established by the Mental Health Systems Act of 1980.

Chapter 2 Questions

Fill in the Blank

1. Three main components of the therapeutic relationship include _____, _____, and _____.
2. The four phases of the therapeutic relationship include _____, _____, _____, and _____.

True or False

3. When interacting with the patient, the nurse needs to be aware of both verbal and nonverbal communications. _____

Matching

1. Patient: "Do you think I should let my mother know?" Nurse: "Do you think you should tell her?"

    A. Advising

2. "Of all the points you have identified, which is the most concerning?"

    B. Restating

3. "Tell me more about what was happening."   C. Focusing

4. "I think you should take your medication."   D. Giving approval

5. "But how is it that you are a world-famous designer?"   E. Silence

6. "I went to school to be a nurse. That's how I know this is right."   F. Challenging

7. Patient: "It's a waste of everyone's time for me to try to talk to them." Nurse: "Do you feel that no one understands you?"   G. Exploring

8. "Isn't that normal?"   H. Presenting reality

9. "I see no one else in the room with us."   I. Indicating the existence of an external source

10. The nurse says nothing, maintaining active listening behaviors.   J. Reflecting

11. Patient: "I stay awake all night. I can't get any sleep." Nurse: "You are having trouble sleeping?"   K. Seeking information

12. Nurse: "That's great I'm glad that you were able to …"   L. Offering self

13. "My name is Sue. I am your nurse today. I would like to spend a few minutes with you to see how things are going."   M. Probing

14. Nurse: "Do you still think that your family wants to harm you?"   N. Voicing doubt

15. Nurse: "The next time you feel stressed out, what might help you manage it better?"   O. Reassuring

16. "Let me make sure that I understand what you said."   P. Testing

17. "Who told you that the doctor wanted to hurt you?"   Q. Verbalizing the implied

18. "Everything will be okay."   R. Defending

19. "You know I need to know this information. Tell me all about that day."   S. Formulating a plan of action

Chapter 2 Answers

Fill in the Blank

1. *Genuineness*, *empathy*, and *positive regard* are the three main components of a therapeutic relationship.

2. The four phases of the therapeutic relationship are *preorientation*, *orientation*, *working*, and *termination*.

True or False

3. True.

It is essential that the nurse make sure that the words spoken and behaviors exhibited are congruent and correctly convey the meanings intended. Awareness of illness symptoms (anxiety, sensorial disturbances) and cultural influences will ensure communication is effective and accurate.

Matching

1. J
2. C
3. G
4. A
5. F
6. R
7. Q
8. N
9. H
10. E

11. B
12. D
13. L
14. P
15. S
16. K
17. I
18. O
19. M

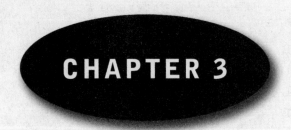

CHAPTER 3

Neurobiologic Theories and Psychopharmacology

3.1 Neurobiology

Causative relations for mental health disorders remain mostly unknown; however, in recent years a greater emphasis has been placed upon the organic basis of mental illness. Neurobiologic research provides for increasing knowledge in the field of psychiatry and impacts daily clinical practice. Much research has been afforded to the functioning of the brain, and this has broadened the appreciation of how the brain functions and possible causes of malfunctions or malformations. Psychiatric and mental health nurses must possess a basic understanding of the brain structure and function, as well as the theories addressing psychiatric disorders, not only to provide the scientific rationale needed for analysis of data and planning of the patient's care but in order to fulfill their role as educators for the patient and family.

Subsequent to the increased knowledge regarding brain functioning, medications have been identified that will address symptoms patients with mental illness experience. The 1990s was designated as the "decade of the brain." Consequentially, several psychiatric disorders began to be considered as a result of brain malfunctions or malformations. Keeping in spirit with the holism found in nursing, it is important to consider that biology, psychology, and sociology are integrated sciences.

There are four types of influences on mental health disorders:

1. Neurophysiological
2. Neurochemical
3. Genetic
4. Endocrine

Psychopharmacology is the study of the action, effects, and development of psychoactive medications (those affecting the mind or mental processes) subsequent to the study of neurobiologic theories.

Though there are several therapeutic approaches in the treatment and management of mental illness, medication is considered an essential and effective intervention in assisting the patient to be best prepared for adjunctive therapies (behavioral and cognitive approaches). This chapter focuses on the role of the nurse, both in the administration of the medication and in education/health teaching of five major categories of medications. Concepts regarding the medications will also be reviewed in the corresponding illness specific chapters.

The foundation of the human neural information system is the neuron (nerve cell). See Figure 3-1. While there are many different types of neurons, classification is by morphology and function. Branching from the cell body is the dendrite tree; this receives signals from other neurons. The end of the axon has branching terminals (axon terminals) that will release the neurotransmitters. Neurotransmitters are required to send information from one neuron to the next across the synaptic cleft (space between the terminals and dendrites).

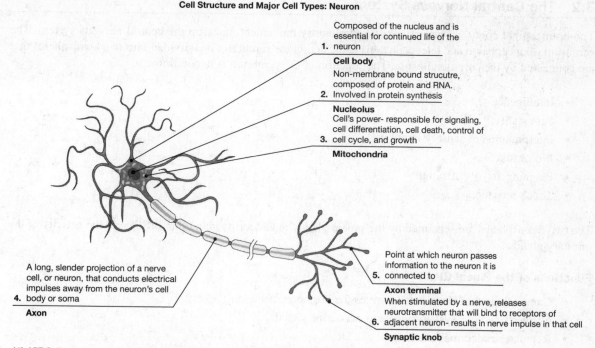

Cell Structure and Major Cell Types: Neuron

1. Composed of the nucleus and is essential for continued life of the neuron
   Cell body

2. Non-membrane bound strucutre, composed of protein and RNA. Involved in protein synthesis
   Nucleolus

3. Cell's power- responsible for signaling, cell differentiation, cell death, control of cell cycle, and growth
   Mitochondria

4. A long, slender projection of a nerve cell, or neuron, that conducts electrical impulses away from the neuron's cell body or soma
   Axon

5. Point at which neuron passes information to the neuron it is connected to
   Axon terminal

6. When stimulated by a nerve, releases neurotransmitter that will bind to receptors of adjacent neuron- results in nerve impulse in that cell
   Synaptic knob

LifeART Collection Images Copyright © 1989-2001 by Lippincott Williams & Wilkins, Baltimore, MD

Figure 3-1 Nerve cell.

Neurotransmitters are chemical messengers. A process referred to as "reuptake" occurs when the neurotransmitters attach to the receptor site and are reabsorbed by the neuron to be reused. Neurotransmitters are an essential component of the body's functioning. There are believed to be over 100 in the body. It is important to consider what effect each of these has on the body and how illness and medication or drugs interfere in their functioning.

Types of Neurotransmitters

- **Acetylcholine** is involved with memory, muscle stimulation (including the GI system), and learning. Alzheimer's disease is associated with a lack of this neurotransmitter.

- **Endorphins** are associated with emotions and pain perception. They are released as a response to fear or trauma, and are similar to opiate medications but are much stronger.

- **Dopamine** is a neurotransmitter associated with thought and pleasure. Deficits in dopamine have been found in Parkinson's disease. Schizophrenia is associated with excessive amounts of dopamine. Two main subgroups of dopamine receptors are D1-like (D1 and D5 receptor subtypes) and D2-like (D2, D3, and D4 subtypes). Many neuroleptic medications, discussed later in this chapter and in subsequent chapters of specific illnesses, are D2 receptor antagonists.

- **GABA** (gamma-aminobutyric acid) is usually an inhibitory neurotransmitter, acting as a brake for the excitatory neurotransmitters. Individuals lacking in GABA experience anxiety disorders.

- **Glutamate**, an excitatory relative of GABA, is the most common neurotransmitter in the central nervous system (CNS). It is associated with memory. This neurotransmitter is known to be toxic to neurons and in excess can kill other neurons. Occurrences of brain damage or stroke can lead to an excess and result in more brain cells dying than from the initial trauma. It is believed that amyotrophic lateral sclerosis (ALS, or Lou Gehrig's disease) is caused by excessive glutamate.

- **Serotonin**, an inhibitatory neurotransmitter, is associated with emotion and mood. Lack of serotonin results in depression, anger management issues, OCD, suicide, increased desire for carbohydrates, and difficulty sleeping. There are also connections to migraines, IBS (irritable bowel syndrome), and fibromyalgia.

- **Norepinephrine** (noradrenalin) is associated with the alert response of the body (increasing heart rate and blood pressure) and is important for forming memories.

3.2   The Central Nervous System

The brain, spinal cord, and nerves affecting voluntary movement make up the central nervous system. The cerebrum (diencephalon and telencephalon) is located in the forebrain. It is divided into two hemispheres that are connected by the corpus callosum. The function of the cerebrum is to determine

- Intelligence
- Personality
- Interpretation of sensory impulses
- Motor function
- Planning and organization
- Touch sensation

The two hemispheres are separated by the pineal gland, an endocrine gland that influences the activity of the pituitary gland.

Functions of the Pineal Gland

- Causes feeling of sleepiness (secretes the hormone melatonin).
- Converts nervous system signals to endocrine signals.
- Regulates endocrine functions.

The left hemisphere controls the right side of the body (logical and analytical functioning), and the right hemisphere controls the left side of the body (creativity, intuition, artistic capabilities).

Four lobes make up the cerebral hemisphere:

- Frontal (decision making, problem solving, and planning)
- Parietal (reception and processing of sensory information from the body)
- Occipital (vision) and temporal lobe (memory, emotion, hearing, and language)

Figure 3-2 defines the lobes and functional areas.

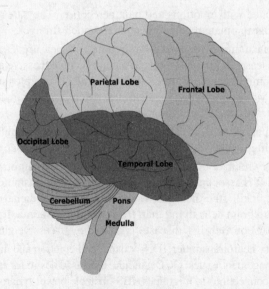

Figure 3-2 Brain.

The cerebellum, located below the cerebrum, controls fine movement coordination, balance/equilibrium, and muscle tone. Post-mortem studies report cellular abnormalities in the limbic system and cerebellum of patients diagnosed with autism. The brain stem, located at the top of the spinal cord, is composed of the following:

- Midbrain (auditory and visual responses, motor function, relaying of signals from brain to the spinal nerves)
- Pons (arousal, controls autonomic functions, sleep, consciousness, awareness)
- Medulla oblongata (respiratory and cardiovascular functioning)
- Nuclei for CN III-XII

The locus ceruleus (associated with stress, anxiety, and impulsivity) was thought to play a significant part in the etiology of anxiety. A stimulus, if perceived as a threat, stimulates a more intense and prolonged discharge of the locus ceruleus, which signals the sympathetic division of the autonomic nervous system. This release of norepinephrine stimulates the nerve endings of the heart, blood vessels, and respiratory center, resulting in the physiologic changes associated with an acute stress response. Research now indicates that anxiety engages a wide range of neurocircuits. This line of study focuses on two key regulatory centers found in the cerebral hemispheres of the brain—the hippocampus and the amygdala (components of the limbic system). They are both thought to activate the hypothalamic-pituitary-adrenocortical (HPA) axis.

The limbic system, referred to as the "emotional brain," is located above the brain stem and includes the following:

- Thalamus
- Hypothalamus
- Hippocampus
- Amygdala

The function of the limbic system is to control

- Emotions
- Emotional responses
- Hormonal secretions
- Mood
- Motivation
- Pain/pleasure sensations

The thalamus is located above the brain stem. It is considered the "sensory switchboard" of the brain. It transmits information from all senses (except olfactory) to the receiving areas in the cortex and sends replies to the cerebellum and medulla. The hypothalamus is located below the thalamus and is responsible for maintaining the body's homeostasis. It regulates basic responses (thirst, hunger, pain) and the functioning of the sympathetic and parasympathetic nervous systems. Responses are dispatched throughout the body via two measures: the autonomic nervous system and the pituitary gland. The hippocampus is located within the temporal lobes. Its function serves to consolidate memories, emotions, navigation, and spatial orientation, and it is involved in learning. Though certainly not solely responsible for the symptoms associated in major depressive disorder, several lines of research have supported the consideration that the hippocampus has a central role in the pathophysiology of this illness.

The amygdala, a walnut shape of neural clusters located deep in the temporal lobe, influences fear (learned and unlearned) and aggression. Experiments have indicated the amygdala's role in rage and fear, as well as perception and processing of emotions. Signals reach the amygdala both directly and indirectly through the thalamus and cortex, and amygdala hyperactivity has been demonstrated in patients with acute depression. Additionally, research has revealed that dual-diagnosis (mental illness and substance abuse) may result from developmental changes in the amygdala. (See Figures 3-3 and 3-4.)

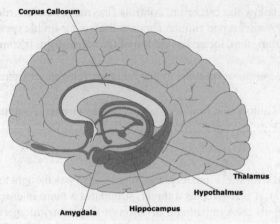

Figure 3-3 Brain.

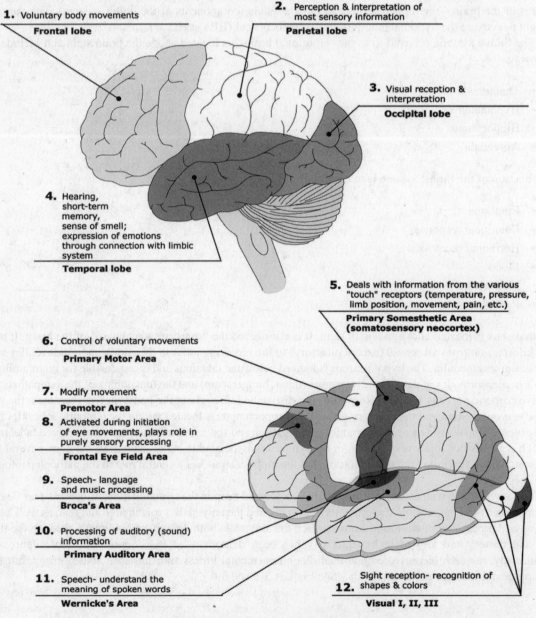

Figure 3-4 Brain and brain functions.

3.3 Psychopharmacology

Psychopharmacology is the study of drug-induced changes in mood, sensation, and behavior. Pharmacological interventions target the actions of neurons, neurotransmitters, and receptors. Most medications either increase or decrease the activity of a certain transmitter-receptor system. Nurses, who administer these medications, are expected to

- Understand how the medications prescribed for their patient's work
- Their side effects
- Contraindications
- Drug and food interactions
- Specific nursing actions necessary to assist the patient manage their medication regimens

Awareness of the indications, mechanisms, actions, and potential side effects of psychopharmacological interventions allows the nurse to individualize the plan of care for each patient. The psychological, physical, and social effects of medications must be identified and discussed with the patient. The ability to recognize the presence of adverse effects will allow prompt interventions to ease the discomfort or, if necessary, discontinue that treatment option.

There are several significant terms that nurses should know in order to comprehend discussions in subsequent chapters on specific disorders related to medication and medication therapy.

Box 3-1: Significant Terms Used in Medication and Medication Therapy	
Efficacy	Maximum therapeutic effect that can be achieved
Potency	Amount of medication needed to achieve the maximum effect
Half-life	Time it takes for half of the medication to leave the blood stream
Off-label use	Use of a drug for a disease that differs from the original testing and FDA approval
Black box warning	Package inserts contain a highlighted box indicating a serious or life-threatening side effect

A medication is selected based on its effect on the target symptoms (delusion, panic, hallucination) and is evaluated by its ability to decrease or eliminate those symptoms. Following are some considerations employed which relate to the selection of medication as a treatment:

1. Many medications used in psychiatric treatment must be administered in adequate dosages for a period of time to reach their full effectiveness (some antidepressants require a period of one to one and a half months for therapeutic benefit).
2. Medication dose is adjusted to the lowest effective dose. Initial dosages may be higher, but once the symptoms have decreased, the dose is adjusted to a lower level.
3. Younger patients require a higher dosage of medication than older patients. Therapeutic effect takes a longer time in older patients.
4. It is usual for psychiatric medications to be tapered (decreased gradually) when stopped due to possible rebound, recurrence of the symptoms, or withdrawal.
5. Follow-up care is an essential support for compliance, to determine need for dosage adjustment, and to manage side effects.
6. Compliance is increased when the number of medications and number of daily doses is minimized.

This chapter reviews the following categories of medications used in the treatment of psychiatric disorders: antipsychotics, antidepressants, mood stabilizing, antianxiety, and stimulants. Included in the review are the mechanism of action, dosage, side effects, patient teaching, and specific nursing considerations.

3.4 Antipsychotic Medications

Antipsychotic medications, also referred to as neuroleptics, are used to treat patients who are experiencing psychotic symptoms (delusions, hallucinations) that are exhibited in illness such as schizophrenia, schizoaffective disorder, and bipolar disorder mania. Off-label uses include treatment of anxiety and insomnia, aggressiveness, and disturbed thought processes that accompany Alzheimer's disease. There are two subcategories of antipsychotics: standard first-generation, and the atypical antipsychotics.

Antipsychotic Medications

TYPE	MEDICATION DRUG NAME	ADVERSE EFFECTS	NURSING CONSIDERATIONS
First generation	Chlorpromazine Fluphenazine Haloperidol Loxapine Mesoridazine Molindone Perphenazine Pimozide Thioridazine Thiothixene Trifluoperazine	Dry mouth, blurred vision, seizures, increased heart rate, decreased blood pressure, constipation, tremor, muscle stiffness, muscle rigidity, involuntary repetitive movements of muscles (tardive dyskinesia), fever, and muscle damage (neuroeliptic malignant syndrome, or NMS)	Increased risk for falls, need for eye examinations when thioridazine is used. Do not discontinue medication abruptly, assess patient for any blood discrepancies, monitor weight and assist with management. Educate patient of possible side effects, monitor elderly patients for dehydration, consult MD regarding advisement of patient/guardian regarding tardive dyskenesia and about dosage reduction or use of anticholenergic for +EPS, monitor blood pressure.
Second generation	Aripiprazole Clozapine Olanzapine Quetiapine Risperidone Ziprasidone	Tremor, muscle stiffness, muscle rigidity, uncontrolled movements of the face and arms (tardive dyskinesia), fever and muscle damage (NMS), drowsiness, weight gain, dizziness	Older patients tolerate atypical antipsychotics better, with less chance of tremor, muscle stiffness, uncontrolled movements, and NMS. Clozapine can stop production of white blood cells, increasing risk for infection. Can also cause seizures. Atypical medications can be effective with patient's resistant to first-generation medications. Clozapine and Ziprasidone may cause abnormalities in the heart's rhythms.

Phenothiazines (Chlorpromazine/Thorazine), thioxanthens (chlorprothixene/Taractan), butyrophenones (Haloperidol/Haldol), and pharmacologically related agents are known as first-generation antipsychotics. First introduced in the 1950s, these medications allowed individuals experiencing psychotic symptoms the opportunity to lead a more "normal" life by decreasing or eliminating their thought and sensory disturbances.

The chemical structure of the various antipsychotics allows them to bind to dopamine receptors without triggering the postsynaptic response that occurs typically with the binding of dopamine, thereby helping to reduce the excess levels of dopamine seen in schizophrenic patients. This helps to address the positive symptoms of the illness. These medications are antagonists for the muscarinic receptors for acetylcholine, a_1 receptors for Norepinephrine, and histamine (H_1) receptors for histamine. This antagonism is noted to be responsible for the adverse effects of this type of medication. See the previous box for the identification of more common antipsychotics. The major action of all antipsychotics is to block receptors for the neurotransmitter dopamine. Antipsychotics are antagonists of D2, D3, and D4, resulting in positive effect on symptoms but producing extrapyramidal side effects. Side effects of antipsychotics include the following:

- Extrapyramidal side effects
- Neuroleptics malignant syndrome
- Tardive dyskinesia
- Anticholinergic side effects and some hormonal and cardiovascular changes

See Figure 3-5 for side effects of antipsychotics.

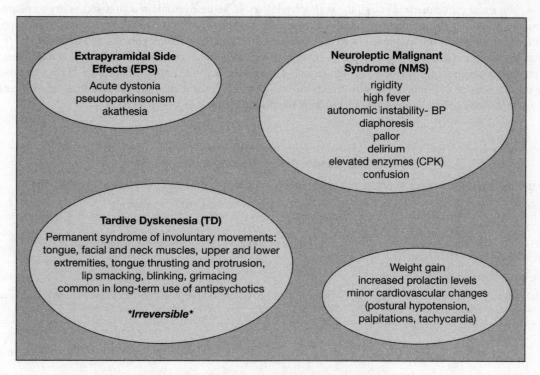

Extrapyramidal Side Effects (EPS)
Acute dystonia
pseudoparkinsonism
akathesia

Neuroleptic Malignant Syndrome (NMS)
rigidity
high fever
autonomic instability- BP
diaphoresis
pallor
delirium
elevated enzymes (CPK)
confusion

Tardive Dyskenesia (TD)
Permanent syndrome of involuntary movements: tongue, facial and neck muscles, upper and lower extremities, tongue thrusting and protrusion, lip smacking, blinking, grimacing common in long-term use of antipsychotics

Irreversible

Weight gain
increased prolactin levels
minor cardiovascular changes
(postural hypotension, palpitations, tachycardia)

Figure 3-5 Adverse reactions of antipsychotics.

The second-generation antipsychotics are weaker antagonists of D2 and inhibit the reuptake of serotonin, therefore decreasing EPS and allowing for treatment of any depressive aspects of schizophrenia. A new generation of antipsychotics is being developed that is assigned the classification of dopamine system stabilizers (DSS), which is reported to be able to preserve or enhance dopamine transmission where it is lacking and reduce it where it is too high.

While several adverse reactions are associated with antipsychotic medications, three of the most significant are as follows:

1. Extra pyramidal side effects (EPS)
2. Neuroleptic malignant syndrome (NMS)
3. Tardive dyskinesia (TD)

Refer to Figure 3-5 for a review of the symptoms associated with these side effects.

Extrapyramidal side effects are neurological symptoms that are the most common side effects of antipsychotic medications. EPS includes acute

- Dystonia (muscular rigidity/cramping, stiff or thick tongue, difficulty swallowing; in extreme cases, can result in laryngospams and respiratory distress)
- Pseudoparkinsonism (symptoms resemble those of Parkinson's disease—stiff and bent-over posture, masklike faces, decreased arm swing, shuffling gait, cogwheel rigidity, drooling, tremors, bradycardia, pill-rolling movement of the thumb and fingers while at rest)

- Akathesia (experienced by patients as a need to move about; they are noted to be restless or with increased anxiety, rigid posture or gait, lack of spontaneous gesture)
- Neuroleptics malignant syndrome (a potentially fatal, idiosyncratic reaction; symptoms include rigidity, high fever, autonomic instability with resulting unstable blood pressure, diaphoresis, and pallor; delirium, elevated enzymes—particularly CPK—mental confusion, mutism. These usually occur in the first two weeks of treatment but can occur at any time).
- Tardive dyskinesia (TD)

Another potential side effect, acute dystonia, is a brief or sustained muscle spasm that is often accompanied by slow, abnormal movements. Though the pathophysiology of acute dystonic reaction secondary to neuroleptics remains unknown, the incidents generally occur at a time when the blood level of the medication is dropping. Acute dystonia occurs more frequently with parenteral medications, in younger patients and in males.

Acute dystonic reactions may increase in severity after the initial occurrence; therefore, it is important that each patient experiencing this side effect be treated. Though the atypical antipsychotics are known to produce fewer occurrences of dystonia, these side effects still do occur with some patients. Anticholinergic medications (see Figure 3-6) are generally prescribed to address the possible dystonic side effects.

Medications Used to Treat Dystonia

Benztropine (Cogentin) 1-2 mg IM/IV (0.2 mg/kg pediatric dose) (may be repeated in 10 minutes)

Diphenhydramine (Benadryl) 1 mg/kg IM/IV max. dose 30 mg (may be repeated in 30 minutes)

Diazepam (Valium) 0.1 mg/kg slow IV (may be repeated in 30 minutes)

Procuclidine (Kemadrin) 5 10 mg IM/IV (0.5 to 2 mg pediatric under age 2, 2-5 mg pediatric over age 2) (may be repeated in 20 minutes)

Lorazepam (Ativan) 1-2 mg po

Trihexaphenidyl (Artane) Initial dose of 1 mg po. If symptoms not controlled progressively increase until control achieved. Not recommended for pediatric use

---

Figure 3-6 Acute dystonic reaction facts.

Antipsychotic medications require that the nurse initiate teaching with the patient to address the possible occurrence of side effects and the risk for noncompliance. Comfort measures, such as the use of sugar-free candy or sugar-free drinks to address the side effect of dry mouth, avoidance of specific foods to decrease interactions, use of stool softeners to ease constipation, and use of sunscreen for photosensitivity, will assist in minimizing the effects for the patient. Following are nursing considerations regarding the use and administration of antipsychotic medications:

- Review all medications prescribed for your patient (including OTC and herbal supplements, vitamins) for possible dangerous drug to drug interactions.
- Ensure evaluation of symptom alleviation or elimination (disturbed thought processes or sensory perceptions, bizarre behaviors).
- Assess and monitor the patient's level of consciousness, especially geriatric patients; sedation may result in ataxia and falls.
- Assess and monitor vital signs. Contact the prescriber regarding any altercations as dosage adjustment, or medication cessation may be indicated
- Assess and monitor the patient's white blood count (WBC) during clozapine therapy, and contact the prescriber for results below 2,000/mm^3, if the absolute neutrophil count falls below 1,000/mm^3, or if the patient develops flulike symptoms or other signs/symptoms of infection.
- Provide patient education to the patient and family/significant others related to compliance, expected effects, use of birth control to prevent pregnancy while taking the medication, risk of hyperthermia, need to reduce/protect from sunlight, and possible drowsiness.

3.5 Antidepressant Medications

According to the World Health Organization (WHO), depression is one of the most common mental health problems in the world. Ten to 20 percent of adults in the United States experience depression at some point in their lives (see Chapter 11). Several drug therapies have been developed to treat depression over the past half century, and many of the second-generation antidepressants have also been approved by the FDA for treatment of mental illnesses other than depression (anxiety, obsessive-compulsive and panic disorders, social phobia, and post-traumatic stress disorder). This chapter will review the following:

- Selective serotonin reuptake inhibitors (SSRIs; recommended first-line pharmacological treatment for depression)
- Selective noradrenaline reuptake inhibitors (used when patients have not responded to SSRIs)
- Monoamine oxidase inhibitors (MAOI)
- Tricyclic antidepressants
- Atypical antidepressants such as venlafaxine (Effexor), bupropion (Wellbutrin), trazedone (Desyrel), and nefazodone (Serzone)

Additional information related to these medications can be found in Chapter 11.

Antidepressant medications affect neurotransmitters primarily, and most importantly, serotonin, norepinephrine, and dopamine. The main group of second-generation antidepressants is referred to as selective serotonin reuptake inhibitors, or SSRIs. These medications are termed "selective" because they single out the neurotransmitter serotonin. Research regarding depression indicates that a disturbance in neurotransmitter levels affects mood and behavior. SSRIs relieve the symptoms of depression through increasing available serotonin by blocking the reabsorption of this neurotransmitter by the brain. An increased level of serotonin improves neurotransmission and subsequently improves the mood.

Consideration must be made when SSRIs are tapered or discontinued. When the shorter-acting SSRIs (short half-life medications, including Effexor, Zoloft, and Luvox) have their dosages changed or discontinued, patients can experience what is called a SSRI discontinuation syndrome (an anticholinergic rebound). See Figure 3-7 for a description of experiences resulting from discontinuation syndrome.

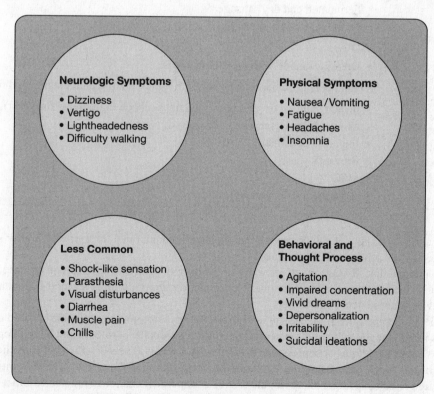

Figure 3-7 SSRI discontinuation syndrome.

Antidepressant medications must be taken for a period of time until full effectiveness is reached. That is an important consideration and must be shared with the patient and family/significant others. Typically, antidepressant medications are used to treat major depressive disorders, anxiety disorders, the depressed phase of bipolar disorder, and psychotic depressions. Additionally, they are prescribed for off-label uses for the treatment of chronic pain, migraines, peripheral and diabetic neuropathies, sleep apnea, dermatologic disorders, panic disorders, and eating disorders.

The other antidepressants work in various ways to affect neurotransmitter levels. Monoamine oxidase inhibitors (MAOIs) were discovered to positively influence the symptoms of depression experienced by individuals in the 1950s. There are potentially lethal dietary and drug interactions associated with MAOIs; therefore, they are typically reserved as a last resort. When they are ingested, MAOIs inhibit the catabolism of dietary amines. When foods containing triamines are consumed, it leads to hypertensive crisis. When foods containing tryptophan are consumed, it can lead to hyperserotonemia (serotonin syndrome).

FOOD CATEGORY	FOODS TO AVOID WHEN TAKING MAOIs
Grains	• Fresh or homemade yeast breads, sourdough breads • Crackers
Vegetables	• Fava beans, Italian broad beans, sauerkraut, Chinese pea pods, fermented pickles and olives
Fruits	• Bananas, overripe fruit, avocados
Milk	• All cheese not on "recommended" list, aged cheese, cheese sauces
Meat and Beans	• Liver • Smoked or dried meats • Smoked, pickled, or dried fish • Meat processed with tenderizers • Meat extracts • Salami • Fermented and dry sausage • Fermented soybean products
Oils	• Olives • Dressings made with aged blue cheese
Beverages	• Tap beer, ale, chianti and vermouth wines, sherry, champagne, and mixed drinks
Other	• Instant soup mixes and bouillon cubes (check ingredients for yeast), miso soup • Cheese-filled dessert and cheesecake • Imported chocolate • Brewer's yeast • MSG • All aged and fermented products

Patient education should include the directive that the diet be maintained for four weeks after stopping MAOIs (or as directed by the physician). See Figure 3-8.

It is understood that MAOIs are effective by preventing the enzyme monoamine oxidase from metabolizing norepinephrine, serotonin, and dopamine. Consequently, the individual's mood is enhanced through the increased levels of these neurotransmitters.

Tricyclic antidepressants influence the neurotransmitters serotonin, norepinephrine, and dopamine. These medications inhibit the reuptake of these neurotransmitters, especially serotonin and Norepinephrine, and result in relieving various symptoms of depression (irritability and anger). The side effects of tricyclic antidepressants are a result of this block of reabsorption. It should be noted that the relapse rate after discontinuing the use of tricyclic antidepressants is large; many run the risk of a 50 percent chance of relapse within a year.

See Figure 3-9 for an overview of the three major groups of antidepressants.

Monoamine Oxidase Inhibitors (MAOIs)

- Hypertensive Crisis- potentially life threatening event that occurs if patients receiving MAOIs eats food containing tyramine (amino acid)

- Potentially Fatal Drug Interactions- MAOIs cannot be given in combination with the following medications:

  + Tricyclic Antidepressants
  + Meperidine (Demerol)
  + CNS depressants
  + many antihypertensives/general anesthetic

- Lethal overdose capability- concern for suicidal patients receiving this medication

Figure 3-8 MAOIs.

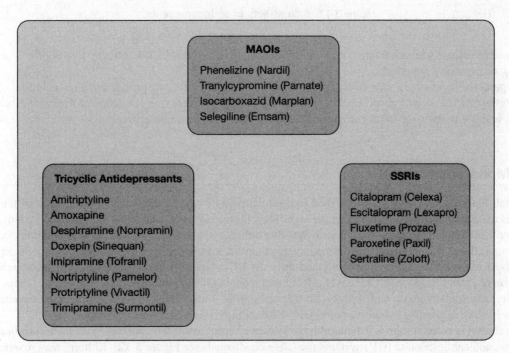

Figure 3-9 Atypical antidepressants.

Atypical antidepressants target other neurotransmitters in addition to serotonin but do not fit into the categories of the other antidepressants. Typically these are medications used when other antidepressants are ineffective or have resulted in problematic side effects (see Figure 3-10).

Atypical Antidepressants

Bupropion	Wellbutrin
Desvenlafaxine	Pritiq
Duloxetine	Cymbalta
Mirtazapine	Remeron
Trazodone	Desyrel
Venlafaxine	Effexor

Figure 3-10 Inhibitors.

MAOIs	Tricyclics	SSRIs
Daytime sedation	Dry mouth	Anxiety
Insomnia	Constipation	Agitation
Weight gain	Urinary	Akathesia
Othostatic	hesitation/retension	Nausea
hypotension	Dry nasal passages	Insomnia
Sexual dysfunction	Blurred near vision	Sexual dysfunction
	Orthostatic hypotension	Weight gain
	Weight gain	
	Tachycardia	

Figure 3-11 Side effects of antidepressants.

Most individuals who are treated with antidepressants will experience side effects. See Figure 3-11 for an overview of these adverse effects.

Atypical antidepressants' side effects are similar to those in the other categories but also include some serious side effects. Patients who abuse alcohol can experience liver problems, an activation of hypomania or mania, seizures, and mydriasis (important recognition for those with narrow-angle glaucoma).

3.6 Mood Stabilizers

Mood stabilizing medications are prescribed in the treatment of bipolar disorders. Stabilization of the mood describes the desired effect of minimizing the significant highs and lows that can be experienced by individuals diagnosed with bipolar disorder. There is evidence that indicates that sodium influences affect human excitation and mania. Lithium is a commonly prescribed medication that influences the flow of sodium through nerve and muscle cells in the body. Lithium has been used since the 1870s, initially for depression, gout, neutropenia, and prevention of cluster headaches. Lithium is effective in reducing the symptoms of elation, flight of ideas (FOI), irritability, manipulativeness, and anxiety. To a lesser extent it also helps to reduce insomnia, psychomotor agitation (PMA), aggressive/assaultive behaviors, distractibility, paranoia, and hypersexuality.

The central nervous system is the major organ system affected by lithium, but the renal, gastrointestinal (GI), endocrine, and cardiovascular (CV) systems may also be affected (see Figure 3-12). Lithium may reverse these actions by acting through G proteins, neurotransmitters, and "second messenger systems" to regulate ion channels, which it is felt in bipolar disorder are open too wide, allowing an increase in ion flow to the inside of the neuron. Lithium is the most effective mood stabilizer in eliminating suicidal ideations. Because of toxicity with risk to both the kidneys and thyroid, regular blood levels are required. It typically requires one to two weeks for the therapeutic level (0.8 to 1.4 mEq/L) to be reached, and lithium levels should be monitored closely during this

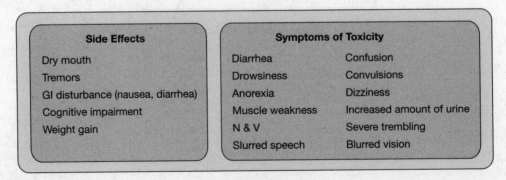

Side Effects	Symptoms of Toxicity	
Dry mouth	Diarrhea	Confusion
Tremors	Drowsiness	Convulsions
GI disturbance (nausea, diarrhea)	Anorexia	Dizziness
Cognitive impairment	Muscle weakness	Increased amount of urine
Weight gain	N & V	Severe trembling
	Slurred speech	Blurred vision

Figure 3-12 Lithium.

time until the therapeutic level is reached. Maintenance levels for lithium treatment should be between 0.4 to 1.0 mEq/L. The effective lithium blood level is close to the toxic blood value levels; therefore, it is common for some individuals to experience symptoms of mild toxicity (especially hand tremors). Treatment of lithium toxicity relies upon the level of lithium in the blood. Gastric lavage and use of medications to prevent absorption are appropriate. However, dialysis is used when levels are very high. If the patient has an acute level of lithium toxicity, how well he or she responds to treatment depends on the amount ingested and promptness of treatment. Those who do not develop CNS symptoms usually have no long-term complications. If serious CNS symptoms occur, the toxicity may result in permanent neurologic problems.

Three anticonvulsant medications—Carbamazepine (Tegretol), Divalproex (Depakote), and lamotrigine (Lamictal)—have shown efficacy in the treatment of individuals with bipolar disorder. Blood level monitoring is required for both Tegretol (4 to 12 mcg/mL) and Depakote (50 to 120 mcg/mL). Depakote (valproic acid) is an anticonvulsant that is approved by the USFDA (United States Food and Drug Administration) for the treatment of acute mania and is frequently prescribed as a mood stabilizer in the treatment of bipolar disorder. It is available in a variety of forms:

1. Capsules
2. Sprinkles
3. Extended release
4. Oral solutions

Depakote helps to prevent the breakdown of GABA (a chemical found in the brain that acts as a calming agent). By allowing the continued presence of adequate GABA, this medication helps to stabilize the electrical nerve activity in the brain and calm the periods of mania. Similar to lithium, Depakote takes a period of time to achieve its full effect, and individuals using this medication must have periodic blood level monitoring. The therapeutic blood level for this medication is 50 to 125 mmol/l.

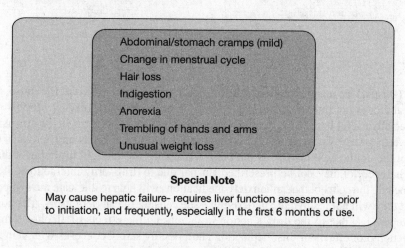

Abdominal/stomach cramps (mild)

Change in menstrual cycle

Hair loss

Indigestion

Anorexia

Trembling of hands and arms

Unusual weight loss

Special Note

May cause hepatic failure- requires liver function assessment prior to initiation, and frequently, especially in the first 6 months of use.

Figure 3-13 Depakote side effects.

3.7 Antianxiety Medications

Anxiolytic medications are prescribed in the treatment of:

- Anxiety and anxiety disorders
- Insomnia
- Obsessive compulsive disorder
- Depression
- Post-traumatic stress disorder
- Alcohol withdrawal

See Figure 3-14 for the list of these medications.

Among the most widely prescribed medications, antianxiety prescriptions hail from various classifications of medications. In this chapter, we will primarily discuss benzodiazepines. Benzodiazepines (Xanax, Klonopin, Ativan) intensify the actions of the amino acid GABA. Though all of these medications have the same pharmacologic makeup and result in similar responses, there is a difference in the course and action. There is a tendency toward dependence on this medication, and there is a risk for patients to experience discontinuation symptoms (a recurrence of the original symptoms requiring treatment) when the medication is discontinued. Withdrawal from this medication can be life-threatening, and discontinuation of any benzodiazepine should be monitored by a doctor.

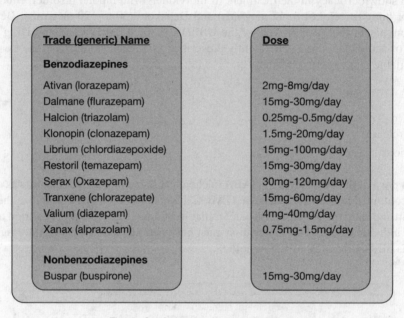

Trade (generic) Name	Dose
Benzodiazepines	
Ativan (lorazepam)	2mg-8mg/day
Dalmane (flurazepam)	15mg-30mg/day
Halcion (triazolam)	0.25mg-0.5mg/day
Klonopin (clonazepam)	1.5mg-20mg/day
Librium (chlordiazepoxide)	15mg-100mg/day
Restoril (temazepam)	15mg-30mg/day
Serax (Oxazepam)	30mg-120mg/day
Tranxene (chlorazepate)	15mg-60mg/day
Valium (diazepam)	4mg-40mg/day
Xanax (alprazolam)	0.75mg-1.5mg/day
Nonbenzodiazepines	
Buspar (buspirone)	15mg-30mg/day

Figure 3-14 Antianxiety medication.

Busperidone (Buspar), an azapirone, does not cause sedation, has no potential for abuse, does not enhance CNS depression, and does not interact significantly with other medications (except MAOIs and haloperidol). It is therefore especially useful in the treatment of anxiety or depression/anxiety. On the downside, effectiveness requires several weeks of use. This can result in noncompliance. Buspar binds and activates the 5HT1A serotonin receptor, not the amino acid GABA as the benzodiazepams are thought to. Patients that are prescribed either MAOIs or haloperidol may not be prescribed Buspar due to drug–drug interactions. It is important that patient teaching include the concept that antianxiety medications will help to alleviate the symptoms experienced by the patient, but they will not resolve the underlying issue causing the anxiety itself. Alcohol is to be avoided during benzodiazepine use due to the drug's action in increasing the effects of alcohol. Emphasis should be placed on the psychomotor effects of this medication and possibly safety concerns with using machinery or in decision-making abilities.

Chapter 3 Questions

Multiple Choice

1. Which of the following should be included in the health teaching for your patient receiving Valium?

    A. Avoid using alcohol (a CNS depressant).

    B. There are no restrictions in activities.

    C. Limit fluid intake.

    D. Beverages like coffee may be used.

2. You are caring for a patient with the diagnosis of major depression. Which of the following medications would not likely be prescribed for your patient?

   A. Prozac

   B. Tofranil

   C. Parnate

   D. Zyprexa

3. Your patient, who is prescribed lithium, has developed diarrhea and vomiting. What is the first thing you should do?

   A. Recognize that this is a drug interaction.

   B. Give the patient Cogentin.

   C. Reassure the patient that these are common side effects of lithium therapy.

   D. Hold the next dose and obtain an order for a stat serum lithium level.

4. You are assigned to a patient who is diagnosed with anxiety disorder. Which of the following medications would most likely be ordered for your patient?

   A. Prozac

   B. Valium

   C. Risperdal

   D. Lithium

5. You are providing health teaching for your patient, who is prescribed Valium. What would you include in your teaching plan?

   A. Avoid foods rich in tyramine.

   B. Take the medication after meals.

   C. It is safe to discontinue this medication any time after long-term use.

   D. Double up on the next dose if one is forgotten.

6. Which of the following should be encouraged for your patient prescribed lithium?

   A. Weigh self once per month.

   B. Restrict fluid intake to prevent edema.

   C. Do not restrict sodium intake.

   D. Avoid eating cheese and bananas and drinking wine.

7. The CNS is composed of all of the following, except:

   A. Brain

   B. Heart

   C. Spinal cord

   D. Nerves

Fill in the Blank

8. Neurotransmitters are manufactured in the neuron and will either _____ or _____ action in a cell.

True or False

9. Major neurotransmitters have been found to play a role in psychiatric disorders, and the actions and side effects of psychiatric medications.

Matching

10. Dopamine	**A.**	An excitatory amino acid implicated in the brain damage caused by strokes, hypoglycemia, and sustained hypoxia/ischemia.
11. Norepinephrine	**B.**	Found in the brain, spinal cord, and peripheral nervous system—affects the sleep/wake cycle and signals muscles to become active.
12. Serotonin	**C.**	A major inhibitory neurotransmitter (calming), it induces relaxation, reduces stress, and increases alertness.
13. Acetylcholine	**D.**	Located in the brain stem, its role is in learning, attention, memory, sleep, wakefulness, and mood regulation.
14. Glutamate	**E.**	Found only in the brain and derived from tryptophan, it plays an important role in anxiety, mood disorders, and schizophrenia.
15. Gamma-aminobutyric acid (GABA)	**F.**	Found primarily in the brain stem, involved in the control of complex movements, regulation of emotional responses, motivation, and cognition.

Chapter 3 Answers

Multiple Choice

1. **The correct response is (A).** Valium is a CNS depressant. Taking it with another CNS depressant, such as alcohol, will potentiate the effects. The client should be told that activities requiring alertness should be avoided. The medication can cause a dry mouth, so fluid intake should be increased, and stimulants must not be taken because they can decrease the effectiveness of Valium.

2. **The correct response is (D).** Zyprexa is an antipsychotic. Prozac is an SSRI, Tofranil is a tricyclic antidepressant, and Parnate is an MAOI antidepressant.

3. **The correct response is (D).** Hold the next dose and obtain an order for a stat serum lithium level. Diarrhea and vomiting are symptoms of lithium toxicity. The next dose is held and the blood test completed to validate the observation. These symptoms are not due to a drug interaction. Cogentin is used to manage EPS side effects of antipsychotics. The common side effects of lithium are fine hand tremors, nausea, polyuria, and polydipsia.

4. **The correct response is (B).** Valium is an antianxiety medication. Prozac is an antidepressant, Risperdal is an antipsychotic, and Lithium is an antimanic (mood stabilizer).

5. **The correct response is (B).** Instruct the patient to take Valium after meals because of the gastrointestinal upset that can occur with antianxiety medications. Tyramine should be avoided for those taking MAOIs because a hypertensive crisis can result. Valium can cause a dependency. It should therefore be discontinued slowly to prevent the occurrence of seizures. Patients should not be told to double up on their doses of Valium due to its CNS depressant effects.

6. **The correct response is (C).** Patients need to maintain adequate sodium intake to prevent lithium toxicity (6 to 10 g/day). Patients prescribed lithium should be instructed to maintain a normal diet, with normal salt and fluid intake (2500 to 3000 ml/day). Lithium decreases sodium reabsorption by the renal tubules, which can cause sodium depletion. Weight gain is a side effect of the medication. Monitoring should occur more frequently than monthly. Tryamine avoidance is required with MAOIs, not lithium.

7. **The correct response is (B).** The heart is part of the cardiovascular system.

Fill in the Blank

8. The correct responses are *excite/stimulate*, and *inhibit/stop*.

True or False

9. The correct response is True. Major neurotransmitters (dopamine, Norepinephrine, epinephrine, serotonin, acetylcholine, neuropeptides, glutamate, and GABA) have all been associated with psychiatric disorders and treatment.

Matching

10. F

11. D

12. E

13. B

14. A

15. C

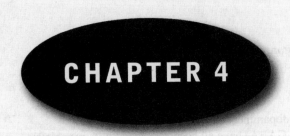

CHAPTER 4

Therapeutic Approaches in Psychiatric Nursing

Many treatment options are available for patients who are experiencing psychiatric disorders. This chapter reviews various treatment settings, psychiatric rehabilitation programs, and the challenges facing the reintroduction into the community that psychiatric patients can experience. We will also discuss the various roles of the multidisciplinary treatment team, with a focus on the role of the psychiatric nurse.

4.1 Medication Therapy

Over the past five decades, there have been significant improvements in the treatment of mental illness. Paramount to these changes was the discovery of medications to treat psychiatric disorders in the 1950s, with chlorpromazine (Thorazine) the first psychotropic medication. The development of medications allowed for a more humane treatment, replacing the previous treatment options. See Figure 4-1 for selected examples of historical treatment options.

Neolithic Age–early 1900s	**Trepanation**—born from the belief that mental illness was a result of demons inside of the skull, a hole was bored to facilitate the escape of said demon. Despite the thought that such treatment would have gone by the wayside, there remains advocates of the continuation of this treatment.
1700–1800	**Mesmerism**—based upon the concept that the gravity of the moon affected the body fluids (as it affected water on the earth), and played a role in mental illness. Magnets were used on different parts of the body as a means to disrupt the effect of gravity and restore "normal" fluid flow.
Early 1800s	**Phrenology**—this intervention is based on the belief that an individual's personality are evidenced in the bumps and crevices in their skull. This approach is considered a pseudoscience, but is part of the history of psychiatric diagnosis and treatment.
Early 1900s	**Hydrotherapy**—guided by a theory that water is a soothing element, psychiatrists used varying methods to apply the liquid as a treatment option. Examples include: warm baths, stimulating sprays, ice-water wraps, even the use of high-pressure jets.
1927	**Insulin Coma Therapy**—discovered by accident, reports a 90% recovery rate for schizophrenia. Not used due to dangerousness of insulin overdose and potential for death.
1930s–1950s	**Lobotomy**—a neurosurgical pocedure (psychosurgery) resulting in the destruction of the connections to the prefrontal cortex (refer to Chapter 2 to see the potential impact). This procedure essentially stopped being performed in the early 1970s.

Figure 4-1 History of psychiatric treatment modalities.

4.2 Therapeutic Approaches

Jean Piaget's belief about the cognitive development in children is centered on an understanding that human intelligence is an extension of the person's ability to adapt psychologically to his or her environment. There are four major stages identified, and each individual must progress successfully through each of these stages (see Figure 4-2).

AGE	STAGE	MAJOR DEVELOPMENTAL TASKS
Birth-2 Years	Sensorimotor	Developed separation of self from the environment as mobility increases; Concept of object permanence
2-6 Years	Preoperational	Expressing self through use of language, increasing understanding of symbolic gestures, achievement of object permanence
6-12 Years	Concrete Operations	Application of logic to thinking, understanding of reversibility and spatial considerations, differentiation and classification, increasing socialization and understanding of rules
12-15 Years	Formal Operations	Thinking and reasoning abstractly, developing and testing hypotheses, logical thinking and reasoning are expanded/refined, achievement of cognitive maturity

Figure 4-2 Piaget's stages of cognitive development.

Cognitive and behavior therapy are typically combined as a therapeutic approach referred to as cognitive-behavioral therapy (CBT). To allow for better understanding of each component, they have been individualized for review.

Cognitive therapy is a relatively short-term, present-oriented psychotherapy that has been clinically demonstrated to be effective for a variety of psychiatric disorders, including depression. It focuses on helping patients reduce their symptoms, solve their problems, and achieve specific goals. It is primarily based upon the belief that psychiatric diseases and subsequent behavioral health issues are classified by a negative distortion in thought processes (self-degradative considerations, decreased self-confidence, etc.). Nurses who participate in providing psychiatric care should have an understanding of how cognition develops to recognize appropriate interventions that will allow individuals to recognize and respond in a healthier manner to their thoughts.

As discussed previously, maladaptive behaviors are considered to evolve when inadequate learning has occurred. Behavior is considered to be maladaptive when it is age-inappropriate, results in impairments in daily functioning, or is perceived as socially unacceptable. In behavior therapy, the focus is on correcting the learned ineffective behavioral responses, based upon the belief that a change can be effected in behaviors and adaptive coping skills can be employed without the individual needing to understand the origin of the behavior. The core principles in this therapeutic approach are based upon the classical conditioning research and operant conditioning. Classical conditioning is a means of associated learning—the individual experiences a response to a specified stimulus. Operant conditioning, the foundation of behavior modification, uses a reward system for desired behaviors. The individual's "operations" are cued by a desired reward. The main concepts of these models were discussed previously. Specific techniques used in behavior therapy are reviewed in Figure 4-3.

The use of the nursing process assists the nurse in his or her role in directing the patient in the use of behavior therapy. An assessment is completed of the patient's current behavior with regard to his or her developmental level. Analysis of the data helps the nurse determine what actual or potential problems exist for the patient, and determine appropriate interventions to assist the patient in the development and utilization of appropriate behavioral responses. The most common example of behavior modification can be seen in the child and adolescent population. The use of tokens or points and level systems provide tangible rewards for positive and appropriate behaviors. As the patient collects the rewards, the individual is able to select an item from the unit "store," or has additional privileges allowed (later bedtime, off-unit activities, etc.). The continuing assessment of the patient's responses to the nursing strategies will help to determine the effectiveness of these actions in the evaluation of care.

Aversion Therapy	The individual, while exposed to a stimulus, experiences an unpleasant / negative response. This conditioning is afforded to result in the person associating a negative response to the stimulus
Contingency Contracting	An arrangement is agreed upon by all parties involved with the expected behavioral change specified. Also identified are the reinforcers (positive and negative). This contract is specific, but must have flexibility for adjustment.
Covert Sensitization	Utilizes the individual's imagination to produce an unpleasant response to the stimulus. Mental imagery can evoke a negative image, preferred in the use of relaxation when an undesirable behavior is considered.
Extinction	A decrease in the behavioral response as a result of the progressive withdrawal of positive reinforcement. Childhood temper tantrums offer the best example of this technique. The behaviors decrease as the parents withdraw their attention to the behaviors.
Flooding/Implosive therapy	Typically used to decrease an individuals sensitivity towards a phobia. The individual is "flooded" with the stimulus until a response is no longer elicited. This therapeutic approach is not recommended for patients who would experience adverse effect from such heightened anxiety.
Modeling	The individual imitates the behaviors demonstrated by the therapist, or other role model. Howard (2000) identifies ideal role models as those individuals who demonstrate the qualities or abilities that the person admires.
Overt Sensitization	An aversion therapy method that will result in an unpleasant or uncomfortable experience as a result of undesired behavior.
Premack Principle	A frequently occurring response acts as a positive reinforcement for a behavior that occurs less frequently (Premack, 1959).
Reciprocal Inhibition	Initiating an adaptive behavior that is incongruent with the undesired behavior resulting in a decrease or elimination of that undesired behavior
Shaping	Positive reinforcements are offered for a progression towards the ultimate behavior.
Systematic Desensitization	An approach to assist Individuals to overcome phobias by progressing through a series of steps towards the ultimate goal of facing the phobia directly.
Time Out	Removal of the individual from the environment in which the undesired behavior is exhibited. Isolation will result in a decrease or elimination of the undesired behavior to avoid removal.
Token Economy	A written or unwritten agreement where reinforcers for appropriate behavior is in the form of an agreed upon token. These tokens are then used to secure a desired item (some type activities, etc.)

Figure 4-3　Behavior therapy techniques.

Cognitive Therapy

Cognitive therapy was originally established for the treatment of depression. It conveys the belief that an individual's thoughts precede moods and that false beliefs about oneself will lead to negative emotions. The goal of this approach is to assist patients in recognizing and reviewing patterns of negativity, replacing them with more positive and reality-oriented thoughts. The use of the nursing process assists the nurse in his or her role in using techniques of cognitive therapy. Many of these tactics are practiced within the scope of practice for a general practitioner is heard/used more often. Assessment of the individual's perception of self and place in the environment helps to provide data necessary for determination of current impairments. Nurses work with the patient to establish patient-centered goals to increase self-esteem and perception of self and to develop skills for identifying negative thoughts and perception. A review of various nursing care plans demonstrates specific interventions that embody the cognitive therapy concept. The following increase feelings of hope and power in one-on-ones:

- Acknowledgment of a patient's feelings (seeking to understand a patient's perception)
- Conveyance of attitudes of the therapeutic relationship (establish rapport and increase understanding of how the patient views his or her environment)
- Use of Socratic questioning and collaborating a plan of action (use of problem-solving techniques, assisting the patient to see past the here and now)

The continuing assessment of the patient's responses to the nursing strategies will help to determine the effectiveness of these actions in the evaluation of care.

Relaxation Therapy

Patient education regarding the use of relaxation techniques is often encouraged for many psychiatric conditions. See Figure 4-4. The body and mind response to real and perceived stress can have a negative influence on functioning. Stress occurs on a daily basis, and many people feel that today's culture and climate encourages a more negative human response to stimuli. Stress management programs and devices have resulted in an entrepreneurial boom, and many places of employment recognize the importance of offering programs and counseling to assist staff in managing stress levels effectively (resulting in decreased absences and illnesses). An assessment of the stress experienced by individuals, in addition to knowledge and use of adaptive coping skills, will help determine the need for relaxation therapy.

The use of the nursing process assists nurses in their role in directing the patient in the use of relaxation techniques. Assessment of the individual's current stressors and responses, previously employed coping skills, and readiness for learning are essential in identifying problems. Working with the patient to establish patient-centered

TECHNIQUE	NURSING INTERVENTIONS
Deep breathing	1. Direct the patient to sit, stand, or lie in a comfortable position 2. Place one hand on abdomen, the other on chest area 3. Inhale slowly, use a count of 4-6, through the nose 4. Exhale slowly, use a count of 4-6, through the mouth Pursing the lips will help maintain control
Progressive relaxation	1. Direct the patient to sit in a comfortable chair, hands opened on lap, eyes closed, feet flat on floor 2. Take 3 breaths (as described in deep breathing exercise) 3. Beginning at the feet and moving up to the face, tense each muscle group for 6-8 seconds and then relax for a count of 20 4. Direct the patient to focus on the feelings between contraction and relaxation 5. Use of soft, relaxing music may facilitate relaxation benefits
Meditation	1. Provide a quiet environment, encourage the patient to sit in a comfortable position (chair, cross-legged on the floor, yoga position, etc.) 2. Instruct the patient to identify a specific word, sound, object to focus 3. Encourage the patient to practice centering attention on the selected focus for 15 minutes per day, over several weeks 4. Reassure the patient that initially intrusive thoughts may interject, but with practice they will exert more control over their focus
Mental imagery	1. Direct the patient to sit or lie in a comfortable position 2. Assist them in selecting a scene, place, or other image that they find enjoyable 3. Instruct the patient to close their eyes and verbally guide them to their selected place 4. Offer very descriptive encouragement to enhance their imagination (the smell of the air, the sound of birds, etc.) 5. Interject words emphasizing how relaxed the patient is feeling, encourage them to return to this place whenever they feel the need for relaxation
Biofeedback	1. Educate the patient regarding the biofeedback equipment to be used 2. Encourage the patient to focus on the results of the measurements provided 3. Encourage the use of relaxation techniques to decrease the signals emitted from the equipment

Physical exercise	1. Encourage the patient to participate in regular physical activity (as directed by their physician)
	2. Provide patient education related to the benefits of different types of activity
	  a. aerobic exercise benefits the cardiovascular system by improving the body's use of oxygen
	  b. low-intensity exercise improves flexibility, helps maintain weight, relieve muscular tension
	  c. Vigorous exercise increases serotonin and endorphins, improving mood

Figure 4-4 Relaxation techniques.

goals to reduce negative influences of their responses to stressors and provide the tools necessary for prevention of future maladaptive responses are focused on assisting the patient in achieving his or her highest level of functioning. Interventions include teaching the patient to develop effective coping skills and improving the patient's self-identification of the presence of increasing stress/anxiety. The continued assessment of the patient's responses to the nursing strategies will help to determine the effectiveness of these actions in the evaluation of care.

4.3   Assertiveness and Self-Esteem

Assertiveness Training

Assertive behavior (protecting personal rights while respecting the rights of others) allows for individuals to have more control over situations through encouraging the use of decisive and confident behaviors in their journey and interactions with others. Differing from aggressive behaviors (these individuals violate the rights of others) and nonassertive behaviors (pleasing others and violating one's personal rights), assertive behaviors allow for an increased self-esteem and foster the formation of satisfying and positive interpersonal relationships. The use of the nursing process assists nurses in their role in directing the patient in the use of assertive behaviors. Assessment of the individual assists the nurses in educating the patient regarding the appropriateness of their behavioral response. During this phase, nurses must allow for recognition/self-assessment of their own responses. Role modeling is an important intervention. Nurses must be able to understand and use assertiveness skills themselves in order to assist their patients in the development and utilization of similar techniques. This data is used to determine the actual and potential problems encountered by the patient.

The next step is to establish patient-centered goals. A primary goal is to assist the individual to establish satisfying and more meaningful interpersonal relationships. Interventions include patient education regarding their individual rights and need to respect themselves and specific assertiveness techniques (verbal cues, body language, cognitive approaches). The continuing assessment of the patient's responses to the nursing strategies will help to determine the effectiveness of these actions in the evaluation of care.

Supporting Self-Esteem

Self-concept includes the perception of physicality (body image), personal identity (who one is), and self-esteem. Self-esteem is the realistic awareness of one's abilities and limitations. It is the recognition and valuing of oneself. This presence of judgment (ability to form such an opinion of oneself) differentiates us from other animals. The development of the self occurs across the life span. As discussed previously, Erikson offers an explanation of how one's self-esteem progresses. An understanding of this concept is important in nursing care, as it offers guidelines for usual and expected human responses. Establishing personal boundaries is important in the development of the self. It is a critical element needed for establishing healthy relationships. The ability to form boundaries demonstrates a healthy self-esteem, shows recognition of one's own needs (self-respect) and the needs of another, and sets limits for others.

- *Rigid boundaries*—Some individuals maintain a very distinct and consistent boundary. Typically, this indicates an individual's inability to consider others or open themselves to alternatives. A person with rigid boundaries is closed or walled off so nobody can get close to him or her either physically or emotionally.
- *Flexible boundaries*—These are the healthiest boundaries. Individuals with this ability are able to allow variances as appropriate. These people are resistant to manipulation and exploitation.
- *Enmeshed boundaries*—This occurs when boundaries become blended, when an individual is no longer able to differentiate his or her needs and desires from another person.

The use of the nursing process assists nurses in their role in directing the patient in establishing personal boundaries. During the assessment phase, the nurse must first ensure self-awareness of his or her own self-esteem and boundaries. Data collected from and about the patient allow for analysis of the presence of self-esteem problems. The nurse then works with the patient to determine patient-centered goals (ability to identify strengths, accept positive feedback from others, accept personal responsibility and try new experiences, etc.). Interventions include a myriad of esteem-boosting strategies, including:

- Establishing a therapeutic relationship
- Conveying acceptance and being nonjudgmental in approach
- Using therapeutic communication techniques to encourage verbalization of feelings
- Assisting the patient to identify positive attributes and personal strengths

The continuing assessment of the patient's responses to the nursing strategies will help to determine the effectiveness of these actions in the evaluation of care.

4.4 Therapeutic Groups

Belonging to a group is an inherent role for human beings. Groups we can be part of include family, friends, work, activity, networking, social, religious, and living. As a member of a group, each of us has a role and responsibility to facilitate the functioning of the group. Nurses participate in various groups throughout the course of their work. There are task groups (policy and procedure committees), interdisciplinary treatment teams (formulating plans of care for patients and unit-specific policy and procedures), as well as specialized groups directed toward the care of their patients. The setting for therapeutic groups may be the inpatient unit, or in the community. To function effectively as a group leader, the nurse needs to be aware of the phases of group development, the roles and motivation of the group members, and how to address problematic behaviors sometimes exhibited during the group sessions.

The concept of therapeutic group differs from that of group therapy. Group therapy has a theoretical base, and the leaders typically have advanced degrees. In therapeutic groups, the focus is not on theory, but on group relations and the interactions among group members. Leaders of both types of groups need to have an understanding of the group process (the roles of group members and how members interact with each other), as well as group content (knowledge of the topic or issue at hand).

There are also self-help groups. These particular groups consist of individuals sharing similar problems, are focused on reducing further emotional distress, and may or may not have a professional leader (such as Alcoholics Anonymous, weight loss groups, bereavement groups, etc.).

Psychiatric and mental health nurses are ideal group leaders due to their holistic approach to patient care and lead various types of psychoeducational and therapeutic milieu groups (patient education, assertiveness training, support groups, transition to discharge, etc.), following the guidelines established by the American Nurses Association, as discussed in Chapter 2. Generalist nurses may lead therapeutic groups; however, the nurse must hold an advanced degree to function as a leader for group therapy.

4.5 Complementary and Alternative Medicine

Allopathic medicine has been the historical focus of treatment learned in medical schools across the United States. Alternative and complementary medicine has been establishing itself as a therapeutic alternative to more conventional approaches to care. Alternative medicine techniques are used to replace customary treatment, and complementary medicine is a combination of interventions with traditional approaches. For a review of the categories of complementary and alternative medicine (CAM), see Figure 4-5.

CATEGORY	EXAMPLE
Alternative Medical Systems	Acupuncture, Homeopathetic medicine, Environmental medicine, Naturopathic medicine
Mind Body Interventions	Art & music therapy, meditation; dance, humor, prayer therapies, biofeedback, hypnotherapy
Biologically Based Therapies	Herbal medicine, antioxidizing agents, chelation therapy, metabolic therapy
Manipulative and Body Based Methods	Acupressure, chiropractic, massage, osteopathy, reflexology, rolfing
Energy Therapies	Blue light treatments, electroacupuncture, electomagnetic fields, electrostimulation/neuromagnetic stimulation

Figure 4-5 Categories of complementary and alternative medicine.

4.6 Indication and Treatment Goals of Psychiatric Settings

There are several potential levels of care in the mental health continuum of care. Important in this decision making regarding appropriate level of care is an understanding of the indications and goals. The environment in which this care is delivered is as varied as the levels occurring within the walls of a hospital, in the community, in a jail facility, in a school, in a church, or on the streets. The goal in determining the level of care for patients is to meet their needs at the least restrictive level. The following are defined from the least restrictive to the most restrictive.

Crisis intervention is a brief (typically not more than six hours) type of care that focuses on stabilization, symptom reduction, and prevention of relapse that will require inpatient care. Nurses respond to crises every day across the practice areas. Identification of and ability to mobilize support systems is a priority focus in crisis care. The nurse is responsible for assessing the precipitating elements of the current situation. This includes

- The event itself
- Assessment of the individual's mental status
- Assessment of current coping mechanisms
- Adequacy of support system
- Accessibility to other support services
- Use or abuse of substances

Analysis of this data will assist the nurse in selecting the most appropriate interventions to resolve the crisis and will help move the individual toward his or her pre-crisis level of functioning. During the evaluation phase, the nurse and individuals involved should review and summarize the events of the treatment based upon this feedback. A referral for continued treatment may be indicated.

Crisis counseling may last up to three months. A crisis response occurs typically when a person experiences normal reactions to an abnormal occurrence. Crisis intervention revolves around the belief that most individuals will be able to recover from a crisis if they have available to them the support, guidance, and resources required. The expectation is that the clinician will develop a rapport with the individual (patient, family, or community), assess and identify the problem, assist the patient in utilizing adaptive coping skills, and formulate/implement a plan of action to address the situation.

Outpatient treatment is the level of care that occurs outside of the hospital setting. The Community Mental Health Act of 1963 demonstrates a fundamental belief that community-centered care was more desirable than inpatient treatment. The least restrictive care environment, these services are less intensive and are for those patients who do not require inpatient, residential, or home-care settings. A main advantage for this treatment option is the ability to maintain direct ties with the community and the preservation of the patient's autonomy. The goal of outpatient treatment is to empower the patient through education and guidance in self-supportive measures.

While it is typical that patients voluntarily pursue outpatient treatment, many states do have a law that can mandate compliance with outpatient treatment (Mandatory Outpatient Treatment, or MOT). New York State has one of the most used and most recognized Assisted Outpatient Laws, *Kendra's Law*. MOT is a court-ordered outpatient service for noncompliant patients based upon a risk assessment of dangerousness. This risk assessment is based upon the patient's history of dangerousness, not on the actual presentation of the patient. The goal is to decrease the danger posed to the community and the patient if he or she were to decompensate due to noncompliance with medication or sessions. These patients, by the fact that they are court-ordered to attend outpatient treatment and/or comply with prescribed therapies, can be hospitalized by the occurrence of noncompliance—no danger to self, others, or inability to care for self needs to be current.

Many patients discharged from inpatient treatment are referred for outpatient treatment. The focus of this treatment is reintegration into the community and home setting, medication management and compliance, and symptom treatment. Nursing care in the community is significantly different than unit-based nursing care. The nurse should have an awareness of community resources and knowledge of and flexibility in problem-solving techniques for the patient and significant others. Additionally, it must be remembered that typically the nurse is a guest in the home of the patient. Though a professional and therapeutic relationship occurs, it is different than the typically authoritarian role in the hospital. Treatment may be provided within one organization or may reach across several organizations, depending upon the needs of the patient and ability of the organization. A good example of the need for multiple organizational involvements would be child and adolescent patients. These patients often require additional services offered in the school setting as well as services at home.

Residential services are a treatment level that is outside of the hospital yet provides for 24-hour/day supervision. Similar to the length of stay for partial programs, patients may participate in residential services for anywhere from 24 hours to several years. Community mental health services in the form of in-home mental health care is an alternative to inpatient care for those patients who can safely be maintained in the home but for whom outpatient services does not meet their treatment needs. Residential services can take place as temporary living arrangements until the patient is prepared to return to living alone or can be longer-term adult homes, halfway houses, group homes, independent living programs, respite housing, and crisis housing. Many challenges come with the establishment of such residential living situations, often involving the immediate community's opposition to having psychiatric patients living in their neighborhood.

Partial hospitalization programs (PHP) or "day hospitals" were developed during the 1980s in response to curtailing the costs associated with inpatient psychiatric treatment. This service helps those patients that are experiencing decompensation in their social or occupational functioning, or those individuals not able to perform independently on a daily basis, who are not deemed an imminent danger to self or others. Typically patients are enrolled in partial programs on a short-term basis (24 hours to 3 to 6 months) or long-term (several months to years). This particular treatment modality is also appropriate for those patients who do not need the strict structure of an inpatient unit but are not yet able to return to the community. It is an excellent transitional opportunity and may assist in preventing, or minimizing, recidivism.

Inpatient treatment is the most restrictive of the treatment modalities and is used for those patients which exhibit one or more of three specific criteria:

- Danger to self
- Danger to others
- Inability to provide basic needs (review Maslow's Hierarchy of Needs)

The focus of treatment in the inpatient setting is typically one-on-one interactions and milieu therapy. Milieu therapy is a term identified by Bruno Bettelheim in 1948 that describes the use of the environment to treat the psychiatric patient. Milieu therapy includes everything in the environment that can influence the individual and is an essential responsibility and intervention of nurses. Examples are providing a safe environment for an aggressive patient, ensuring the safety of a patient experiencing disturbed thought process, advocating for patients, and referring patients to appropriate community resources.

Historically, patients could (and would) be hospitalized for months and even years. Since the deinstitutionalization movement of the 1970s and 1980s, the goal is to minimize these hospitalizations and return patients to the community as soon as is feasible. The Americans with Disabilities Act (ADA) holds that mental illness is a form of disability, and in 1999 the United States Supreme Court made a decision based upon this inclusion that the institutional isolation of an individual with mental illness is a form of discrimination. Inpatient psychiatric care can occur in a psychiatric hospital, in a psychiatric unit in a general hospital, or in a state operated psychiatric facility.

Additionally, some patients who meet criteria for discharge from inpatient care but are not yet prepared to return to the community may continue to reside at state-run facilities, and there are forensic services for the incarcerated population. Inpatient psychiatric hospitalizations are on a voluntary or involuntary basis. Please refer to your specific state mental hygiene laws regarding involuntary psychiatric admissions. An involuntary hospitalization is a good example of a legal/ethical issue in psychiatric nursing, as discussed in Chapter 2. Initiating an involuntary hospitalization could infringe upon an individual's self-determination, as well as lead potential charges of false imprisonment.

4.7 The Role of the Nurse and Trends of the Profession

Milieu therapy (therapeutic community, or therapeutic environment) is the application of the concept that the environment can serve to influence all aspects of the patient's hospital experience in a therapeutic (helpful) manner. This approach can be applied to the inpatient and outpatient setting. The idea of the therapeutic community originates with B. F. Skinner and holds the belief that we need to focus not solely on the difficulties a patient is experiencing but assess and emphasize his or her strengths. The multidisciplinary treatment team in the psychiatric setting can include the following:

- Psychiatrist
- Psychologist
- Psychiatric nurse practitioner
- Psychiatric and mental health nurse
- Psychiatric social worker
- Occupational, recreational, and art therapists
- Psychiatric aides

Not all settings have a representative from each discipline available, and some have only part-time staff.

Each clinician involved in the care of a patient needs to recognize that every interaction with a patient (verbal and nonverbal) is an opportunity for a positive and therapeutic event. It is important that the patient is encouraged to be responsible and accountable for the environment in which he or she operates. The use of community meetings is effective in establishing such an attitude toward the unit or therapeutic setting. As important to responsibility for his or her environment, each patient is to be held responsible and accountable for his or her behaviors. Peer pressure is a positive influence in the therapeutic community. Feedback from a peer can, at times, be more effective than from an authority figure on the treatment team. Managing the occurrence of inappropriate or acting-out behaviors is paramount. It is essential that such behaviors are addressed at the time of the occurrence. This allows for an introspective approach and encourages the evaluation of behaviors upon others in the group. A core belief in milieu therapy is refraining from punishment.

Chapter 1 discussed the history of psychiatric nursing and identified a few well-regarded leaders in this practice area. Hildegard Peplau is considered the "mother of psychiatric nursing." Emphasizing the nurse–patient relationship, she focused on the importance of patient participating and independent nursing actions. Peplau's approach embraces the concept of the shared experience, with the nurse facilitating this experience through the nursing process. Nurses gather both objective and subjective data and formulate a professional opinion about their patient's situation. Validation of the nurse's perception is done with the patient. Once the nurse and patient have agreed upon the current issue, selection of appropriate interventions occurs.

This collaborative approach to care allows for the shared experience. The psychiatric and mental health nurse works with patients who are experiencing mental health issues across their life spans. The main focus is to promote and maintain optimal functioning, prevent the occurrence of mental illness/further decompensation, and assist in the development and utilization of adaptive coping skills to manage the various stressors experienced. This book provides specific responsibilities with regard to the application of the nursing process in the psychiatric setting for each disorder discussed.

As with medical nursing, psychiatric nursing will continue to gravitate toward the community level of care. It will be important for nurses to review and improve case management skills (one of the roles of the nurse discussed previously). The current focused trends in psychiatric and mental health nursing revolve around the following:

- Violence and self-inflicted injuries
- The aging population
- Increase in cultural/ethnic diversity and improvements in technology

Nurses can and will be expected to provide both preventative and post-event care for those individuals exposed to violent situations (murder, assaults, wars, suicides, gang-related events, etc.). As the population ages, consideration for age-related cognition problems (senility, Alzheimer's disease, and other dementias) as well as issues related to belonging and loss will require attention. The expansion in cultural diversity demands that all nurses attend to their competency in providing appropriate care recognizing various beliefs, attitudes, and health-care practices. The introduction of technological studies (MRIs, CT scans, PET scans, etc.) in support of biological theories, and the use of other technology in care (internet, intranet, PDAs, computer documentation, medication administration, etc.) require that nurses keep current in accessing and utilizing these methods of communication and information.

One of the most important roles that nurses have and must remain focused on is the role of a patient advocate. As discussed, the care of the psychiatric patient extends far past the confines of the hospital walls. Nurses must be aware of the legal and ethical issues, aware of community resources and accessibility, and interested in and involved in legislative activities regarding mental health issues and concerns. When the economy experiences difficulties, often the more vulnerable and less represented populations face dire cutbacks.

The Roles of the Psychiatric Nurse

Nurses take on various roles in their care of the psychiatric patient. The nurse is a caregiver, care encourager, teacher, role model, surrogate of a significant person to the patient, counselor, authority figure, and "friend." The term friend is highlighted as a means of emphasizing the importance of maintaining professional and therapeutic boundaries while striving to make a connection. Many novice nurses become confused by what appears as a "friendship" between the nurse and his or her patient, as this caring relationship can appear as a friendship to the untrained eye. Bronislaw Malinowski coined the phrase "phatic communication" in 1923 to describe the small talk that occurs during a professional relationship. As discussed previously, continual therapeutic communication can have an adverse effect on the establishment of positive rapport with a patient by maintaining an unemotional relationship. The skill of social chat is an essential element for the psychiatric nurse, offering the flavor of social interaction, yet maintaining professional boundaries. The goal is the provision of nursing care to assist the patient in reintegration into the community through the art of a positive rapport and a supportive and therapeutic relationship.

Chapter 1 reviewed the American Nurses Association's Standards of Psychiatric Mental Health Clinical Nursing Practice. This defines the specific actions of the psychiatric nurse. As a psychiatric nurse, you will apply the same nursing process (the basic framework of nursing) in your

- Assessment
- Diagnosing
- Outcome planning
- Intervening
- Evaluation of care as in any other practice area

As with the other practice areas, you will use the standardized classification system of the North American Nursing Diagnosis Association (NANDA) to define your identified problems.

In addition to ensuring familiarity with the nursing process and NANDA diagnostic labels, you will be expected to be familiar with the *Diagnostic and Statistical Manual of Mental Disorders* (DSM-IV) produced by the APA (2000), and the International Statistical Classification of Diseases and Related Health Problems issued by the World Health Organization (1993). Knowledge of the medical diagnosis, signs and symptoms of illnesses, prevalence and other relevant health issues allows for professional communication of the nurse as a member of the multidisciplinary treatment team.

The focus of care in psychiatric nursing is on counseling, an intervention supported by the American Nurses Association (see Standards of Psychiatric Mental Health Clinical Nursing Practice in Chapter 1). While formal counseling does require education above the generalist level (diploma, ADN, BSN), nurses must possess a basic knowledge of counseling techniques and skills. The establishment of the therapeutic relationship (discussed in Chapter 2) and the establishment of a positive and professional rapport depends upon this ability.

4.8   The Influence of Theoretical Knowledge and Models on Nursing Practice

Chapter 1 reviewed several leading theories regarding psychiatric illness and treatment. There are many theories available that try to describe and explain human behavior in response to mental health and mental illness. Clinicians use the concepts behind these theories to guide their practice. As a nurse, knowledge of these theories will assist you in

- Determining relevant aspects for assessment data
- Assisting in the analysis of data to identify appropriate nursing impairments/problems
- Selecting applicable nursing strategies to achieve identified outcomes
- Evaluating the effectiveness of your plan of care

These theories provide frameworks for understanding human behavior and responses to illness, and as a means for assessing interactions with patients, families, and colleagues. Additionally, they provide direction in accessing our highest level of functioning, and that of patients.

Sigmund Freud

As discussed earlier, Sigmund Freud developed the psychoanalytic theory. Integral to his theory are ego defense mechanisms. He believed that human behavior is motivated by subconscious thoughts and feelings. He identified three components of the personality's structure: the id (innate desires), the superego (morality), and the ego (mediator of the id and superego). He described the use of ego defense mechanisms as the means which the ego uses to protect itself and manage basic drives or emotional issues. The ego acquires these protections to minimize the experience of anxiety by impeding the conscious awareness of the ominous feelings.

Important to note is that ego defense mechanisms are believed to operate at the unconscious level—most individuals are unaware of their use and require reality orientation by the clinician. They serve to distort reality to minimize the perception of threat to an individual. Defense mechanisms are important and are called into use by all individuals. In some instances when such a disruption in reality occurs, it impedes adaptive coping and thwarts personal growth. (We will discuss defense mechanisms further in our review of anxiety and anxiety disorders.) See Figure 4-6 for a list of defense mechanisms.

Henry Stack Sullivan

Sullivan's theory on interpersonal relationships lies at the core of Hildegard Peplau's nursing theory of interpersonal relationship. He felt that most mental illness was a response to difficulties with interpersonal relationships. The responsibility of the nurse, in relation to the formation of a therapeutic relationship, embraces the ideals of the interpersonal theory. It is through the formation of these positive and therapeutic relationships with the nurse that the patients will gain confidence in establishing positive relationships with others.

Abraham Maslow

Abraham Maslow encouraged assessment of an individual's strengths versus weaknesses. In contrast to theories which embrace negative aspects in relationships and self-regard, Maslow focuses on love, compassion, happiness, and well-being. He identified motivation as a hierarchy of needs essential for all humans to attain. Nursing uses the needs that have been determined by Maslow in prioritization of nursing care and as a means of recognizing human potential/strengths. The most basic human needs are the physiological; the most advanced are self-transcendent.

The Holistic Approach of Nursing

The ideas of behavioral theorists such as Ivan Pavlov, John Watson, and B. F. Skinner also developed as a result of the belief that, contrary to Freud's determination that an individual's future is destined at a young age, the personality is composed of learned behaviors. The nursing profession incorporates this principle to support the interventions of behavior management and behavior modification programs.

The biological model with respect to psychiatric disorders holds that there is a neurological, chemical, biological, and/or genetic etiology, and that the ensuing abnormal behaviors are part of the disease process. Psychiatric medications are found to target specific parts of the brain. It is the belief that such illnesses are a result of a biological imbalance, and medications (such as the advent of chlorpromazine) can target the illness and address the symptoms. In addition to medication, there is support for nutritional implications, surgery, and other biological interventions. The continued advancements in medical research demand that nurses remain aware and knowledgeable of all research and new findings in the psychiatric field. Nursing actions address the physical needs of a patient (medications, sleep, nutrition, food and fluid, exercise, elimination, and other bodily needs and functions), as well as prepare the patient for somatic therapies (such as electroconvulsive therapy).

It is essential that the nurse recognize and embrace ideas of researchers without absolutely discarding other components of care. Nurses will need to continue to incorporate interventions focused on the biological needs of patients, as well as the essential consideration of establishing a therapeutic relationship, as the biological theory continues expanding its position in psychiatric care. A holistic profession, nursing will continue to incorporate these concepts of physicality with the emotional needs of the patient, recognizing that society and the environment play a part in the patient's response to illness.

EGO DEFENSE MECHANISM	DEFINITION	EXAMPLE
Altruism	Individual manages internal conflict/stressors through actions dedicating self to meet needs of others	Mother of a child who was killed in a drunk driving accident forms a local chapter of anti-impaired while driving group
Avoidance	Evasion of events, activities, objects or persons who symbolize unconscious impulses	Person who has a fear of heights navigates road trips to bypass bridges
Compensation	Overemphasis in one area to balance perceived deficits in another	Nurse offers to chair several committees so her supervisor will like her.
Conversion	Use of a physical symptom to express an emotional discord	An individual who threatened to hit someone suddenly becomes paralyzed in his arm.
Denial	Inability to recognize an unbearable situation; reality of implications and consequences of behaviors	A patient with diabetes who eats candy
Devaluation	The assignment of negative qualities to self or others to manage an emotional conflict or stressor	Person who overindulges on sweets and then describes themselves as weak or fat
Displacement	Directing emotional component from one object to another less threatening one	A person who got a poor evaluation comes home and has a fight with their spouse
Dissociation	Separating a thought or activity from the consciousness	A young woman has no memory of a sexual assault that occurred as a child
Identification	An unconscious modeling of self by another or even group of people. Occurs as the individual is establishing their identify or aspiring to reach a goal.	Nursing student decides to enter practice as a critical care nurse because her favorite clinical instructor is one.
Intellectualization	Use of abstract thinking to separate and control or minimize emotions of a painful experience	Woman focuses on arranging the funeral of her mother instead of embracing her feelings of sadness and grief
Introjection	Assimilation of another's beliefs, attitudes and values as one's own.	An individual, who has no inclination to exercise, joins the gym like her best friend
Passive Aggression	Individual manages internal conflict/stressor by circuitously expressing aggression towards others under the facade of compliance.	Nurse who agreed to work a weekend when asked by their supervisor, calls in sick
Projection	Ascribing unacceptable inclinations on another object or person	A prejudicial person loudly accuses others of being racist
Repression	Blocking of emotionally painful or conflicting thoughts, impulses or memory from conscious awareness	Individual has no recall of events before the age when removed from parents care due to abuse
Rationalization	Identification of socially acceptable behaviors to explain behavior.	Student who fails a test states "The teacher doesn't know how to teach"
Reaction Formation	A means of excusing one's self to avoid guilt, responsibility, conflict, or loss of respect.	Nurse who feels her supervisor is an ineffective leader tells her colleagues "She's the best manager I have ever had"
Sublimation	Behavior in opposition of thoughts and feelings; overcompensation for unacceptable impulses	A person who experiences aggressive impulses becomes a boxer
Suppression	Debilitating unacceptable thoughts and impulses through substitution of socially acceptable acts. A conscious expulsion of thoughts or feelings from the conscious self	A nurse comes to work, despite the recent death of her father, stating "The unit is too busy now, I don't have time to think about my Dad."
Undoing	Exhibiting behavior as a means of negating unacceptable behavior.	The doctor who had yelled at the unit staff the day before brings in coffee and bagels for everyone.

Figure 4-6 Ego defense mechanism.

4.9　The Patient Population of Psychiatric Nursing

As mentioned, psychiatric and mental health nurses provide care across the life span. Psychiatric nursing interventions occur across the mental-health continuum and include individuals (children, adolescents, adults), families, and communities. Psychiatric nurses work with those patients who have a chronic mental illness, those individuals who are experiencing transient functional difficulties, and those who are not actively experiencing problems. In addition to providing psychiatric nursing care to those individuals experiencing acute and chronic mental illness, the nurse will be expected to care for those patients who are medically ill, dying or grieving, homeless, incarcerated, and developmentally disabled.

When caring for a medically ill patient, it is essential that the nurse attend to both the physical and psychosocial needs of the patient. Patients respond emotionally to physical illness, and the psychological stress can exacerbate the signs and symptoms of their medical illnesses. Mentally healthy individuals faced with psychosocial difficulties due to a situational or maturational problem may experience a crisis that requires a time-limited approach. When that problem is a life-threatening or disabling illness or disease, the patient may require long-term interventions. The nurse can ensure a comprehensive approach by maintaining safe and compassionate care, assisting patients in coping more effectively. Addressing both the physical and psychosocial needs of the patient will facilitate compliance with treatment, improve quality of life, and contribute to enhanced healing. There is an enhanced diagnostic category "Psychological Factors Affecting Medical Condition" (PFAMC) in the DSM-IV that specifically identifies factors that can impede medical treatment, pose health risks, or cause stress-related pathophysiological changes. Expected psychological responses to serious medical illnesses include the following:

- Depression
- Anxiety
- Substance abuse
- Grieving
- Denial
- Fear of dependency

A psychosocial assessment is an essential component of all patient care, not just the psychiatric patient. It is important that the nurse is able to appreciate how the illness is affecting the patient's perception of quality of life. Included in this assessment are the identification of current coping skills, support system, health practice and beliefs, and the patient's perceived impact of the illness/disease.

Nurses are in an ideal position to assess these components and provide education related to coping skills, healthy living, and stress reduction activities. Typically the information is included in assessment tools employed by facilities, but if not, the nurse should advocate for inclusion of biological and psycho-social-spiritual needs of the patient.

Care of the terminally ill and their significant others can be a demanding yet fulfilling charge. It has the potential of affecting the nurse on a professional and personal level as the nurse develops the ability to accept end-of-life for their patients. The goal for the nurse is to ensure dignity during the death process for the patient and significant others. This focus allows for a positive experience for all those involved.

The Implications of Hospice and Palliative Care

Hospice and palliative care allow for a personal and comfortable end-of-life experience. Hospice care allows patients to die in their own homes versus the hospital. The ability to be maintained at home offers flexibility in final arrangements for the patient and allows the patient to remain in the comfort of familiar surroundings for as long as possible. Hospice care is available to everyone regardless of age, illness, and ability to pay. What is required is the identification by a physician that the patient has a life expectancy of six months or less due to a terminal illness, and the patient has opted for hospice instead of curative care. Palliative care is an upcoming specialty that has advanced in response to the hospice movement and the recognition of the need for improved treatment of the dying. The focus of care is to ensure minimal pain to be experienced by the dying individual.

4.10   Grief

The Grief Response

It is understood that each person will, at one point or another during his or her existence, experience death, grief, and mourning. Loss is a unique and individually defined experience, and grief is a normal response to this loss. It can be due to separation or lost possession of an item or individual. It can be a failure (actual or self-identified), life situation that alters the individual or family composition, or other life experiences as identified by the person. Loss through death can result in a significant crisis for many individuals.

The Theories Addressing the Human Response to Grieving

Though often used interchangeably, the clinician must distinguish between the following terms associated with grief:

- *Loss* is the state of being without something that one once had.
- *Grief* is the emotional distress related to the loss.
- *Bereavement* is being in a position where someone has been parted from something—usually by death.
- *Mourning* is the conventional manifestation of sorrow experienced by one, especially related to death.

Though each individual responds to loss personally, there has been sufficient research to identify expected behaviors. Psychological states experienced during times of loss and grieving include shock, denial, and longing for the deceased. Among theorists of human response to grief, nurses are most familiar with Elisabeth Kubler-Ross; however, John Bowlby and George Engel are also renowned in this field. Though each of the theorists applies his or her own specific perspective to the human response to grieving, the core experiences are universal, including:

- Consternation and denial
- Awareness of corporal unease
- Obsession with a representation of the deceased
- Feelings of regret and guilt
- Feelings of anger
- Alteration in attitude
- Refocus of behavior

The Identification of a Maladaptive Response to Grief

It is important to remember that each person requires an independent period of time to process loss. The acute phase of the grief process can continue for a period of months, and the resolution of the entire process may extend for years without being considered an abnormal response. Recognition of the cultural belief and practices held by those mourning are essential considerations to minimize the possibility of interrupting their individual grieving process. An individual's response to loss is considered dysfunctional if the individual is unable to employ adequate cognitive and emotional responses in his or her grieving process and there is a delayed, exaggerated, or prolonged reaction. Several researchers have noted that a significant occurrence in maladaptive grieving is related to the loss of self-esteem. The nurse can expect to assess the following in the patient experiencing maladaptive grieving:

1. Communication of feelings related to distress or denial and inhibited grieving before completion of the process
2. Exaggerated or prolonged grieving for the person's cultural expectation

The individual may also report inability to maintain adequate daily functioning, self-destructive behaviors, self-neglect, and social isolation. He or she might experience sustained depressive or anxiety symptoms, or even experience suicidal ideations.

Psychiatric Nursing Care of the Dying Patient

The nursing care of a dying patient and his or her significant others requires a holistic, compassionate attitude. An important consideration is the occurrence of anticipatory grieving. An individual who is dying may experience feelings of loneliness and social isolation due to the subconscious separation initiated by family/significant others as they experience anticipatory grieving and begin distancing from the dying individual.

The basis of nursing is a caring approach, which is essential in the determination of perceived quality of care by the patient (individual, family, and community). Nursing care for the bereaved occurs through active listening, assisting in the facilitation of communication processes, educating individuals and significant others/communities in the dying process, and promoting effective bereavement through recognizing situations that can enhance health and allow grieving individuals to move past the loss. The nurse must have cultural competency and excellent communication skills to manage the flow of information between the patient/family and other members of the multidisciplinary team. Various aspects related to loss and death must be assessed. Cultural rituals, beliefs, and attitudes can pertain to:

- Dying and care of the body
- Afterlife
- Expectation of normal expressions of grief
- Family members roles
- Tolerance related to age of the deceased and cause of death (suicide, substance-induced illness, virus related death, etc.)

Equally important is the nurse's ability for self-care. Nursing care of the dying is a physically and emotionally taxing practice. The nurse must be able to recognize the impact and ensure the ability to recharge him- or herself. When health-care providers experience loss in their practice, it can revive the clinicians' past grief response. Nurses who have unresolved issues related to death, dying, and grief may be ineffective in their role of providing care for others experiencing loss. The need for critical debriefing is a recognizable staff support in the event of grief/loss in preventing the clinician's own maladaptive reactions. The intervention of education is always paramount in nursing.

This nursing action plays an even greater role in palliative and comfort-focused care for the patient and significant others. Increasing awareness of the disease process, the need to keep the health-care providers informed, and expected emotional, physical, and psychological responses to the impending loss are essential components in this type of care situation.

Expected Grieving Behaviors Common to Persons at Various Stages across the Life Span

During the assessment phase of the nursing process, it is necessary for the nurse to have an understanding of the age/developmental perception and response toward death/loss, and any cultural or religious beliefs or practices associated with loss/death. This knowledge will assist the nurse with gathering objective and subjective data related to death/loss and analyzing these data.

Behavioral and emotional responses to grieving are as individual as the time required for the person to progress through the stages of the grieving process. The primary emotional responses to loss and grief are as follows:

1. Anger
2. Depressed mood
3. Guilt
4. Anxiety

These responses are demonstrated throughout the grieving process, though the intensity and frequency in exhibition will vary. Nursing interventions should include meeting the spiritual needs of the grieving individual. Individuals differ in their personal values and perceptions of life's purpose. These attitudes are important to assess in order to determine actions required to assist the person in coping effectively with the event.

Behavioral responses to grief and loss are more readily observable by the nurse. Effective assessment of these behaviors will allow for appropriate selection of nursing interventions to assist the individual in managing his or her loss/grief effectively. Deep-felt crying, increased psychomotor agitation, visually searching for the deceased, irritability, hostility, frustration, and disorganization are only some of the behaviors which may be demonstrated. These individuals may also have physiological responses, such as:

- Change in sleeping pattern (hypersomnia or insomnia)
- Change in appetite (increased or decreased)
- Physiological responses to anxiety (increased heart rate, palpable heart rate, dizziness, fainting, etc.)

It is recognized that individuals experiencing a normal grieving process will encounter both physical and psychological responses. While each person responds to loss/death individually, there are typical markers that have been identified indicating the progress of the grief process.

- *4 to 8 weeks*—Acute grief, the first phase, generally is resolved
- *3 to 6 months*—Active symptoms of grief (depressed mood, changes in sleep or appetite), presence of anxiety, social isolation, and preoccupation with the loss)
- *1 to 2 years*—The complete mourning process

Cultural beliefs and practices play a large role in the response to loss and death for both the patient and the caregiver. Most individuals experience the general responses of grieving discussed earlier (shock, denial, disorientation, anger, and sadness), but there are specific responses influenced by cultural background. Generalizations for every culture and ethnic origin are reviewed during your nursing education, but it is important that you be able to identify and research specific populations in the geographical areas in which you practice. Some cultures express their loss in a visible and noted manner; some are more reserved and private. Many cultures have rituals associated with death and dying, from the death process to burial considerations. Awareness of expected behaviors will assist you in appropriately analyzing your data and developing the most appropriate plan of care.

Signs and Symptoms of Dysfunctional Grieving

Dysfunctional grieving is an exaggerated, prolonged, or inappropriate response to the loss. Characteristics of concerning behaviors associated with ineffective grieving include suppression/repression of emotions or obsession preoccupation with the loss. There are some life situations which may increase a person's vulnerability for dysfunctional grieving. These are important considerations for assessment by the nurse:

- The loss involves a child, significant other, spouse, or parent
- The loss was sudden, untimely (suicide, murder, manslaughter)
- Multiple losses were experienced
- Presence of unresolved conflict between the deceased and survivor
- Dependent or interdependent relationship existed between deceased and survivor, issues of low self-esteem or trust issues
- Survivor has history of psychiatric illness (chronic or acute), substance abuse, or depression, ineffective coping skills
- Survivor is medically ill

In addition to determining the presence of the above situations, the nurse must determine the grieving individual's perception of the loss and the presence of support system, and identify any barriers to learning. The use of therapeutic communication techniques (open-ended questions) will facilitate exploration of these topics.

Nursing Diagnosis

Nursing diagnoses identified by the North American Nursing Diagnosis Association includes the following:

- *Acute grief reaction*—Focuses on the devastating and often overwhelming pain people experience upon the death of someone they care about and who was an integral part of their lives.

- *Dysfunctional grieving*—Extended unsuccessful use of intellectual and emotional responses by which patients (individuals, families, communities) attempt to work through the process of modifying self-concept based upon the perception of loss.
- *Anticipatory grieving*—Related to the intellectual and emotional responses and behaviors by which individuals, families, and communities work through the process of modifying self-concept based on the perception of potential loss.

4.11   Psychiatric Illness and the Homeless Population

Historically, treatment of mental illness was not recognized. It was believed that psychiatric disorders were incurable and that those individuals were a danger to themselves and society as a whole. The focus was on removal to warehouse-type facilities, a place to meet only the very basic needs for survival. Many changes occurred that improved the humane and progressive approaches to psychiatric treatment. The Community Mental Health Centers Act of 1963 initiated to move toward deinstitutionalization (the closing of those warehouse-type facilities). Despite the attention given toward improving community-based treatment options, this movement was not effective in preventing a large population of mentally ill persons who are homeless.

Self-esteem is an important component for mental health. Incidences of homelessness can have a significantly negative influence on one's esteem, and there is a strong correlation between homelessness and the presence of a mental illness. Deinstitutionalization has resulted in a significant number of mentally ill individuals now trying to function within the community setting. Many have little or no support services. This may be due to societal lack of services, the patient's own inability to comply, lack of sufficient follow-up by social services, and lack of stable interpersonal relationships. Access to the patient is severely impacted by the lack of a permanent residence, follow-up appointments are difficult to manage, and everyday activities become increasingly disorganized and unmanageable.

It is reported that 20 to 40 percent of the homeless population suffers from severe mental illness. Individuals who have mental illness are homeless for longer periods of time, have an increased relationship with law enforcement, have a poorer level of physical health, and experience severe financial difficulties. The impact on their bio-social-psycho functioning is significant, and makes for a most challenging care issue. Frequently the mentally ill homeless are involved with law enforcement (misdemeanors, complaint calls, etc.), often resulting in removal from the community to hospitals or correctional facilities.

The establishment of a therapeutic and working relationship with a case manager is important in the stabilization of the homeless mentally ill. This relationship, maintained upon the client's return to the community (typically the shelter system, sometimes a group or adult home), can help in preventing decompensation and recidivism.

4.12   Forensic, Correctional, and Psychiatric Nursing

Forensic nursing is the practice area where nursing science, forensics, and criminal justice are intertwined. The role of the nurse in the forensic setting is on the identification, collection, documentation, and preservation of potential evidence while using the nursing process to identify and treat various nursing diagnoses evidenced through assessment of subjective and objective data. An example of this type of nursing is the SANE (Sexual Abuse Nurse Examiner) nurse who is called in to gather data when a sexual abuse is alleged. The forensic nurse provides direct care to the patient and consultation services to nursing, medical, and legal agencies. They can provide expert court testimony in areas of trauma, investigations of death, delivery of services, and nursing care.

Psychiatric forensic nursing focuses on the patient's mental status and behaviors before, during, and after a criminal act. The essence of the practice is that of a psychiatric and mental health nurse; however, the relationship is significantly different from the traditional relationship. The roles of the psychiatric forensic nurse include the following:

- Forensic examiner
- Competency therapist
- Consultant
- Profiler

Though frequently the source of confusion, there is a difference between correctional health nursing and forensic nursing. Both settings focus on the care of an incarcerated individual. However, correctional health nursing does not provide interventions related to the legal status of the inmate/prisoner. The correctional health nurse frequently is not even advised of the nature of the crime committed.

The correctional mental health nurse provides nursing care within a jail, prison, or ward of a forensic hospital. A more traditional nurse–patient relationship, the focus is on the activities of daily living and nursing care addressing the actual or possible responses to the disease process, not on the cognition and behaviors associated with the crime. Expert communication and interpersonal skills are fundamental in forensic mental health nursing. Additionally, a nonjudgmental and open-minded attitude is required in providing care to this unique population. Caring, the core element in nursing, can be a difficult behavior to maintain if you are not comfortable in your setting.

Chapter 4 Questions

Multiple Choice

1. Which of the following most significantly impacted the ability to transfer psychiatric care to the community setting?
   A. Theories of personality development
   B. Advent of psychotropic medications
   C. Group therapy sessions
   D. Deinstitutionalization

2. Which of the following is an appropriate patient-centered goal for a psychiatric patient being treated in the community setting?
   A. The patient will comply with prescribed medications within one month.
   B The patient will accept goals developed for his or her care within one month.
   C. The patient will participate in care planning strategies and tolerate guidance and direction of the case manager within one month.
   D. The patient will accept increased social isolation as a result of the presence of mental illness within one month.

3. The following are examples of various community treatment facilities:
   A. Psychiatric unit, partial hospitalization program, group home
   B. Jail, group home, residential treatment facility
   C. State hospital, correctional facility, residential treatment center
   D. Supervised apartment, adult home, residential treatment facility

4. All of the following are members of the multidisciplinary psychiatric community treatment team, except:
   A. Social worker
   B. Psychiatric nurse
   C. Psychologist
   D. Vocational therapist
   E. Medical doctor
   F. All except E
   G. All of the above

5. The id is defined as:
   A. One's sense of self, mediator
   B. Values, ideals, moral standards—the moral arm of the personality
   C. Desires, drives, instincts

6. The superego is defined as:

    A. One's sense of self, mediator

    B. Values, ideals, moral standards—the moral arm of the personality

    C. Desires, drives, instincts

7. The ego is defined as:

    A. One's sense of self, mediator

    B. Values, ideals, moral standards—the moral arm of the personality

    C. Desires, drives, instincts

8. The use of which of the following is used to manage basic drives or emotionality issues:

    A. Therapeutic relationship

    B. Medications

    C. Group therapy

    D. Defensive mechanisms

9. Hospice and palliative care allows for patients:

    A. To receive specialized care in the hospital

    B. To receive curative measures

    C. To remain in their homes as long as possible

    D. Who are too elderly to receive care

10. An individual is said to be experiencing dysfunctional grieving if his or her response is

    A. Shock, denial, and longing for the deceased

    B. Anger, depression, guilt, and anxiety

    C. Increased psychomotor agitation, sobbing, hostility

    D. Delayed, exaggerated, or prolonged

11. Many individuals experience general responses to grieving, more specific reactions can be influenced by

    A. Culture

    B. Age and developmental level

    C. Support systems

    D. Presence of mental illness

12. The difference between forensic psychiatric nursing and correctional mental health nursing is

    A. Educational preparation of the nurse

    B. The role of the forensic nurse is in the collection, documentation, and preservation of potential evidence, focusing on the patient's mental status and behaviors

    C. The focus of correctional mental health is on the patient's activities of daily functioning and nursing problems associated with their psychiatric disorders

    D. B and C

13. You are the group leader for a medication group for schizophrenic patients. The group will last for eight weeks, and new patients will be welcomed throughout the group. This group is

    A. Open and ongoing

    B. Closed and ongoing

    C. Open and time-limited

    D. Closed and time-limited

14. John has been attending your group for a month but has yet to participate. One intervention you, as the leader, may use to encourage him to speak is

   A. "John, why do you come to the group if you are not going to talk?"

   B. "John, what do you have to say about what was just said?"

   C. "John, you should be feeling comfortable enough to contribute to the group."

   D. "Tell us what you are thinking, John."

15. During your group, one of the patients states, "I hear someone telling me that the medication the nurse is trying to give me is poisoned. When I looked around to see who it was, there wasn't anyone around." Another patient responds, "I used to hear voices, too. I found out that the voices I was hearing weren't real. The ones you hear aren't real either." Which of the therapeutic factors in groups is this an example of?

   A. Ventilation

   B. Altruism

   C. Group cohesiveness

   D. Symptom management

16. During community meeting, one of the patients threatens to hit another patient. The best response by you, the group leader, would be to

   A. Get the other members out of the area.

   B. Direct the threatening patient to leave the group.

   C. Call for assistance.

   D. Validate the anger experienced by the patient, but set limits on aggressive behavior or threats to others.

17. Soon after the death of her husband, the wife confides that, "Joe was my everything. I can't go on without him." The best response is:

   A. "Every day it will get a little easier for you."

   B. "You have your children to live for."

   C. "His death is a big loss for you."

   D. "Keep in mind that he is no longer in pain; that will help you feel better.

18. Since you work as a hospice nurse, a colleague asks you who is an appropriate referral for hospice services. The best response would be:

   A. "Hospice care is for terminally ill cancer patients."

   B. "Any patient in the end stage of their illness is appropriate."

   C. "We provide care for end-stage renal failure patients."

   D. "Patients whose families are no longer able to care for them are admitted for hospice care."

19. One day your hospice patient's husband says to you, "Whenever Lisa talks about dying I never know what to say." He asks you what would be the right thing. You would encourage him to say:

   A. "Don't talk about dying, I need you to be strong and fight to live."

   B. "I don't feel comfortable when you say that. Let's not talk about it."

   C. "Dying is a long time off. Let's just be happy for today."

   D. "I feel sad when I think about not having you with me."

20. You are assigned to care for a hospice patient diagnosed with cancer. Which of the following interventions ensures protection of your patient's rights?

   A. Providing choices and fostering self-governance

   B. Reinforcing that the prognosis is good

   C. Providing nursing actions that convey respect and genuineness

    D. Supporting the patient's spirituality

    E. A, C, and D

    F. C and D

21. You are the evening nurse in the county jail. One responsibility is to complete an assessment on newly admitted inmates to the facility who are known to have a psychiatric treatment history or demonstrate behaviors indicative of behavior health disorders. Which of the following skills would be a priority for you to have?

    A. Knowledge of and access to community resources

    B. Ability to make a suicide risk assessment

    C. Ability to establish chain-of-custody evidence

    D. Ability to provide spiritual support

22. A high degree of credibility is required if a nurse gives testimony as a(n):

    A. Fact witness

    B. Expert witness

    C. Correctional health nurse

    D. Nurse

True or False

23. ____Crisis intervention can be expected to require 72 hours, focusing on facilitating inpatient hospitalization.

24. ____Crisis counseling should be concluded within six hours.

25. ____ The Community Mental Health Act of 1963 supports the idea that outpatient treatment is the optimal level of care.

26. ____The goal of outpatient treatment is to empower the patient through education and self-supportive measures.

27. ____Outpatient treatment is voluntary only.

28. ____ Day hospitals were developed to meet the needs similar to a daycare setting.

29. ____Inpatient treatment is considered the most restrictive level of treatment.

30. ____Using the environment as part of treatment is called Milieu therapy.

31. ____Deinstitutionalization encourages inpatient hospitalization.

32. ____Involuntary hospitalization can be considered an infringement of a person's autonomy.

33. ____Forensic psychiatric nursing and correctional mental health nursing both require the nurse to have expert communication skills and a nonjudgmental attitude.

Fill in the Blank

34. Every _____ with a patient is an opportunity for a therapeutic event.

35. The focus of nursing care in the psychiatric setting is to promote _____ functioning.

36. Current trends in psychiatric and mental health nursing include violence towards self and others, the aging population, cultural diversity, and _____.

37. The term used to define "small talk" that occurs between a patient and clinician is _____ communication.

38. As a psychiatric nurse, you are expected to use the _____ in the assessment, diagnosing, planning, intervention, and evaluation of care.

Chapter 4 Answers

1. **B.** The development of medications allowed for more humane treatment, replacing previous treatment options.

2. **C.** The goal of outpatient treatment is to empower the patient; active involvement in treatment planning allows and encourages this control.

3. **D.** This is the only answer that included only community-based agencies. Inpatient units, state hospitals, and jails are not considered community levels of care.

4. **G.** All of the identified professionals, including the medical doctor, are participants in the multidisciplinary treatment team.

5. **C.**

6. **A.**

7. **B.**

8. **D.** Ego defense mechanisms are the means the ego uses to protect itself and manage basic drives.

9. **C.** Hospice and palliative care allow for a personal and comfortable end-of-life experience, allowing the patient to die in his or her own home versus the hospital. The focus of care is to ensure minimal pain to be experienced by the dying individual.

10. **D.** A, B, and C are expected responses to loss/grief. Grief is viewed as dysfunctional when the process is inhibited, exaggerated, or prolonged.

11. **A.** Rationale: Cultural beliefs and practices play a large role in an individual's response to loss/death. Specific responses influenced by cultural background can influence emotionality levels, care of the body, final arrangements, and so on.

12. **D.**

13. **C.** An open group is a group that adds members throughout the length of the group. A closed group does not add new members. Time-limited refers to a group that meets for a specific number of sessions.

14. **D.** Asking the patient what he is thinking is the least threatening. It is important, as the leader of the group, that your approach be slow and encouraging to facilitate participation.

15. **D.** Symptom management is taught by peers through validation of the other's perception of reality. Also, group members can help symptom management through monitoring reactions of others and providing feedback. Ventilation describes expression of feelings, altruism offers a feeling of reward from giving support to others, and group cohesiveness occurs in mature groups when each member feels connected to each other and the leader.

16. **D.** The best response would include reinforcement of appropriate behaviors. A and B may be appropriate if the patient continues to escalate, but other interventions need to be attempted first. Setting limits would include informing the patient he or she will need to leave the group if he or or she is unable to manage the behavior.

17. **C.** The most appropriate response includes a validation of the patient's feelings. The other responses minimize the feeling of loss experienced and will not facilitate him or her to communicate more.

18. **B.** Hospice services are provided for any terminally ill patient.

19. **D.** The best response would be one that offers an honest recognition of the feelings the spouse is experiencing and facilitates a discussion about both of their emotions and responses to this life event. The other responses debilitate communication.

20. **E.** All of the interventions except B support the rights of a patient. B provides false reassurance.

21. **B.** Individuals newly incarcerated are often experiencing a crisis and may be suicidal. Assessing for potential for violence directed to self is an essential skill. The chain of custody of evidence is not a skill needed for this situation. It begins when an item of evidence is collected, and it is maintained until the evidence is disposed. If not properly maintained, an item may be inadmissible in court.

22. B. An expert witness is someone recognized by the court as having a specific level of skill/expertise in a designated area. To establish credibility as an expert witness, the nurse must have academic preparation, professional training, occupational/life experience, and involvement in professional organizations. Additionally, dress, manner, performance, and the ability to communicate effectively are required.

True or False

23. F

24. F

25. T

26. T

27. F

28. F

29. T

30. T

31. F

32. T

33. T

Fill in the Blank

34. Interactions

35. Optimal

36. Improvements in technology

37. Phatic

38. Nursing process

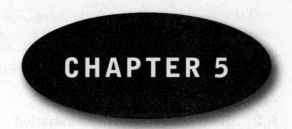

CHAPTER 5

Assessment Tools and Strategies

5.1   Assessment

The assessment interview, which requires effective communication skills, interviewing, behavioral observation, record review, and a comprehensive assessment of the client and relevant systems, enables the psychiatric mental health nurse to make sound clinical judgments and plan appropriate interventions with the client. This process is often referred to as a psychosocial assessment, which includes a mental status examination. This assessment is also a clinical baseline used to evaluate the effectiveness of the treatment and interventions, and can also be a measure of the client's progress.

The assessment interview can be conducted in a variety of settings including but not limited to:

- Psychiatric or medical emergency rooms
- Crisis centers
- Medical-surgical units
- Intensive care units
- Maternity units
- Community mental health centers
- Private practice
- Schools
- Homes

Self-Awareness and Personal Considerations

Before the nurse begins to assess a client's mental health status, the nurse must be knowledgeable and aware of factors that can influence the assessment process and its outcome. The nurse cannot let personal feelings and beliefs influence treatment of the client.

Both the nurse and client bring their life experiences and backgrounds to a professional relationship. These experiences include religious beliefs and attitudes, cultural biases and beliefs, and values. The nurse has to be acutely aware of his or her own body language, facial expressions, communication skills, and interviewing techniques. These techniques are acquired and improve through practice, supervision by a more experienced clinician, and observation and modeling of more experienced clinicians.

If the client perceives that the nurse may be judging him or her, disapproves of his or her answers, or is rushing through the questions to complete the interview, the patient may respond superficially or omit discussing certain problems altogether. The nurse must be aware of his or her own feelings and responses, and approach the assessment professionally.

The mental health nurse must also be aware of countertransference issues, which occurs when the nurse responds to the client based on personal and/or unconscious needs, problems, and conflicts. These reactions are inappropriate and can cause conflict in the nurse–patient therapeutic relationship. Sharing your feelings with a more experienced clinician can assist the nurse in recognizing biases and value judgments.

5.2 The Mental Status Examination

The mental status examination (MSE) is the basis for understanding the client's presentation and the extent of the person's mental impairment. This examination focuses on the client's cognitive functions at the time the evaluation takes place, which include the following:

- Sense of time
- Sense of place
- Personal identity
- Appearance
- Speech
- General intellectual level
- Ability to interpret proverbs
- Memorization and short-term recall
- Mathematical ability
- Insight, judgment
- Reasoning
- Problem-solving ability
- Thought patterns

The nurse should conduct this exam and record its findings in an objective, nonjudgmental manner. If a client is acutely disturbed or psychotic, it is not unusual to see an MSE administered daily by a mental health clinician, which can include the nurse or psychiatrist.

The MSE is an important part of the differential diagnosis of dementia and other psychiatric symptoms or disorders. An MSE can also be given repeatedly to monitor or document changes in a patient's condition. The most commonly used test of cognitive functioning is the Folstein Mini-Mental Status Examination (MMSE), a brief 30-point questionnaire developed in 1975. It is a simplified scored form of the mental status exam that consists of 11 questions and takes only 5 to 10 minutes to administer, making it easy to use routinely and quickly.

The actual categories of the mental status examination are seen in Figure 5-1.

Conducting the Interview

Initially, the nurse should use *open-ended questions* to start the assessment process. Examples of open-ended questions can include the following:

- How can we help you?
- What brings you here today?
- What has been happening to you?

If the patient is having difficulty focusing, or organizing his or her thoughts, the nurse may have to use more direct and focused questions to obtain needed information. These questions should be clear and simple, and focus on one specific symptom or behavior. These types of questions are called *close-ended questions*. Following are examples of close-ended questions:

- Are you feeling suicidal?
- How many packs of cigarettes do you smoke daily?

- How many hours do you sleep daily?
- What prescribed medications do you take?
- What street drugs do you use?

Ideally, the interview should be conducted in a quiet, private area, but be aware of the client's current behavior, body language, and reports from family and friends who may have accompanied the client to the facility before choosing an area. **The nurse should never conduct an interview in an isolated area.** Utilize the perceptions of the client's behavior and emotional state from family members, friends, caregivers, and anyone

Personal Information
- name
- age
- sex
- race
- marital status
- significant other
- occupation
- educational level
- living arrangements
- religious preference

Appearance
- grooming and dress
- hygiene
- posture
- height, weight, nutritional status
- facial expression
- level of eye contact
- tattoos, body piercings, scars
- relationship between age and appearance

Motor Activity
- tremors
- tics
- gestures and mannerisms
- hyperactivity
- balance and gait
- abnormal movements (tardive dyskinesia)
- restlessness or agitation
- aggressiveness
- rigidity
- echopraxia (imitation of movements & gestures of others)
- psychomotor retardation

Speech
- rate: slow, rapid, normal
- volume: loud, soft, normal
- pressure of speech
- intonation
- disturbances: slurring, stuttering, mumbling
- aphasia

Affect
- congruence with mood
- flat
- bland
- animated
- constricted

Mood
- sad
- depressed
- irritable
- labile
- euphoric
- elated
- anxious
- fearful
- blunted

Thought Processes
- disorganized
- coherent
- flight of ideas
- neologisms (made up words that have meaning to a psychotic person)
- thought blocking
- circumstantiality
- concrete thinking
- clang associations
- perseveration
- word salad
- poverty of speech
- mutism
- ability to concentrate
- attention span

Thought Content
- delusions: grandiose, persecutory, reference, somatic, nihilistic, control suicidal or homicidal ideation
- paranoia/suspiciousness
- religiosity
- magical thinking
- phobias

Perceptual Disturbances
- hallucinations: auditory, visual, tactile, olfactory, gustatory
- illusions
- derealization
- depersonalization

Cognitive Ability
- orientation: time, person, place
- level of consciousness: (e.g. alert, confused, stuporous, unconscious)
- comatose memory: immediate, recent, remote
- attention
- capacity for abstract thought
- insight
- judgement

Figure 5-1 Mental status examination.

else who may have accompanied the client. Be aware that the client and/or family members may or may not feel comfortable being interviewed in the presence of one another. Always seek permission from the client if possible to conduct separate interviews with family members or friends. If physical or sexual abuse is suspected, the nurse should make every effort to assess the client in privacy. Observe and record the client's interaction with you during the course of the interview. Are they cooperative, hostile, suspicious, or defensive? The nurse should inquire if the client is upset or irritated about something, and if his or her observation is accurate.

Appearance

When conducting the MSE, take notice of the client's appearance. Does the client appear to be his or her stated age? Does he or she appear younger or older? Is the client dressed neatly or disheveled? Has the client attended to their grooming and hygiene? Is clothing age-appropriate and is the client dressed appropriately for the weather? Is makeup excessive or garish?

Motor Activity

The nurse will take notice and record the client's physical movements. Is the client lethargic, restless, or agitated? Are there any unusual mannerisms or gestures observed? Are there excessive body movements, tics, grimaces, or tremors? Are there repeated movements or compulsions, or involuntary movements such as tongue protrusion, lip smacking, chewing, grimacing, blinking, choreiform (resembling the rapid jerky movements associated with chorea) movements of limbs and trunks, and foot tapping that are indicative of tardive dyskinesia?

Speech

The nurse will assess the client's speech in terms of rate, volume, amount, and any abnormalities. Is there stuttering, slurring of words, mumbling, or accents? Does the client speak nonstop or is there poverty of speech? Does the client use clang associations (rhyming of words) or neologisms (invented words that only have meaning to the client)?

Mood and Affect

A client's mood refers to his or her self-report of the prevailing emotional state. Mood can be evaluated by asking the simple question, "How are you feeling today?" The client may report feeling sad, hopeless, helpless, euphoric, or anxious. The nurse can also ask the client to rate his or her mood on a scale from 1 to 10. For example, the nurse may ask the client who states he is depressed, "On a scale from 1 to 10, one being the least depressed and ten being the most depressed, where would you place yourself at this moment?"

If a client is suspected of being suicidal, self-destructive, or homicidal, those thoughts must be addressed immediately. Ask the client if he or she feels like harming him- or herself or others. Have there been any previous attempts to cause harm, and under what circumstances? The nurse must assess the client's plans, ability to carry out those plans, and the accessibility of weapons. Assess the client's attitude regarding death and the availability of support systems.

If a client makes a specific threat or has a plan to harm another person, health-care providers are legally obligated to warn that targeted person. This is one of the few situations in which the nurse must breach the client's confidentiality in order to protect the targeted person.

Affect refers to the client's outward expression of his or her emotional state. The nurse will assess if the client's affect is appropriate to his or her mood. For example, the client may be talking about the recent loss of a loved one while smiling and laughing.

Clients can also experience **lability** in expression by shifting from one affect to another very quickly. The client may be laughing and smiling one moment, and within minutes become irritable and angry.

Following are common terms used in assessing affect:

- Blunted affect
- Flat affect

- Broad affect
- Inappropriate affect
- Restricted affect

Thought Process and Content

The client's thought process refers to how the client thinks, and the thought content refers to what the client says. The nurse will assess if the client's verbalizations are based in reality and are making any sense. The nurse will assess and record if the client is easily distracted, or if he or she appears to be responding to internal stimuli. Is the client able to focus and answer the questions being asked? If the client appears to be having difficulties in thought process and content, the nurse may use very focused questions requiring short answers. The following are common terms utilized to assess thought process and content:

Process

- Circumstantial thinking
- Flight of ideas
- Loose associations
- Tangential thinking
- Thought blocking
- Perseveration
- Word salad

Thought Content

- Delusions: paranoia, grandiose, religious, somatic
- Thought broadcasting
- Thought insertion
- Ideas of reference
- Depersonalization
- Magical thinking
- Hypochondriasis
- Nihilistic ideas
- Phobias
- Obsession

Perceptual Disturbances

Some clients may experience perceptual problems, which include hallucinations and illusions. Hallucinations are false sensory impressions or experiences. Hallucinations can involve the five senses and body sensations:

- Auditory (sound/hearing voices) are the most common hallucination
- Visual (sight) the second most common hallucination
- Tactile (touch)
- Gustatory (taste)
- Olfactory (smell)

Command hallucinations are the types that tell the person to do something, such as harm or kill another person, or harm or kill oneself. The nurse can assess the client's perceptions by asking, "Do you ever see or hear things? Do you ever have strange experiences?"

Illusions are misperceptions of actual environmental stimuli. For example, a person is walking along a path and believes she sees a snake, but upon further investigation discovers it is only a large branch. Reality corrected this illusion. Hallucinations have no basis in reality.

Cognitive Ability

Level of Consciousness

The client's orientation to person, place, and time should be assessed. The nurse will determine this by a few simple questions:

- What is your name? What month or year is it?
- Do you know where you are? What building are you in?
- What is today's date? What month or year is it?

Level of consciousness should be determined. Terms used to describe this include alert, confused, sedated, or stuporous.

Memory

The client should be assessed for memory problems. Areas to be assessed include

- Remote memory
- Recent memory
- Immediate memory

Remote memory can be assessed by reviewing information from the client's history, asking questions about place of birth, schools attended, dates of marriages, and so on.

Recent memory can be assessed by asking the client to recall information of events over the past 24 hours, such as "What did you do yesterday?" The nurse must be able to verify this information.

Immediate recall can be assessed by asking the client to repeat a series of numbers either forward or backwards within a 10-second interval.

Ability to Concentrate

The nurse can assess the client's ability to concentrate by asking the client to perform simple tasks:

- Spell a word backwards
- Repeat the names of the months backwards
- Start with the number 100 and continue to subtract 7

Abstract Thinking and Intellectual Abilities

The nurse can assess the client's ability to use abstract thinking by asking the client to interpret common proverbs. If the client gives a literal translation, this is evidence of concrete thinking. Abstract thinking is lacking if the client cannot interpret its meaning. Following are examples of common proverbs:

- People who live in glass houses shouldn't throw stones.
- A stitch in time saves nine.
- A rolling stone gathers no moss.
- A bird in the hand is worth two in the bush.

If a client has an educational level below the eighth grade, the nurse can assess intellectual functioning by asking the client to identify similarities between pairs of objects. Examples of paired objects often used for this purpose include the following:

- Apple and orange
- Bicycle and bus
- Newspaper and television

The nurse needs to consider that the information in this category is highly influenced by the client's sociocultural background and the treatment setting.

Judgment and Insight

Judgment refers to the ability to interpret one's environment and situation correctly and to adapt one's decisions and behavior accordingly. If a client reveals that he is unemployed, but is spending large amounts of his unemployment money on frivolous items, or having unprotected sex with multiple partners, this client is exhibiting poor judgment.

Insight is the client's understanding of the nature of the illness or problem. An example of a client with poor insight is one who blames others for her own behavior.

5.3 Psychosocial Assessment Description

As stated earlier in this chapter, the mental status exam aids in collecting objective data. The Psychosocial Assessment is focused on the client's subjective data. This assessment focuses on the client's psychosocial history, which includes the following:

- Personal background
- Social background
- Coping strategies utilized
- Strengths and weaknesses
- Cultural practices and beliefs that may interfere with traditional treatments
- Spiritual beliefs and practices

Conduction of the Psychosocial Assessment

The nurse conducting the interview must be culturally competent, have fundamental knowledge of growth and development, and be competent in psychopathology, pathophysiology, and pharmacology. Some nurses may find it uncomfortable to question clients about their religious practices and beliefs. Many health-care professionals believe that religious and spiritual needs should be a part of assessments and that religious resources should be available to those who request it.

Following are some questions that can assist with a spiritual assessment:

- Do you practice or belong to any religion or spiritual group?
- What role does religion or spirituality play in your life?
- Do you find that your religion helps you in stressful situations?
- Has your illness affected your religious practices?

As stated earlier, cultural competence and an awareness of individual cultural health-care practices are very important, since nurses are taking care of an increasingly culturally diverse population. Following are some questions the nurse can ask to assess a client's cultural and social background:

- How would you describe your cultural background?
- What is your primary language?
- Who do you live with? Describe your family.
- What is a typical day like for you?
- Who do you go to when you are medically or mentally ill?
- How does your culture view mental illness? Is it viewed as a taboo, curse, or something negative?
- Do you eat any special foods?

In assessing a client's coping skills, the following questions can be helpful:

- What do you do when you get upset?
- What usually helps you to relieve the stress?

Ask clients about any substance use and abuse, as well as any prescribed medications they may be taking.

After completion of the assessment, always summarize the data with the client to ensure accuracy of the information. This is also a good time to validate data with secondary sources such as family or friends. Inform the client, and any significant others who may have accompanied the client, what will happen next and who the client will be seeing.

5.4   Formulation of the Nursing Diagnosis

As you have already learned, a nursing diagnosis is a clinical judgment about individual, family, or community responses to actual and potential health problems or life processes. A nursing diagnosis provides the foundation for the selection of nursing interventions and therapeutic outcomes for which the nurse is accountable.

The psychiatric-mental health nurse uses nursing diagnoses and standard classifications of mental disorders (DSM-IV-TR), as well as the standard international classification of diseases (ICD–10), to develop a treatment plan based on assessment data and theoretical premises. The nursing diagnosis has three structural components:

1. *Problem process*—This describes the patient at present. The nursing diagnostic title states what should change.

   Example: Impaired social interaction

2. *Etiology (related to's)*—This includes the probable cause or factors that contribute to or are related to the development or maintenance of the nursing diagnosis title. Stating the etiology tells what needs to be done to effect change and identifies causes that the nurse can treat through interventions.

   Example: Impaired social interaction *related to* impaired thought processes (hallucinations or delusions)

3. *Supporting data (as evidenced by's)*—This refers to signs and symptoms, and states what the condition is like at present. Supporting data validates the nursing diagnosis.

   Example: Impaired social interaction *related to* impaired thought processes *as evidenced by* dysfunctional interaction with peers.

Medication Assessment Tool

The assessment tool for obtaining a drug history can be used by staff nurses admitting patients to the hospital, or by nurse practitioners who may use it with their prescriptive privileges. It can also be used when obtaining a patient's signature of informed consent prior to pharmacological therapy.

Information to gather includes the following:

- Current and past use of prescription drugs, including:
  - Dosage
  - How long used
  - Prescribed by whom and why
  - Any side effects experienced/results
- Current and past use of over-the-counter drugs such as herbal supplements, including:
  - Dosage
  - How long used
  - Prescribed by whom and why
  - Any side effects experienced/results

- Current and past use of street drugs, alcohol, nicotine, and/or caffeine including:
  - How long used
  - Amount used
  - How often used
  - When last used
  - Effects produced
  - Overdoses
  - Any rehabilitation programs utilized, where, and for how long
- Allergies to food or drugs
- Any special diet considerations
- History of any medical problems
- Pregnant or breastfeeding
- Recent lab work or referrals

AIMS (Abnormal Involuntary Movement Scale)

Tardive dyskinesia, a late-appearing side effect of antipsychotic medications, is characterized by abnormal, involuntary movements. This permanent movement disorder will be discussed in more detail in Chapter 9. This tool helps to detect and assess the level of possible dyskinesia in patients taking antipsychotic medications. The patient is observed in several positions, and the severity of symptoms is rated from 0 to 4. The AIMS can be administered every three to six months. If the nurse detects an increased score on the AIMS, indicating increased symptoms of tardive dyskinesia, the physician must be notified so that the dosage or drug can be changed to prevent the advancement of tardive dyskinesia. The AIMS examination procedure is as follows:

Either before or after completing the examination procedure, observe the patient unobtrusively at rest (e.g., in the waiting room).

The chair to be used in this examination should be a hard, firm one without arms.

1. Ask the patient whether there is anything in his or her mouth (such as gum or candy) and, if so, to remove it.
2. Ask about the "current" condition of the patient's teeth. Ask if he or she wears dentures. Ask whether teeth or dentures bother the patient "now".
3. Ask whether the patient notices any movements in his or her mouth, face, hands, or feet. If yes, ask the patient to describe them and to indicate to what extent they "currently" bother the patient or interfere with activities.
4. Have the patient sit in chair with hands on knees, legs slightly apart, and feet flat on floor. (Look at the entire body for movements while the patient is in this position.)
5. Ask the patient to sit with hands hanging unsupported—if male, between his legs, if female and wearing a dress, hanging over her knees. (Observe hands and other body areas.)
6. Ask the patient to open his or her mouth. (Observe the tongue at rest within the mouth.) Do this twice.
7. Ask the patient to protrude his or her tongue. (Observe abnormalities of tongue movement.) Do this twice.
8. Ask the patient to tap his or her thumb with each finger as rapidly as possible for 10 to 15 seconds, first with right hand, then with left hand. (Observe facial and leg movements.)
9. Flex and extend the patient's left and right arms, one at a time.
10. Ask the patient to stand up. (Observe the patient in profile. Observe all body areas again, including hips.)
11. Ask the patient to extend both arms out in front, palms down. (Observe trunk, legs, and mouth.)
12. Have the patient walk a few paces, turn, and walk back to the chair. (Observe hands and gait.) Do this twice.

Scoring Procedure

Complete the examination procedure before making ratings.

For the movement ratings (the first three categories below), rate the highest severity observed. 0 = none, 1 = minimal (may be extreme normal), 2 = mild, 3 = moderate, and 4 = severe. According to the original AIMS instructions, one point is subtracted if movements are seen **only on active movement**, but not all those performing the assessment follow that rule.

Facial and Oral Movements:

1. Muscles of facial expression

   e.g., movements of forehead, eyebrows, periorbital area, cheeks. Include frowning, blinking, grimacing of upper face.

   0 1 2 3 4

2. Lips and perioral area

   e.g., puckering, pouting, smacking.

   0 1 2 3 4

3. Jaw

   e.g., biting, clenching, chewing, mouth opening, lateral movement.

   0 1 2 3 4

4. Tongue

   Rate only increase in movement both in and out of mouth, **not** inability to sustain movement.

   0 1 2 3 4

Extremity Movements:

5. Upper (arms, wrists, hands, fingers)

   Include movements that are choreic (rapid, objectively purposeless, irregular, spontaneous) or athetoid (slow, irregular, complex, serpentine). Do **not** include tremor (repetitive, regular, rhythmic movements).

   0 1 2 3 4

6. Lower (legs, knees, ankles, toes)

   e.g., lateral knee movement, foot tapping, heel dropping, foot squirming, inversion and eversion of foot.

   0 1 2 3 4

Trunk Movements:

7. Neck, shoulders, hips

   e.g., rocking, twisting, squirming, pelvic gyrations. Include diaphragmatic movements.

   0 1 2 3 4

Global Judgments:

8. Severity of abnormal movements.

   0 1 2 3 4

   based on the highest single score on the above items.

9. Incapacitation due to abnormal movements.

   0 = none, normal

   1 = minimal

   2 = mild

   3 = moderate

   4 = severe

10. Patient's awareness of abnormal movements.
    0 = no awareness
    1 = aware, no distress
    2 = aware, mild distress
    3 = aware, moderate distress
    4 = aware, severe distress

Dental Status:

11. Current problems with teeth and/or dentures.
    0 = no
    1 = yes
12. Does patient usually wear dentures?
    0 = no
    1 = yes

Personality and Intelligence Tests

The clinician should discuss personality and intelligence tests with the patient. Following is a description of each.

Personality Tests

Personality tests reflect the client's personality in areas such as self-concept, impulse control, reality testing, and major defenses. Personality tests may be objective (constructed of true-or-false or multiple-choice questions). The nurse compares the client's answers with standard answers or criteria and obtains a score or scores.

Other personality tests, called projective tests, are unstructured and are usually conducted by the interview method. The stimuli for other tests, such as pictures or Rorschach's ink blots, are standard, but patients may respond with answers that are very different.

Below is a list of commonly used objective personality tests:

- *Minnesota Multiphasic Personality Inventory (MMPI)*—566 multiple-choice items; provides scores on 10 clinical scales such as hypochondriasis, depression, hysteria, paranoia; 4 special scales such as anxiety and alcoholism; 3 validity scales to evaluate the truth and accuracy of responses.
- *MMPI–2*—Revised version of MMPI with 567 multiple-choice items; provides scores on same areas of MMPI.
- *Milton Clinical Multiaxial Inventory (MCMI) and MCMI-II (revised version)*—175 true-false items; provides scores on various personality traits and personality disorders.
- *Psychological Screening Inventory (PSI)*—103 true-false items; used to screen for the need for psychological help.
- *Beck Depression Inventory (BDI)*—21 items rated on scale of 1 to 3 to indicate level of depression.
- *Tennessee Self-Concept Scale (TSCS)*—100 true-false items; provides information on 14 scales related to self-concept.

Following is a list of commonly used projective personality tests:

- *Rorschach test*—10 stimulus cards of ink blots; client describes perceptions of ink blots; narrative interpretation discusses areas such as coping skills, interpersonal attitudes, and characteristics of ideation.
- *Thematic Apperception Test (TAT)*—20 stimulus cards with pictures; clients tell a story about the picture; narrative interpretation discusses themes about mood state, conflict, quality of interpersonal relationships.
- *Sentence Completion Test*—client completes a sentence from beginnings such as "I often wish," "Most people," and "When I was young."

Intelligence Tests

Intelligence tests are designed to evaluate the client's cognitive abilities and intellectual functioning

Both intelligence tests and personality tests are frequently criticized as being culturally biased. Needless to say, it is important to consider the client's culture and environment when evaluating the importance of scores or projections from any of these tests. They can provide useful information but may not be appropriate for all clients.

Chapter 5 Questions

Multiple Choice

1. Which of the following is an example of an open-ended question?

    A. Have you gained any weight recently?

    B. Who is the current president of the United States?

    C. What concerns do you have about your current health status?

    D. Where do you reside?

2. Which of the following is an example of a closed-ended question?

    A. How is your relationship with your family?

    B. Have you had any recent health problems?

    C. Where do you go to college?

    D. What are you feelings about your diagnosis?

3. The patient's belief that the television broadcast is directed at him or her is an example of:

    A. Ideas of reference

    B. Thought broadcasting

    C. Circumstantial thinking

    D. Thought insertion

4. The nurse can assess the patient's ability to concentrate by instructing the patient to do which of the following?

    A. Name the last three presidents.

    B. Spell a word backwards.

    C. Explain the expression, "a stitch in time saves nine."

    D. Explain what his or her typical day at work is like.

5. The patient who believes the FBI is out to get him or her is experiencing

    A. A hallucination

    B. Thought blocking

    C. Tangential thinking

    D. Delusion

Matching Column

Column A	Column B
6. _____Hallucination	**A.** Overproductive speech with rapid shifting, fragmented ideas and topics
7. _____Mood	**B.** Outward expression of the client's emotional state
8. _____Neologisms	**C.** A group of words that are put together randomly, without any logical connection
9. _____Flight of ideas	**D.** False sensory perceptions arising from any of the five senses
10. _____Loose associations	**E.** False belief not shared by others or based in reality
11. _____Delusions	**F.** Self report by client of his/her prevailing emotional state
12. _____Tangential thinking	**G.** Unrelated topics introduced without ever getting to point of the communication
13. _____Word salad	**H.** The psychotic person invents new words that are meaningless to others, but have symbolic meaning to the psychotic person
14. _____Thought blocking	**I.** Thinking is characterized by speech in which ideas shift from one unrelated subject to another
15. _____Affect	**J.** Stopping abruptly in the middle of a sentence or thought, and sometimes unable to continue the idea

Chapter 5 Answers

Multiple Choice

1. C
2. C
3. A
4. B
5. D

8. H
9. A
10. I
11. E
12. G
13. C
14. J
15. B

Matching Column

6. D
7. F

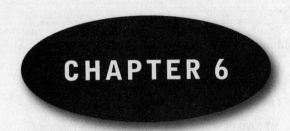

CHAPTER 6

Childhood and Adolescent Psychiatric Disorders

6.1 Psychiatric Disorders in Children and Adolescents

Risk factors associated in psychiatric disorders of children and adolescents are genealogy, biochemistry, pre- and postnatal factors, psychosocial development, and personal attitudes. As the child grows, he or she develops appropriate coping mechanisms to manage life stressors more effectively and reduces the risk for development of psychiatric and physical health problems. A child or adolescent who is unable (due to various bio-psycho-social influences) to achieve these markers is considered an "at risk" individual and requires closer observation to enable early detection and intervention to minimize the potential for the development of an illness. According to the U.S. Surgeon General, about 20 percent of children are estimated to have mental disorders with a mild functional impairment, and 5 to 9 percent of children ages 5 to 17 have a serious mental disorder.

Children and adolescence experience similar psychiatric illnesses as adults, and the diagnostic criteria used for adults are used for children and adolescents. Typical childhood disorders include the following:

- Pervasive developmental disorders (PDD)
- Attention-Deficit Hyperactivity Disorder (ADHD)
- Autism spectrum disorders
- Anxiety disorders
- Bipolar disorders
- Depression
- Schizophrenia
- Disruptive behavior disorders (conduct disorder)

Though many eating disorders, particularly anorexia, originate in adolescence and continue into adulthood, not all mental disorders identified in childhood and adolescence persist into adulthood. This chapter will focus on the psychiatric disorders that are diagnosed in infancy, childhood, or adolescence.

The Role of the Psychiatric and Mental Health Nurse in Child and Adolescent Psychiatric Treatment

The roles of the nurse in the child and adolescent psychiatric treatment setting are those of care provider, parent, role model, teacher, counselor, milieu specialist, and multidisciplinary treatment team member. Hospitalization of children and adolescents is typically a result of dangerousness (self and others) and the inability of the parent/legal guardian to safely manage the individual in the home/residential setting.

The nurse can have a pivotal and influential influence intervening with children and adolescents. The nurse's role is to champion and advocate the environmental supports that will cultivate the characteristics and attitudes required by the at-risk child or adolescent to minimize or prevent the occurrence of a psychiatric problem. The benefit of a therapeutic and supportive environment fostered by psychiatric treatment and interventions on these developing individuals is to assist them in evolving to their optimal functioning emotionally, physically, and psychiatrically. It is essential that the nurse working in this area have a solid understanding of developmental theories, communication skills, age-appropriate therapeutic interventions (limit-setting, restraints, etc.), ability to facilitate a positive rapport with the patient and family, and observational abilities.

Risk Factors, Characteristics, and Family Dynamics in Child and Adolescent Psychiatric Disorders

There are many risk factors associated with the presence of psychiatric illness in children and adolescents. Many biological influences result in the presentation of symptoms related to impaired functioning in children, including:

- Fetal alcohol syndrome (FAS)
- Lead poisoning
- Malnutrition
- Substance addiction at birth
- Presence of viruses (such as HIV)

Often interventions are delayed until it becomes apparent that the symptoms exhibited are not self-corrective with medical interventions and will not be "outgrown." Once interventions are initiated, they need to be from a varied perspective. Multiple resources must be energized to address the needs from a biological, spiritual, psychological, emotional, and environmental perspective.

Genetic influences are associated in several of the psychiatric disorders (autism, bipolar disorders, schizophrenia, ADD/ADHD, mental retardation). Variations in neurotransmitters have a role in the presence of mental illness. Several sources discuss the role of an individual's temperament in mental illness. Temperament is the combination of mental, physical, and emotional traits (natural disposition) of an individual. There has been speculation that this tendency of a person is genetically influenced but can be altered by the interpersonal relationships and environmental experiences in development.

There are many social and environmental stressors that can negatively affect a person and increase vulnerability for psychiatric illness. Interpersonal discords, financial difficulties (with possible legal implications as a result), overcrowding (large families or multiple families residing in the same home), domestic violence, physical or sexual abuse, or placement outside of the related family are all stressors that may contribute to the development of a mental illness. Cultural and ethnic considerations are important, especially for those who are newly integrated into society. Assimilation issues can result in great stress and misidentification of possible disorders.

Fortunately, children are quite resilient. Many children who are identified as at-risk individuals will be able to successfully navigate life without developing a psychiatric disorder. With proper assessment and intervention, they may be able to integrate positive learned behaviors and decrease the impact of psychiatric disorders.

6.2 Mental Retardation

A diagnosis of mental retardation is found on Axis II of the psychiatric diagnosis, and as identified in the *DSM-IV-TR*, three criteria must be met:

1. An IQ less than 70
2. Significant limitations in two or more areas of adaptive behavior (measured by an adaptive rating scale)
3. Evidence these limitations were present before the age of 18

The degree of mental retardation ranges from mild to profound, is determined by the individual's IQ, and influences their functional abilities:

1. Mild retardation: IQ 50–70
2. Moderate retardation: IQ 35–50
3. Severe retardation: IQ 20–35
4. Profound retardation: IQ less than 20

Etiology

The DSM-IV-TR indicates that the cause of mental retardation is primarily biological or psychosocial, or a combination of the two. Some genetic conditions that can be the cause of mental retardation are:

- Down syndrome
- Fragile X syndrome
- Prader-Willi syndrome
- Neurofibromatosis
- Phenyletonuria (PKU)

Other causes of mental retardation are problems during pregnancy (such as use of alcohol), problems at birth (hypoxia), exposure to disease or toxins with delayed medical interventions (whooping cough, measles, meningitis, lead or mercury poisoning), and iodine deficiency (malnutrition).

Assessment

The severity of mental retardation is specific to the patient's IQ. The nurse is expected to assess both the individual's weaknesses and strengths. Interviewing the family and caregiver are essential in determining the level of functioning of the individual. Areas to assess include self-care abilities, cognitive/educational capabilities, social skills, communication capabilities, and psychomotor abilities. It is important to include in the assessment episodes of violence toward self or others. Some individuals with mental retardation are calm, passive, and directable. Others exhibit aggressive behavior and impulsivity and do not respond to limits.

Diagnosis

Analysis of the data will assist in determining the appropriate diagnostic labels for the individual with mental retardation. The severity of the mental retardation will guide appropriate selection of diagnosis. Following are the most common nursing diagnoses for this disorder:

- Risk for injury
- Self-care deficit
- Impaired verbal communication
- Impaired social interaction

Planning/Outcome Criteria

Control aggressive and impulsive behaviors.

Interventions

- Assess and monitor for signs and symptoms of developmental delays.
- Administer prescribed medications (anticonvulsants for impulsivity, stimulants for comorbid ADHD).
- Provide a safe and nonthreatening environment (ensure dangerous items are removed and possible injurious items, such as side rails, headboard, etc., are appropriately padded).

- Perform supportive and active listening for family members to allow for expression of concerns related to disability.

- Maintain consistency among assigned staff and try to anticipate/meet needs until communication patterns are established. Gather communicative information from family/caregivers to facilitate communication of needs.

- Support the child through introduction to inpatient unit if admitted. Offer explanation of behaviors to others (nonverbal gestures and signals), and use behavior modification to reward appropriate behaviors and discourage inappropriate ones.

- Promotion of optimal functioning through encouragement of self-care goals, integrating general needs of a child (play, socialization, and parental limit setting). Allow the individual to master one skill at a time. If it is noted the patient is not able to negotiate the task, intervene to prevent increased frustration.

- Encourage self-care abilities by supporting participation in early stimulation programs, developing a self-feeding and independent toileting and grooming program. Identify aspects of self-care that are within the client's abilities.

- Assist the family in planning for future needs of the child (introduce talk of alternate housing as indicated).

- Make referrals to community supportive resources.

Education for the Child and Family

- Identify normal developmental milestones and appropriately stimulating activities to encourage socialization, communication, and self-care activities.

- Discuss the importance of calmness, continuity, and consistency in approach. Offer information related to how to maintain a patient and caring approach.

- Provide information related to appropriate stimulation, safety, and motivational tactics.

- Keep education related to appropriate discipline that is easy to understand, consistent, and maintainable. Give direction for assistance as the child increases in size and strength.

- As the child ages, review the adolescent's need for information and guidance related to sexual activity.

- Emphasize the importance of fostering self-worth, self-confidence, and self-value.

- Discuss alternate learning opportunities that can make use of the child's concrete approaches.

Provide Information Related to Prevention of Mental Retardation

- Timely and effective prenatal care
- Support for high-risk situations
- Administration of immunizations (rubella)
- Education regarding injury prevention

Evaluation

The evaluation of effectiveness of care for the patient with mental retardation should focus on positive behavioral responses. The evaluation of care determines if the interventions selected were appropriate for the goals. As necessary, the nurse will reassess and select alternate interventions if the goals have not been obtainable.

6.3   Developmental Disorders

Autistic disorders, Rett's disorder, Asperger's Syndrome, and childhood disintegrative disorders are the four classifications of pervasive developmental disorders (PDD). Pervasive developmental disorders are noted by severe and diffuse impairments in social interactions and communicative abilities. Typically these disorders are comorbid with mental retardation.

Autistic disorders are uncommon occurrences, affecting males four to five times more frequently than females and are evident before the age of three. The primary signs of symptoms of autism include impaired communication, impaired social interactions, and the presence of repetitive behaviors. Typically first observed by the caregiver, the child fails to interact or engage with others in their environment. It can occur that the child, who presents as normally developing, inexplicably becomes socially isolative, nonverbal, self-abusive, or seemingly unaffected by environmental stimuli.

While there has been much controversy over the influence of vaccinations contributing to the development of late-onset autism, there is evidence that there is a genetic link with this disorder. Typically the characteristics of autism do improve as the child develops better communicative skills. Adolescence can evidence a regressiveness, possibly due to hormonal changes, or the increasingly complex nature of social interactions. The prognosis of autism is that it will remain into adulthood and the individual typically has some dependency issues.

Asperger's disorder is an autism spectrum disorder. This disorder occurs more frequently in males than females. It differs from autism in age of recognition, typically between the ages of five and nine (later than autism), and in that linguistic and cognitive development is not affected. Children with autism are viewed as socially removed from others; children with Asperger's disorder would like to be socially involved, but they lack the skills required to make these relationships. Development of repetitive and restricted patterns of behaviors, interests, and activities similar to autistic disorders is noted. School age is when defining characteristics become most noticeable, with significant difficulties related to social interactions and possibly motor skill delays (child described as "clumsy"). Children with Asperger's typically border on obsessiveness with their areas of interest.

Rett's disorder is a neurodevelopment disorder that is classified as an autism spectrum disorder by the *DSM-IV-TR*. The cause of this disorder is associated with genetic malfunctioning and subsequent erroneous messaging to the "on" and "off" switches that control complex expression patterns of other genes. This disorder has only been observed in females, with the onset before age four (typically between birth and five months of age), is a rare occurrence, and does result in mental retardation and developmental degeneration. Prenatal and perinatal development gives the appearance of normalcy, psychomotor growth is within normal limits until the age of five to six months, and head circumference is normal at birth. Between five and six months head circumference growth slows, there is a marked social withdraw, motor skills evidence significant awkwardness, significant delays in expressive and receptive skills become apparent, and there is a loss of purposeful hand movements between the ages of 5 to 30 months.

Childhood disintegrative disorder is classified as an autism spectrum disorder in which normal development occurs until the age of three or four, and then evidences a significant and severe loss of social, communication, and relational skills. The onset can be sudden or occur over time, and is usually combined with severe mental retardation. Children diagnosed with this disorder experience similar social and communication impairments as seen in the autism disorder. Children diagnosed with this disorder typically experience loss in the following areas:

- Expressive language (ability to speak)
- Receptive skills (comprehension of verbal and nonverbal communication)
- Elimination (bowel and bladder control)
- Motor skills (self-control of movement)
- Adaptive behaviors (coping skills)

Impairment in functioning is also present in at least two of these areas:

- *Relationship skills*—Disruption in nonverbal behaviors, difficulty developing peer relations, lack of social reciprocity
- *Communication skills*—Absence or delay in spoken language, failure to initiate or maintain conversation with others, patterned and repetitive use of language
- *Repeated patterned behaviors, interests, and movements*—Typically hand flapping, rocking, spinning, resistance in flexibility of routine, catatonia, and obsessiveness with objects

6.4   Attention-Deficit and Disruptive Behavior Disorders

Attention-deficit hyperactivity disorder (ADHD) is a common childhood disorder that can persist through adulthood. The characteristics of ADHD are inattention, increased physical and mental activity, and most significantly, increased impulsivity. Occurring more frequently in males than females, this disorder is generally not recognized until the child enters school. Though it is difficult to diagnose a child under the age of four, infants who are irritable and experience poor sleep patterns and "energetic" toddlers have been known to meet criteria for diagnosis of ADHD at a later age. It is difficult to connect characteristics to younger children due to variances in "normal toddler behavior." Additionally, cultural considerations are essential to assess in order to accurately determine perception of the child's behavior.

In a social setting, the characteristics of the disorder (impulsivity, increased psychomotor activity, distractibility, and impaired cooperation) significantly influence the child's ability to form meaningful friendships and the perception authority figures have of them. Many children who are diagnosed with ADHD carry that disorder into adolescence. The behaviors associated at that age continue to reflect their impulsivity (acting-out behaviors), high risk-taking behaviors, failed interpersonal relationships, and school-related disciplinary problems. It is now accepted that children and adolescents do not "grow out" of ADHD. This disorder can persist into adulthood. Similar behaviors accompany this diagnosis in adulthood (impulsivity, risky behaviors, social ineptness, legal problems).

ADHD has been linked with biological factors (genetics, biochemical, anatomical, prenatal, and perinatal and postnatal events), environmental influences (chemical toxins, dietary considerations), and psychosocial consequences (altered family processes, impaired living environment, preexisting learning disabilities).

Application of the Nursing Process

Assessment

The collection of information is made through interview of the parents, guardians, and significant others in the child's life. Interviewing the child both independently and with the parents and observing the child's interactions within a peer group can offer relevant data. The following is included in the assessment data:

- Nursing history
- Mental status exam (see Chapter 5; ensure assessment of impulsive and dangerous behaviors)
- Roles and relationships (focus on self-concept and socialization with others)
- Physical assessment
- Self-care abilities

Nursing Diagnosis

Analysis of the data collected may support the following nursing diagnoses:

- Risk for injury
- Impaired communication
- Impaired social interactions
- Compromised family coping
- Caregiver role strain
- Disturbed self-esteem
- Noncompliance

Planning and Implementation

Treatment outcomes and selection of appropriate interventions may include those shown in Figure 6-1.

Disruptive Behaviors

The *DSM-IV-TR* defines conduct disorder as a repetitive and persistent pattern of behavior in which the basic rights of others or major age-appropriate societal norms or rules are violated. Characteristics of this disorder include the following:

- Impairment in functioning in social, academic, or occupational areas
- Engaging in bullying behaviors
- Aggressiveness toward people and animals

- Destructiveness toward property
- Lying and stealing (shoplifting, burglary, etc.)
- Involvement in the judicial system (arrests, probation, etc.)

The disorder can begin during the preschool years but typically is evident from middle adolescence to middle adulthood. Childhood-onset types occur before the age of 10, particularly in males who present as more physically aggressive. Paradoxical to the aggression they exhibit, these children experiences feelings of impaired self-esteem. Behavioral indications include irritability, impulsivity, and low frustration tolerance. The prognosis of those children that have this subcategory of conduct disorder is for the disorder to remain throughout their adolescent period and ultimately develop into antisocial personality disorder as an adult. Adolescent-onset types are less aggressive and experience routine relationships with peers. Their acting-out behaviors typically are regulated to peer group activities, with males displaying aggressive behaviors (fighting, stealing, school disturbances) and females experiencing truancy, sexual acting-out behaviors, and deceptiveness.

NURSING DIAGNOSIS	NURSING INTERVENTION
Risk for injury	1. Provide a safe and nonthreatening environment 2. Identify intentional behaviors that may put the child at risk 3. Employ behavior modification techniques to decrease inappropriate behaviors 4. Provide adequate supervision and assistance, offer simple and clear explanations
Impaired social interactions	1. Establish a trusting and therapeutic relationship with the child to increase self-worth 2. Educate child regarding acceptable and unacceptable behaviors focusing on positives but identifying consequences 3. Facilitate group experiences for the child to allow for essential feedback from peers
Compromised family coping	1. Encourage family to express concerns and feelings regarding child's diagnosis 2. Assess the family's understanding of the child's disorder, assisting a realistic approach and facilitating an understanding of future implications 3. Actively involve the family in implementing strategies to assist problems experienced by the child 4. Explain therapeutic approaches used to the family to help reduce their anxiety and encourage compliance 5. Encourage family to identify and contact support systems and resources to decrease feelings of being overwhelmed 6. Coordinate referrals to ensure continuity of care and clear communication among care providers
Caregiver role strain	1. Assist caregiver in identifying stressors to evaluate risk of caregiver role strain 2. Facilitate discussion of current coping skills to reinforce confidence in managing situation 3. Assist identification of support systems to plan for respite needs 4. Identify formal support services and initiate referrals as needed to lessen risk of strain 5. Encourage caregiver to schedule time for self-care and relaxation to diminish stress
Disturbed self-esteem	1. Provide goals that are realistic for the child to decrease risk for failure 2. Develop activities that will offer success to build self-esteem 3. Provide positive reinforcement for success and for attempts to increase desired behaviors
Noncompliance	1. Arrange that the environment for tasks is distraction free to minimize interruptions 2. Ensure adequate time to allow for 1:1 directions in a clear and concrete manner 3. Establish tasks as multilayer—this allows for partial completion, positive reinforcement, and breaks

Figure 6-1 Nursing diagnosis and intervention.

Assessment

Gathering relevant data from the parents, significant others, and child or adolescent, the nurse should determine the level of disruptive behaviors (initiation of behaviors, attempts at management of behaviors). Etiological factors of this disorder include biological, psychosocial, and family predispositions. An assessment of the child or adolescent's behavioral responses (anxiety, aggressiveness, anger, danger toward others) and his or her ability to control impulses is paramount. It is usual during the assessment phase that data will evidence disturbed peer relationships as a result of aggressiveness exhibited by the individual. During the interview, interjecting appropriate questions to determine the child's or adolescent's perception of right and wrong, morality, and interpretation of the effect of their actions on others will offer insight into their moral development.

In addition to determining the presence of physically aggressive behaviors, the nurse should also investigate if alcohol and substance use or abuse, disruption of self-esteem, and poor school performance (despite intelligence) are present.

Diagnosis

Analysis of the data gathered from interviewing the patient and family and other collaborative participants in care will lead to these potential nursing diagnoses for the patient with conduct disorder:

- Disturbed self-esteem
- Coping, ineffective individual
- Coping, defensive
- Social interaction, impaired
- Risk for other-directed violence

Planning and Intervention

Treatment outcomes and selection of appropriate interventions may include those in Figure 6-2.

Evaluation

The evaluation phase of the nursing process allows for determination of the effectiveness of the selected interventions in assisting the patient to achieve the identified goals.

Oppositional Defiant Disorder

Oppositional defiant disorder (ODD) is also characterized under disruptive behaviors. A pattern of negativism, defiance, disobedience, and hostile behaviors toward authority figures is demonstrated without the presence of major antisocial violations. While during some developmental ages there are expectations for a degree of defiant behaviors ("terrible two's," early teens), the spectrum of such behaviors in the patient diagnosed with ODD are more extreme. This diagnosis is assigned when the patient's behaviors' frequency and effect on functioning become apparent and significant. The prevalence of this disorder is equal among female and males, though it occurs more often in males before early adolescence. It occurs in about 5 percent of the population and is typically diagnosed before the age of eight.

Assessment

Signs and symptoms that are assessed in the patient diagnosed with ODD include the following:

- Passive-aggressive behaviors (limit testing, resistance to directives, procrastination, recklessness, unwillingness to work together, etc.)
- Truancy
- Elopement behaviors
- Anger management issues
- Functional underachievement

Oppositional behaviors typically focused on parents may not be obvious in other social settings. Individuals diagnosed with ODD employ ineffective coping mechanisms (examples: projection, denial, displacement). There is usually relationship drama with peers and others related to their behaviors.

NURSING DIAGNOSIS	INTERVENTION
Noncompliance (specify)	• Verbal interaction to allow patient to express rationale for noncompliance using a nonjudgmental approach • Assist the patient in identifying specific noncompliant behaviors • Assist the patient to identify precipitating facts of noncompliance with emphasis on positive impact of compliant behaviors • Guide patient in clarification of personal values, validate ability of self-determination related to treatment goals • Establish a contract with patient to promote appropriate behaviors
Disturbed self-esteem	• Establish therapeutic relationship • Employ therapeutic communication techniques to foster trust and encourage expression of feelings • Arrange situations that will encourage social interactions with peers • Offer positive feedback for behaviors that indicate increase in self-esteem • Assess mental status each day • Keep the focus on behaviors versus individual • Encourage the use of a journal to allow adequate expression of feelings while decreasing perception of vulnerability
Coping, ineffective individual defensive	• Encourage self-evaluation using journal • Provide a structured, safe environment • Encourage active participation in treatment planning • Facilitate socializing opportunities to allow for observation of techniques • Try to facilitate continuity of care and establishment of a therapeutic relationship through consistent staff assignment • As the patient improves in ability to appropriately express feelings, focus on the relationship between feelings and behaviors • Limit-setting for manipulative behaviors, set clear expectations and outline consequences • Assist the patient to identify and accept responsibility for behaviors/actions • Patient education related to the development and utilization of adaptive coping skills
Social interaction, impaired	• Assign consistent staff (as able) for continuity and to promote establishment of the therapeutic relationship • Provide honest and timely feedback for behaviors to increase awareness and facilitate prompt modifications • Initiate verbal interaction for at least 15 minutes each shift to allow opportunity for expression of feelings and ability to collaborate on plan of care • Allow opportunities for socialization with peers, monitor and provide feedback of assessment • Patient education related to appropriate social skills • Role model appropriate social skills
Risk for other-directed violence	• Provide a safe, structured, nonthreatening environment • Assess need for increased observational monitoring • Maintain continuity in approach by all members of the multidisciplinary treatment team • Construct a behavioral contract with the patient to clarify expectations of both the staff and the patient • Patient education to improve self-evaluation of agitation levels, techniques to manage feelings prior to out of control situations • Positive feedback for managing stressful situations effectively, for identifying behaviors and employing self-control

Figure 6-2 Planning and intervention.

Diagnosis

Analysis of the data collected will lead to the formulation of these priority nursing diagnoses:

• Noncompliance (specify)
• Coping, ineffective individual
• Defensive

- Disturbed self-esteem
- Impaired social interaction

Planning and Interventions

Refer back to Figure 6-2 for a plan of care for the diagnosed with ODD using priority nursing diagnoses.

Evaluation

The evaluation phase of the nursing process allows for determination of the effectiveness of the selected interventions in assisting the patient to achieve the identified goals.

6.5 Eating and Feeding Disorders of Infancy and Early Childhood

This section will review pica, ruminations disorder, and feeding disorders as occurrences whose etiologies are not a result of medical conditions.

Pica is an abnormal appetite or craving to ingest items that are not suitable for consumption (clay, paint chips, dirt, hair, etc.). It is a behavior that is commonly observed in younger children, those with mental retardation, and on some occasions, pregnant women (typically a first pregnancy occurring in late adolescence). Presence of this behavior occurs after a medical issue results (bowel issues, toxicity such as lead, or parasitic infestations).

Rumination disorder is diagnosed when an individual purposefully regurgitates food to rechew and reswallow, or spits it out. Also known as "merycism," this disorder is common in infants and mostly associated with mental retardation. The regurgitation is not a result of a medical condition; however, it has been noted that a precipitating event of developing this disorder is having an illness including vomiting. Behavior modification is a treatment modality involved in the care of a patient diagnosed with rumination disorder. Typically, if the disorder begins in infancy, the disorder will resolve on its own.

A *feeding disorder* is characterized when an infant or child persistently fails to consume adequate nutrition, resulting in significant issues with body weight (failure to gain, or loss). As a psychiatric condition, the feeding disorder must not be the result of a medical condition.

6.6 Tic Disorders and the Role of the Nurse Providing Care

A tic is a sudden, spasmodic, pain-free, involuntary muscular contraction or vocalization. A tic can present in any body part, most commonly seen as blinking, sudden movement of the neck, shoulder shrugs, facial movements, or coughing. Vocal tics are those that involve the involuntary expression of sounds, grunts, coughs, sniffing, barking, and snorting. Generally aggravated by increased stress experienced by an individual, they usually are minimized during rest or when the person is focused on distracting activities. Though most tics are minimally noticeable, the frequency and intensity can negatively influence a child's life.

Tourette's disorder is characterized by multiple muscular tics and one or more vocal tics that have been occurring for greater than one year. It is a rare disorder that is known to affect boys more, presenting before the age of seven. The individual who has been diagnosed with Tourette's disorder experiences varied tics over their lifetime. These tics have a significant impact on life experiences and functioning, resulting in a disruption of all areas of living (social, academic, occupational).

A chronic tic disorder differs from Tourette's disorder in that either a motor or vocal tic is present, not both.

Treatment modalities for tic disorders include the use of medications in conjunction with psychosocial therapy, which will assist the patient in addressing the impact of the disorder on the person, family, and everyday functioning. The medication that has been identified as the most effective is haloperidol (Haldol). It is important that the nurse be knowledgeable of the doses administered for control of the tics (0.05 to 0.075 mg/kg per day in two or three divided doses. Additionally, ongoing assessment should occur for adverse effects of the medications (discussed previously in Chapter 3). Other neuroleptic medications have also been prescribed in the treatment of tics in Tourette's disorder. These include Pimozide (Orap)—not recommended for children less than 12 years old, Clonidine (Catapres), Risperidone (risperdal), olanzapine (Zyprexa), and ziprasidone (Geodon).

6.7   Elimination Disorders in Children and Adolescents

Following are the two most recognized elimination disorders present in children:

1. Encopresis (repeated defecation into inappropriate places by a child at least fours years of age (chronological or developmental age)
2. Enuresis (repeated urinary voiding of a child at least five years of age (chronological or developmental age)

These events occur regardless of time of day and are mostly involuntary, but they can be intentional. The passage of feces can be the result of psychological constipation (involuntary), or it may be the direct result of ODD or conduct disorder (intentional). Enuresis has similar presentations.

These disorders are more frequent in males. Encopresis can persist intermittently for years, while enuresis typically resolves by adolescence. The effect of elimination disorders is directly related to the individual's social activities. The impacts are disturbed self-esteem, social isolation, anger management issues, feelings of rejection, and potential for dangerous behaviors towards self or others related to feelings associated with these disorders and perception of those in the individual's life.

Treatment modalities for these disorders include the administration of medication (medications with the side effect of urinary retention) and behavioral modifications to serve as a warning that elimination is occurring (such as bed-pad alarms). Treatment of the underlying oppositional disorder will assist in diminishing elimination disorders if the behavior is intentional.

6.8   Separation Anxiety Disorder, Selective Mutism, Reactive Attachment Disorder, and Stereotypic Movement Disorder

Separation anxiety disorder is characterized by anxiety exceeding that expected for the developmental level related to separation from the home or those to whom the child is attached. The resulting anxiety has a significant influence on the child's ability to function appropriately in academic, social, occupational, or other areas of daily living. This disorder is more often seen in females and is exhibited before the age of 18. It is believed that this disorder is a result of a combination of temperament and parenting behaviors.

Assessment

The disorder onset can be during preschool age. Typically it does not occur in adolescence. Interview and observational assessment will include a report of difficulty separating from the caregiver. Though this disorder generally is focused on the mother, it can be the separation from the father, siblings, or other caregiver that is a precipitant. Behaviors displayed in anticipation of the separation may include temper tantrums, clinginess, somatic complaints, crying, and screaming. Difficulty getting the child to attend school is common. Younger children will closely follow around the individual they are fearful of separating from. Older children may avoid age-expected sleepovers or school trips. The child may be described as demanding, intrusive, attention-seeking, or even very compliant and eager to please. As they age, they experience great difficulty leaving the parents' home. Impairments in social skills are not demonstrated in individuals experiencing this disorder. Typically they are able to form age-appropriate relationships without evidence of difficulty. Descriptions of worry are common in relation to concern of harm to self or the caregiver. In addition to a depressed mood, other fears are voiced (spirits, the dark, etc.).

Nursing Diagnosis

- Anxiety (severe)
- Ineffective coping, individual
- Impaired social interaction

Planning and Interventions

Treatment outcomes and selection of appropriate interventions may include those in Figure 6-3.

NURSING DIAGNOSIS	NURSING INTERVENTION
Anxiety (severe)	• Provide a safe and nonthreatening environment • Establish a therapeutic relationship with a calm, trustful, and genuine approach • Explore with the child their perception of the separation and concerns surrounding this action • Explore with the parents (caregiver) concerns/fears they may be experiencing regarding impending separation from the child • Assist the patient and family in formulating realistic goals • Offer positive reinforcement for behaviors exhibited in attaining the goals
Ineffective individual coping	• Identify with the child and parent (caregiver) situations/events which result in distressing situations and their perception of response to these situations • Assist the child to be realistic of self-expectations, help to correlate experiences of not meeting self-demands with episodes of increased anxiety • Patient education related to the development and utilization of adaptive coping skills to manage stressors • Convey a belief in the child's ability to develop appropriate coping skills • Assess the child's knowledge of the disorder, educate about illness, treatment, and prognosis • Encourage the child and parent (caregiver) to actively participate in treatment planning
Impaired social interaction	• Develop the establishment of a trusting and caring relationship through continuity of staff assignments (as able) • Provide opportunities for the child to attend and participate in groups • Provide positive reinforcement for participation in socializing treatments, support efforts to interact with others • Assist the child initially to attend groups, through support and reinforcement • Encourage progressive involvement in the groups activities • Assist the child in establishing realistic goals to improve socialization techniques

Figure 6-3 Planning and intervention.

Evaluation

The evaluation phase of the nursing process allows for determination of the effectiveness of the selected interventions in assisting the patient to achieve the identified goals.

Selective mutism is characterized by persistent failure to speak in social situations where speaking is expected. Communication is accomplished nonverbally via gestures, nodding, or shaking of the head. Rarely one-word utterances are made, which will be in a voice other than the child's "normal tone." Assessment will evidence shyness, social isolation, and episodes of anger in the form of temper tantrums. The prevalence is rare and more common in females than males. While typically lasting for a brief period (one month or so), it can last for years.

Reactive attachment disorder, also referred to as detachment or attachment disorder, typically begins before the age of five, is associated with pathogenic care (parental neglect), and displays as a disturbed or developmentally inappropriate social relatedness. The child can either be inhibited (responds with apparent indifference, a mixed approach-avoidance, and resistance to comforting) or disinhibited (attachments are diffuse, the child is overly familiar with strangers and lacks selectivity). The behaviors exhibited are not a result of any developmental delay (such as mental retardation) and do not fit criteria for pervasive developmental disorder. Treatment focuses on safety and therapy with the child and caregiver (if able). Prognosis with early identification and intervention is good.

Stereotypic movement disorder is often comorbid with mental retardation and is associated with genetic, metabolic, and neurologic disorders. Repetitive, nonfunctional behaviors which interfere in daily functioning and may lead to self-injury require medical attention. Movements assessed include the following:

• Rocking
• Twirling objects
• Head banging
• Picking at skin

- Self-hitting
- Biting oneself

The more severe the mental retardation, the greater the risk for self-injurious behavior. While there are no specific treatments for this disorder, the administration of certain medications may be effective for certain behaviors. The registered nurse must ensure a safe and nonthreatening environment while providing care for these individuals. The use of a monitoring status, medications to decrease behaviors, and priority nursing actions for comfort and care are paramount.

Chapter 6 Questions

Multiple Choice

1. Communication disorders

    A. May be expressive

    B. May be receptive

    C. Involve stuttering or articulation

    D. A and B

    E. A, B, and C

2. A priority goal in providing nursing care for children and adolescents experiencing psychiatric disorders is

    A. Establish a trusting relationship by accepting the patient and their limitations.

    B. Provide information related to the diagnosis and prognosis.

    C. Assess the patient's growth and development levels.

    D. The patient will communicate thoughts and feelings about self-concept.

3. The diagnosis of mental retardation would be found on which axis?

    A. Axis I

    B. Axis II

    C. Axis III

    D. Axis IV

    E. Axis V

4. An example of a nursing intervention in the care of a child with mental retardation is

    A. Promote optimal level of functioning in activities of daily living and enhance self-esteem.

    B. The patient will remain free from injury.

    C. Assess the patient's strengths and abilities.

    D. Self-care deficit.

5. During the assessment phase, you determine that the child has difficulty forming interpersonal relationships. As an infant, she was resistant to hugs from her parents, and her mother reports that communication with others has been difficult. She displayed repetitive and stereotyped behaviors when her routine was disrupted (body swaying, hand clapping, etc.). Based upon your understanding of disorders in children, this patient diagnosis is

    A. Mental retardation

    B. ADHD

    C. Conduct disorder

    D. Autistic disorder

6. A seven-year-old has been diagnosed with enuresis after testing has revealed no medical cause for bedwetting. The parents are upset, and the father states to the mother, "This is your fault. I told you that you are not strict enough." Your initial response is:

   A. "Why do you think that?"

   B. "It's a disorder; nobody is to blame for this."

   C. "Who did the toilet training?"

   D. "You seem to be upset by this information."

7. Key interventions for a patient with a conduct disorder include all of the following except:

   A. Observation of the patient's behavior during routine activities and interactions

   B. Conveying unconditional acceptance and positive regard

   C. Changing staff assignments at the patient's request

   D. Using limit-setting techniques to decrease inappropriate behaviors

8. Medications used in the treatment of ADHD are effective in decreasing hyperactivity and impulsiveness and in improving attention. The most common side effects include

   A. Increased energy, stimulation of growth

   B. Somnolence, weight gain, increased appetite

   C. Insomnia, weight loss, loss of appetite

   D. All of the above

Scenario: Mrs. Smith has brought her four-year-old son, Adam, for an evaluation after it was reported by his preschool teacher that he is disruptive in the classroom (tapping pencils on the desk, answering out of turn, not following directions, easily distracted). Mrs. Smith reports that Adam was "fussy" as a baby and did not sleep well. She adds, "He has always been very energetic and active." Considering the above data, answer these questions:

Questions 9 to 12 are based on the above scenario. Select the answer that is most appropriate.

9. During the assessment of Adam, the mother reports that his teacher sent home a note indicating, "Adam is very fidgety in the class. He doesn't play appropriately with the other children." This is an example of:

   A. Subjective data

   B. Objective data

   C. Analysis of the data

   D. Evaluation

10. Assessing Adam's memory, you tell him three objects, and when you ask him to repeat them to you, he responds, "I don't know." You consider the reason for this response to be

   A. Adam has a poor memory.

   B. Adam is oppositional.

   C. Adam is unable to respond due to his symptom of ADHD.

   D. Adam is psychotic.

11. It is reported that Adam has been exhibiting behaviors that are potentially dangerous. Adam's mother tells of one episode when he attempted to jump down a flight of stairs. What is an appropriate response you could suggest to his mother to address this kind of behavior?

    A. "Adam, it is not safe to jump down stairs. You are to walk down the stairs one at a time."

    B. "Adam, do you think that is safe to jump down the stairs?"

    C. Inform the mother that due to Adam's diagnosis of ADHD, there is no way to stop dangerous behavior.

    D. "Adam, what is the matter with you? Do you want to break your leg?"

12. In developing the treatment plan for Adam, the following individuals are involved:

 A. The patient

 B. The treatment team

 C. The parents

 D. A and B

 E. A, B, and C

13. A 15-year-old patient is admitted to your unit with a diagnosis of anorexia nervosa. You have been assigned to monitor her during the evening meal. The patient states, "I don't know why you don't trust me to eat my food. Sally (the regular evening RN) lets me eat by myself." Your best response to this statement would be:

 A. "Really? OK, let me know when you are done eating so I can check your tray."

 B. "Sally is not here tonight."

 C. "I trust you, but the charge nurse told me to sit with you."

 D. "It sounds as if you are trying to manipulate me."

14. A child with conduct disorder has a nursing diagnosis of risk for other-directed violence. An appropriate goal for this patient would be

 A. The patient will accept responsibility for his or her behaviors.

 B. The patient will not harm others or the property of others.

 C. The patient will verbalize feelings of increased self-worth.

 D. The patient will interact appropriately with others.

15. In developing your plan of care for your patient diagnosed with conduct disorder, you have established the goal "client will not harm others or others' property." What are the most appropriate nursing actions to assist the patient to achieve this goal?

 A. Convey acceptance and positive regard.

 B. Observation of the patient's behaviors and interactions with others.

 C. Encourage appropriate expression of anger, acting as a role model.

 D. Set forth a structured plan of therapeutic activities.

 E. Remove objects from the environment that the patient may use to harm others.

 F. Use limit-setting techniques to reinforce the expectation that the patient will act in a responsible and self-controlled way.

 G. B, C, E, F

 H. All of the above

16. Your nursing history of a patient diagnosed with conduct disorder may include all of the following symptoms, except:

 A. Difficulty or inability forming relationships with peers

 B. Feelings of remorse over behaviors towards others

 C. Use of manipulation to meet own needs

 D. Persistent violation of rules

17. During the assessment of an eight-year-old child, you learn that he has impaired verbal skills and uses acting-out behaviors to express his needs. Which of the following level of mental retardation is indicated for this child?

 A. Mild

 B. Moderate

 C. Severe

 D. Profound

18. You are the nurse on a child unit in a psychiatric facility. Your patient has a diagnosis of severe autistic disorder. Which of the following interventions would be the most appropriate for this patient?

    A. Social skills training

    B. Therapeutic group activities

    C. Neuroleptic medications

    D. Play therapy

Scenario: Your patient has been diagnosed with Tourette's disorder. During the admission assessment, you note that he frequently blinks his eyes and intermittently repeats words that you have said.

Questions 19 and 20 are based on the above scenario. Select the answer that is most appropriate.

19. The correct terminology for the repeating of what someone else has said is

    A. Palilalia

    B. Echolalia

    C. Word salad

    D. Paraphilias

20. The following classification of medications is commonly used in the treatment of tics associated with Tourette's disorder:

    A. Benzodiazepines (Xanax, Ativan, Klonopin)

    B. Neuroleptic (haloperidol, Pimozide, risperidone)

    C. Mood stabilizers (Lithium, Depakote, Tegretol)

    D. Anticholenergic (benapryzine, Benzhexol, orphenadrine, and bornaprine)

Matching

21. Pica	A. Urinary incontinence (bedwetting) after the age of 5, not caused by a medical disorder
22. Tic	B. An abnormal appetite or craving for substances not fit for consumption (chalk, clay, etc.)
23. Anorexia nervosa	C. An abnormally voracious appetite or constant state of hunger; also known as a binge-purge syndrome, characterized by frequent episodes of eating excessive amounts of food followed by self-induced vomiting
24. Impulsivity	D. Disorder that has restricted and repetitive patterns of behavior but no significant delay in cognitive and language development
25. Negativism	E. A sudden, spasmodic, painless, involuntary muscular contraction
26. Autistic disorder	F. Interrupted rhythm of speech related to repetition, blocks or spasms, or prolonged sounds or syllables
27. Mental retardation	G. Characterized by a pathological fear of gaining weight, often accompanied by a persistent unwillingness to eat
28. ADHD	H. Group of disorders characterized by impairments in development, socialization, communication, or the presence of repetitive, stereotypical behaviors

29. Temperament

    I.   Characterized by a pattern of negativistic, defiant, disobedient, and hostile behavior toward authority figures

30. Conduct disorder

    J.   Actuated by emotional or involuntary responses geared toward immediate gratification

31. Therapeutic holding

    K.   Involuntary defecation not related to a medical condition

32. Play therapy

    L.   The combination of mental, physical, and emotional traits of a person (natural predisposition) evident at a very early age, or even from birth

33. Adjustment disorder

    M.   Category used for emotional responses to an identifiable stressor, beginning three months from the stress and lasting no more than six months

34. Asperger's disorder

    N.   A behavioral syndrome usually first observed before the age of three that the child is not demonstrating interest in others or being socially responsive

35. Oppositional defiant disorder

    O.   An intervention employed to control destructive behaviors through the prompt, firm, and nonretaliatory protective restraining to help reduce distress and assist in the maintenance of self-control

36. Enuresis

    P.   Overt or covert opposition to suggestions or ideas

37. Ancopresis

    Q.   An intervention that encourages symbolic expression of feelings

38. Pervasive developmental disorder

    R.   Deficits in general intellectual functioning and adaptive functioning

39. Stuttering

    S.   Characterized by persistent pattern of behaviors that violate the rights of others and disregard social norms

40. Bulimia nervosa

    T.   A disorder occurring before the age of seven that includes increased motor activity, inattention, distractibility, and impulsivity

Chapter 6 Answers

Multiple Choice

1. **E.** Communication disorders may be expressive or receptive and expressive. They primarily involve articulation and stuttering.

2. **D.** Answer A and B are nursing interventions; C is assessment.

3. **B.** Axis I is for clinical disorders, Axis III medical diagnoses, Axis IV psychosocial and environmental issues, and Axis V GAF.

4. **A.** Answer B is a patient-centered goal, C is an assessment, and D is a nursing diagnostic label.

5. **D.** Autistic disorder is characterized by a withdrawal into self, abnormal or impaired development of socialization skills, and impaired verbal and nonverbal communication abilities.

6. **D.** "Why" questions are nontherapeutic, causing a defensive response. The father is upset over the news and using the defense mechanism projection to manage his emotional response. As the registered nurse, you want to acknowledge the feelings experienced by the parent and facilitate further expression of feelings.

7. **C.** Patients diagnosed with conduct disorder use manipulation to gain control over their environment and others in the environment as a means to address self-esteem issues. It is important not to reward or reinforce manipulative behavior by providing the desired effect.

8. **C.** The medications used to treat ADHD are stimulants, and the most common side effects of these medications include insomnia, anorexia, and weight loss.

9. **B.** Objective data (signs or overt data) are obtained by observation or physical examination.

10. **C.** Assessing Adam's memory may be difficult due to impaired attention or inability to manage racing thoughts.

11. **A.** Expectations should be clearly stated, as the child may not be aware of acceptable behavior, and the explanations should be short and clear. A punitive or belittling attitude in the tone of voice is to be avoided.

12. **E.** Including the parents in planning and providing care for a child with ADHD is important, encouraging feelings of empowerment for the parents and providing specific strategies that can help them and the child be successful.

13. **D.** Patients who are diagnosed with eating disorders typically experience difficulty with trust. Addressing the patient's manipulation is therapeutic, assisting him or her to deal with ineffective coping.

14. **B.** A characteristic of conduct disorder is the use of physical aggression in violating the rights of others. A priority goal for this problem is ensuring the safety of others. While the other goals mentioned may be appropriate for this clinical situation, they are not addressing the diagnosis of other-directed violence.

15. **H.** Each of the interventions listed will assist the patient in achieving the goal of safety on the unit. Acceptance and positive regard are essential elements in the establishment of the therapeutic relationship. A basic intervention is to observe the behaviors and interactions of the patient and how he or she manages in his or her environment. It is essential that the environment be checked to ensure there are no weapons that can be used to inflict harm to self or others. Role modeling is an important intervention in teaching adaptive skills for managing life situations. Structured activities and the use of limit setting help to maintain a safe and nonthreatening environment.

16. **B.** Patients diagnosed with conduct disorder are known to experience poor peer relationships, exhibit a repetitive pattern of disregard for the rights of others or societal norms, and intimidate or persuade the responses of others to meet their own perceived needs and desires. Typically, the child or adolescent diagnosed with conduct disorder does not display any feelings of guilt or remorse related to his or her behaviors/actions.

17. **C.** Persons with severe mental retardation have impaired verbal skills. Typically they use nonverbal acting-out behaviors to convey needs.

18. **D.** In autistic disorder, the child typically withdraws into him- or herself and into a fantasy world of his or her own making. Social interaction and communication skills are significantly impaired. A therapeutic relationship may be achieved through the use of a one-on-one approach, such as play therapy.

19. **B.** Echolalia is parrotlike repetition of the words spoken by another. Palilalia is the repeating of one's own words. Word salad is a group of words put together randomly without a logical connection. Paraphilias is repetitive behaviors or thoughts of a sexually nature that involve nonhuman objects, real or simulated humiliation/suffering, or nonconsenting partners.

20. **B.** Haloperidol (Haldol), pimozide (Orap), and risperidone (Risperdal) are neuroleptic medications that have been used effectively in the treatment of tics. Caution is advised regarding the use of Haldol in children related to adverse effects, and Orap is not recommended for use in children under the age of 12.

Matching

21.	B	**31.**	O
22.	E	**32.**	Q
23.	G	**33.**	M
24.	J	**34.**	D
25.	P	**35.**	I
26.	N	**36.**	A
27.	R	**37.**	K
28.	T	**38.**	H
29.	L	**39.**	F
30.	S	**40.**	C

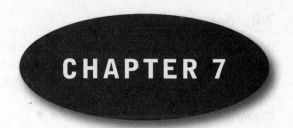

CHAPTER 7

Anxiety and Anxiety Disorders

7.1 Anxiety

Anxiety is a normal emotional response to threatening situations. It is a feeling of dread or apprehension, and a response to internal or external stimuli that can manifest into cognitive, behavioral, emotional, and physical symptoms. Anxiety is different from fear, which is a cognitive process in which the individual intellectually appraises the threatening stimulus. Fear is a reaction to a specific danger. Stress refers to a condition produced by a change in the environment that can be perceived by the individual as threatening, challenging, or detrimental to the person's well-being. Stress often leads to anxiety.

Anxiety is a human experience that is felt universally. Individuals have experienced anxiety throughout the ages, and currently, anxiety disorders are the most common of all psychiatric illnesses resulting in considerable functional impairment and distress.

Hildegard Peplau, a nursing theorist discussed in Chapter 1, had an extensive impact in shaping psychiatric mental health nursing. She also identified anxiety as one of the most important concepts in psychiatric nursing and developed an anxiety model useful in the nursing practice. She identifies four levels of anxiety:

1. *Mild anxiety*—A feeling that something is different, and the person is more alert and their perceptual field is increased. The person may exhibit some physical symptoms such as restlessness, irritability, or mild tension-relieving behaviors. This type of anxiety is associated with everyday living and often motivates people to make changes or engage in more goal-directed activity.

2. *Moderate anxiety*—A disturbing feeling that something is definitely wrong. The person is still able to process information and solve problems, which is greatly enhanced by the support of another. The person may exhibit physical symptoms such as a pounding heart, increased pulse and respiration, perspiration, headache, and gastric discomfort. This type of anxiety can still be constructive, by informing the person that something in his or her life needs attention.

3. *Severe anxiety*—Often causes the person to focus on a specific detail and ignore everything else. Cognitive skills decrease, and learning and problem solving are no longer possible. Behavior becomes automatic and focused on reducing or relieving anxiety. Symptoms include increased somatic symptoms, trembling, and a pounding heart. The person may describe a feeling of impending doom or dread.

4. *Panic-level anxiety*—The most extreme form of anxiety, this involves a disorganization of personality and disturbed behavior. The person is unable to process what is taking place in his or her environment and may lose touch with reality. The behavior exhibited may include confusion, shouting, withdrawal, or hallucinations. Physical behavior may be erratic and impulsive. This level of anxiety cannot persist indefinitely because it is not compatible with life and can lead to exhaustion or death if not safely and effectively treated.

7.2 Anxiety Disorders

Prevalence: Anxiety disorders have the highest prevalence rates of all mental disorders in the United States. Nearly one in four adults is affected, with a similar number among young people. Anxiety disorders are more prevalent among women, people under the age of 45, people who are divorced or separated, and people of low socioeconomic status.

Comorbidity: Both clinicians and researchers have shown that anxiety disorders often co-occur with other psychiatric disorders. Several studies have suggested that 90 percent of people with an anxiety disorder develop another psychiatric disorder in their lifetime.

Etiology: Anxiety may have a genetic component, because first-degree relatives of individuals with increased anxiety have higher rates of developing anxiety. Studies indicate a genetic component to both panic disorder and obsessive-compulsive disorder.

Some biological findings include the GABA benzodiazepine theory. These recently discovered receptors are linked to a receptor that inhibits the activity of the neurotransmitter GABA. The release of GABA slows neural transmission, which has a calming effect. Binding of the benzodiazepine medications to the benzodiazepine receptors facilitates the action of GABA. This theory suggests that abnormalities of these benzodiazepine receptors may lead to unregulated anxiety levels.

Anxiety disorders are diagnosed when anxiety is no longer working as a signal of danger or motivating the individual to make a much needed change. Instead, the anxiety becomes chronic and interferes with personal, occupational, or social functioning. This often results in emotional disability and maladaptive behaviors.

Figure 7-1 shows the *DSM-IV-TR* criteria for symptoms of anxiety disorders.
Following is the *DSM-IV-TR* (APA, 2000) diagnostic criteria for Anxiety Disorders.

DISORDER	SYMPTOMS
Panic disorder without agoraphobia	Recurrent unexpected panic attacks, with at least one of the attacks followed by a month (or more) of persistent concern about having additional attacks, worry about the implications of the attack or its consequences, or a significant change in behavior related to the attacks. Also the absence of agoraphobia.
Panic disorder with agoraphobia	Meets the above criteria. In addition, includes the presence of agoraphobia.
Specific phobia	Marked and persistent fear that is excessive and unreasonable, cued by the presence or anticipation of a specific object or situation (such as flying, heights, animals, receiving an injection, or seeing blood). Exposure to the phobic stimulus almost invariably provokes an immediate anxiety response. The person recognizes the fear is excessive, and the distress or avoidance interfere with the person's normal routine.
Social phobia	A marked and persistent fear of social or performance situations in which the person is exposed to unfamiliar people or to possible scrutiny by others. The person fears that he or she will act in a way that will be humiliating or embarrassing. Exposure to the feared situation almost invariably provokes anxiety. The person recognizes the fear is excessive, and the distress or avoidance interferes with the person's normal routine.
Obsessive-compulsive disorder	Either obsessions or compulsions are recognized as excessive and interfere with the person's normal routine.
Post-traumatic stress disorder	The person has been exposed to a traumatic event in which both of the following were present: The person has experienced, witnessed, or been confronted with an event that involved actual or threatened death or serious injury, or a threat to the physical integrity of oneself or others. The person's response involved intense fear, helplessness, or horror. The traumatic event is re-experienced in the mind, and there is an avoidance of stimuli associated with the trauma and a numbing of general responsiveness.
Acute stress disorder	Meets the criteria for exposure to a traumatic event and person experiences three of the following symptoms: sense of detachment, reduced awareness of one's surroundings, derealization, depersonalization, and dissociated amnesia.
Generalized anxiety disorder	Excessive anxiety and worry, occurring more days than not for at least 6 months, about a number of events or activities. The person finds it difficult to control the worry and experiences at least three of the following symptoms: restlessness or feeling keyed up or on edge, fatigue, difficulty concentrating or mind going blank, irritability, muscle tension, sleep disturbance.

Figure 7-1 Symptoms of anxety disorders.

7.3   Panic Disorder

Panic disorder is characterized by recurrent, unexpected panic attacks, about which the individual is persistently concerned.

Diagnostic Criteria for 300.01 Panic Disorder without Agoraphobia
(cautionary statement)

A. Both (1) and (2):
  (1) Recurrent unexpected panic attacks
  (2) At least one of the attacks has been followed by 1 month (or more) of one (or more) of the following:
    (a) Persistent concern about having additional attacks
    (b) Worry about the implications of the attack or its consequences (i.e., losing control, having a heart attack, "going crazy")
    (c) A significant change in behavior related to the attacks
B. Absence of agoraphobia is characterized by intense, excessive anxiety or fear about being in places or situations from which escape may prove difficult or embarrassing, or which help may not be available if a panic attack were to occur.
C. The panic attacks are not due to the direct physiological effects of a substance (i.e., a drug of abuse, a medication) or a general medical condition (i.e., hyperthyroidism).
D. The panic attacks are not better accounted for by another mental disorder, such as Social Phobia (i.e., occurring on exposure to feared social situations), Specific Phobia (i.e., on exposure to a specific phobic situation), Obsessive-Compulsive Disorder (i.e., on exposure to dirt in someone with an obsession about contamination), Post-traumatic Stress Disorder (i.e., in response to stimuli associated with a severe stressor), or Separation Anxiety Disorder (i.e., in response to being away from home or close relatives).

Application of the Nursing Process

Assessment
In this first step of the nursing process, the nurse must not make assumptions about the patient's abilities or limitations based solely on the medical diagnosis of panic attacks with or without agoraphobia.

The onset of panic attacks is unpredictable and its symptoms arrive unexpectedly. They do not occur immediately before or on exposure to a situation that usually causes anxiety (such as a specific phobia).

At least four of the following symptoms must be present to identify the presence of a panic attack. A discrete period of intense fear or discomfort, in which four (or more) of the following symptoms developed abruptly and reached a peak within 10 minutes:

  (1) Palpitations, pounding heart, or accelerated heart rate
  (2) Sweating
  (3) Trembling or shaking
  (4) Sensations of shortness of breath or smothering
  (5) Feeling of choking
  (6) Chest pain or discomfort
  (7) Nausea or abdominal distress
  (8) Feeling dizzy, unsteady, lightheaded, or faint
  (9) Derealization (feelings of unreality) or depersonalization (being detached from oneself)
  (10) Fear of losing control or going crazy
  (11) Fear of dying
  (12) Paresthesias (numbness or tingling sensations)
  (13) Chills or hot flushes

The average age of onset of a panic disorder is the late 20s. Frequency and severity of panic attacks vary widely. Some individuals have attacks of moderate severity weekly, while others may have fewer severe attacks several times a week. Still others may experience attacks separated by weeks or months. Sometimes the individual experiences periods of remissions and exacerbations. Panic disorders may or may not be accompanied by agoraphobia.

Panic Disorder with Agoraphobia

This type of panic disorder will severely restrict the individual from any type of travel, causing him or her to become nearly or completely homebound unless there is someone available to accompany the individual. Common agoraphobic situations include leaving the home alone, being in crowds; traveling in a car, bus, or train; or being on a bridge.

7.4   Generalized Anxiety Disorder

Generalized anxiety disorder is characterized by at least six months of chronic, unrealistic, excessive anxiety and worry.

Diagnostic Criteria for 300.02 Generalized Anxiety Disorder

(cautionary statement)

A. Excessive anxiety and worry (apprehensive expectation), occurring more days than not for at least six months, about a number of events or activities (such as work or school performance).

B. The person finds it difficult to control the worry.

C. The anxiety and worry are associated with three (or more) of the following six symptoms (with at least some symptoms present for more days than not for the past six months). Note: Only one item is required in children.

(1) Restlessness or feeling keyed up or on edge

(2) Being easily fatigued

(3) Difficulty concentrating or mind going blank

(4) Irritability

(5) Muscle tension

(6) Sleep disturbance (difficulty falling or staying asleep, or restless unsatisfying sleep)

D. The focus of the anxiety and worry is not confined to features of an Axis I disorder, i.e., the anxiety or worry is not about having a panic attack (as in panic disorder), being embarrassed in public (as in social phobia), being contaminated (as in obsessive-compulsive disorder), being away from home or close relatives (as in separation anxiety disorder), gaining weight (as in anorexia nervosa), having multiple physical complaints (as in somatization disorder), or having a serious illness (as in hypochondriasis), and the anxiety and worry do not occur exclusively during posttraumatic stress disorder.

E. The anxiety, worry, or physical symptoms cause clinically significant distress or impairment in social, occupational, or other important areas of functioning.

F. The disturbance is not due to the direct physiological effects of a substance (i.e., a drug of abuse, a medication) or a general medical condition (i.e., hyperthyroidism) and does not occur exclusively during a mood disorder, a psychotic disorder, or a pervasive developmental disorder.

Assessment

As seen above in the diagnostic criteria, anxiety and worry are associated with three or more of the six symptoms of generalized anxiety disorder. This disorder can begin in childhood or adolescence, but is not uncommon after the age of 20. Depressive symptoms are common, often accompanied by numerous somatic complaints. Generalized anxiety disorder tends to be chronic, with frequent stress-related exacerbations and fluctuations seen in the course of this illness.

Predisposing Factors for Panic and Generalized Anxiety Disorders

Genetics: Panic disorder has a strong genetic component. The concordance rate for identical twins is 30 percent, and the risk for the disorder in a close relative is 10 to 20 percent.

Neuroanatomical: Structural brain imaging studies in patients with panic disorders have implicated pathological involvement in the temporal lobes, particularly the hippocampus.

Biochemical: Abnormal elevations of blood lactate have been noted in clients with panic disorder. Likewise, infusion of sodium lactate into clients with anxiety neuroses produced symptoms of panic disorder. Several laboratories have replicated these findings of increased lactate sensitivity in panic prone individuals, but no specific mechanism that triggers the panic symptoms can be explained.

Medical conditions: There are medical conditions associated to a greater degree with individuals who suffer panic and generalized anxiety disorders as compared to the general population. They include the following:

1. Acute myocardial infarction
2. Substance intoxication and withdrawal (cocaine, alcohol, marijuana, opioids)
3. Hypoglycemia
4. Pheochromocytomas (neuroendocrine tumor of the medulla of the adrenal glands)
5. Caffeine intoxication
6. Mitral valve prolapse
7. Complex partial seizures

Diagnosis

An analysis of the assessment data will assist in determining the priority of problems and help formulate the plan of care. Common nursing diagnosis for the patient with panic and generalized anxiety disorder include the following NANDA nursing diagnoses:

- Anxiety
- Powerlessness
- Ineffective coping
- Disturbed thought process

Planning/Implementation

See Figure 7-2 for appropriate plan of care for the patient diagnosed with panic or generalized anxiety disorder.

NURSING DIAGNOSIS	NURSING INTERVENTION
Anxiety	• Stay with patient and provide a safe, calm environment • Encourage verbalization of feelings • Reframe the problem in a way that is solvable • Identify thoughts and feelings prior to the onset of anxiety • Teach relaxation techniques
Powerlessness	• Allow patient to take as much responsibility as possible in performing their ADL's • Include patient to set realistic goals • Help identify areas of life situations that patient can control
Ineffective coping	• Monitor and reinforce patient's use of positive coping skills and healthy defense mechanisms • Teach new coping skills to replace ineffective ones • Teach proper breathing techniques
Disturbed thought process	• Explore with patient thoughts that led up to anxious feelings and relief behaviors • Teach patient behavioral techniques that can interrupt intrusive, unwanted thoughts • Teach client to recognize triggers of anxiety • Refer patient to support groups in the community

Figure 7-2 Nursing diagnosis and intervention.

Evaluation

In evaluating the outcomes of the nursing interventions in the care of the patient with panic disorder or generalized anxiety disorder, the following questions should be asked:

- Is the patient able to recognize and identify signs of escalating anxiety?
- Is the patient able to utilize positive coping skills and healthy defense mechanisms to prevent panic-level anxiety?
- Is the patient able to practice daily relaxation techniques?
- Is the patient amenable to exercising three times a week?
- Is the patient able to perform independent activities of daily living (ADLs)?
- Is the patient able to participate in decision making and have control over his or her own life?
- Is the client able to verbalize acceptance of areas of their life over which he or she has no control?

7.5 Phobias

A phobia is an illogical, intense, persistent fear of a specific object or a social situation that causes extreme distress and interferes with normal functioning. Phobias are usually not the result of a past negative experience, and in fact, the person may never have had contact with the object of the phobia. People with phobias usually recognize that their fear is unusual and irrational but feel powerless to stop it.

There are three categories of phobias:

1. *Agoraphobia*—Characterized by intense, excessive anxiety or fear about being in places or situations from which escape may prove difficult or embarrassing, or which help may not be available if a panic attack were to occur.
2. *Social phobia*—An excessive fear of situations in which a person might do something embarrassing or be evaluated negatively by others. The person has extreme concerns about being exposed to possible scrutiny by others and fears social or performance situations in which embarrassment may occur.
3. *Specific phobia*—A marked, persistent, and excessive or irrational fear when in the presence of, or when anticipating an encounter with, a specific object or situation.

The *DSM-IV-TR* identifies subtypes of the most common specific phobias:

- *Animal type*—Identified as part of the diagnosis if the fear is of animals or insects.
- *Natural environment type*—Includes objects or situations that occur within the natural environment, such as heights, storms, or water.
- *Blood-injection-injury type*—A fear of seeing blood or an injury or of receiving an injection or other invasive medical or dental procedure.
- *Situational type*—The fear involves a specific situation, such as public transportation, tunnels, bridges, elevators, flying, or enclosed places.
- *Other type*—Covers all excessive or irrational fears. It may include phobic avoidance of situations that may lead to choking, vomiting, or contracting an illness; in children, it can be the avoidance of loud sounds or costumed characters.

The diagnosis of phobic disorder is made only when the phobic behavior significantly interferes with the individual's personal, social, and occupational functioning.

Assessment

The nurse should be aware that the phobic person may be no more or less anxious than anyone else until he or she is exposed to the phobic object or situation. This exposure will produce overwhelming symptoms that the nurse must respond to, including panic, palpitations, diaphoresis, dizziness, and hyperventilation. When assessing the patient who suffers from phobias, the nurse must ask the patient about his or her specific symptomology.

Predisposing Factors to Phobias

Psychoanalytical Theory

Freud believed that phobias develop when a child experiences normal incestual feelings toward the opposite-sex parent (Oedipal/Electra complex) and fears aggression from the same-sex parent (castration anxiety). To protect themselves, these children repress this fear of hostility from the same-sex parent and displace it onto something more neutral, which becomes the phobic stimulus.

Contemporary psychoanalysts believe in the same concept of phobic development but believe that castration anxiety is not the only source of phobias; other unconscious fears may also be expressed in a symbolic manner of phobias.

Learning Theory

Some learning theorists believe that fears are conditioned responses and are therefore learned by imposing rewards for appropriate behaviors. When it comes to phobias, the person avoids the phobic object and escapes fear, which in itself is a powerful reward.

Cognitive Theory

Cognitive theorists believe that some individuals engage in negative and irrational thinking that leads to anxiety reactions. This individual will begin to seek out avoidance behaviors to prevent the anxiety reactions, and phobias result.

Biological Aspects

Children experience fears as part of normal development. Most infants are afraid of loud noises; toddlers and preschoolers share a common fear of strangers, darkness, or being separated from their parents. Social rejection and sexual anxieties are common adolescent fears.

Life Experiences

Certain early experiences may eventually lead to phobias later in life. Examples include the following:

- A child who falls down a flight of stairs may develop a phobia of heights.
- A young person who survives a plane crash in childhood may develop a fear of flying.

Criteria for Agoraphobia

(cautionary statement)

Note: Agoraphobia is not a codable disorder. Code the specific disorder in which the agoraphobia occurs (i.e., Panic Disorder with Agoraphobia or Agoraphobia without History of Panic Disorder).

A. Anxiety about being in places or situations from which escape might be difficult (or embarrassing) or in which help may not be available in the event of having an unexpected or situationally predisposed panic attack or panic-like symptoms. Agoraphobic fears typically involve characteristic clusters of situations that include being outside the home alone, being in a crowd or standing in a line, being on a bridge; and traveling in a bus, train, or automobile. *Note*: Consider the diagnosis of Specific Phobia if the avoidance is limited to one or only a few specific situations, or Social Phobia if the avoidance is limited to social situations.

B. The situations are avoided (i.e., travel is restricted) or else are endured with marked distress or with anxiety about having a panic attack or panic-like symptoms, or require the presence of a companion.

C. The anxiety or phobic avoidance is not better accounted for by another mental disorder, such as Social Phobia (i.e., avoidance limited to social situations because of fear of embarrassment), Specific Phobia (i.e., avoidance limited to a single situation like elevators), Obsessive-Compulsive Disorder (i.e., avoidance of dirt in someone with an obsession about contamination), Post-traumatic Stress Disorder (i.e., avoidance of stimuli associated with a severe stressor), or Separation Anxiety Disorder (i.e., avoidance of leaving home or relatives).

Diagnosis

An analysis of the assessment data with background knowledge regarding predisposing factors to the disorder will assist in determining the priority of problems and help formulate the plan of care. Common nursing diagnosis for the patient with phobias includes the following NANDA nursing diagnoses:

- Fear
- Social isolation

Planning/Implementation

Appropriate nursing interventions are to be selected to address specific problems identified for the patient experiencing phobias. These priority interventions include

- Reassure the patient that he or she is safe.
- Discuss patient's perception of the threat.
- Discuss the reality of the situation.
- Include patient in decision making related to the selection of alternative coping skills.
- Encourage patient to explore underlying feelings that may contribute to irrational fears, and the possibility of facing them.
- Attend group activities with patient if it is too frightening or overwhelming for them.
- Be cautious about touching. Give patient enough space to exit if feeling overwhelmingly anxious.
- Give positive feedback for voluntary interactions with others.

Evaluation

In evaluating the outcomes of the nursing interventions in the care of the patient with phobias, the following questions should be asked:

- Can the patient discuss the phobic situation or object without becoming anxious?
- Is the patient able to function in the presence of the phobic situation or object without experiencing panic anxiety and demonstrate techniques he or she can use to prevent the anxiety from escalating?
- Is the patient able to identify the signs and symptoms of escalating anxiety?
- Does the client voluntarily leave his hospital room or home to attend group activities?

Obsessive-Compulsive Disorder

The *DSM-IV-TR* describes obsessive compulsive disorder (OCD) as recurrent obsessions or compulsions that are severe enough to be time-consuming (take more than 1 hour per day), or to cause marked distress or significant impairment.

Obsessions: Unwanted, intrusive, and persistent thoughts, impulses, or images that are experienced, at some time during the disturbance, as intrusive and inappropriate and that cause great anxiety or distress. Examples of obsessions include the following:

- Concerns about contracting an illness
- Fear of germs or dirt
- Fear of being burglarized or robbed

Compulsions: Unwanted repetitive behaviors (i.e. hand washing, checking) or mental acts (i.e., praying, counting) that the person feels driven to perform in response to an obsession. These behaviors are aimed at preventing or reducing distress. Examples of common compulsions include the following:

- Excessive hand washing
- Hoarding objects
- Repetitive checking of windows and doors

TABLE 7-3 Yale-Brown Obsessive Compulsive Scale (Y-BOCS)

Patient's name _____	
Date _____	

Item None Mild Moderate Severe Extreme

1. Hours/day spent on obsessions 0 0 to 1 >1 to 3 >3 to 8 >8	Score 0 1 2 3 4
2. Interference from obsessions None Mild Definite but manageable Impaired Incapacitating	Score 0 1 2 3 4
3. Distress from obsessions None Mild Moderate but manageable Severe Near constant, Disabling	Score 0 1 2 3 4
4. Resistance to obsessions Always resists Much resistance Some resistance Often yields Completely yields	Score 0 1 2 3 4
5. Control over obsessions Complete control Much control Moderate control Little control No control	Score 0 1 2 3 4

Obsession Subscale (0–20)

6. Hours/day spent on compulsions 0 0 to 1 >1 to 3 >3 to 8 >8	Score 0 1 2 3 4
7. Interference from compulsions None Mild Definite but manageable Impaired Incapacitating	Score 0 1 2 3 4
8. Distress from compulsions None Mild Moderate but manageable Severe Near constant, Disabling	Score 0 1 2 3 4
9. Resistance to compulsions Always resists Much resistance Some resistance Often yields Completely yields	Score 0 1 2 3 4
10. Control over compulsions Complete control Much control Moderate control Little control No control	Score 0 1 2 3 4

Comments: Compulsion Subscale (0–20)

Total Score (0–40)

Date:

Total previous score:

Range of severity: 0–7 Subclinical 8–15 Mild 16–23 Moderate 24–31 Severe 32–40 Extreme

Ratings include observations during interviews as well as average occurrence for each item during the last 7 days.

Source: Adapted from Wayne K. Goodman, L. H. Price, S. A. Rasmussen, et al.: "The Yale-Brown Obsessive Compulsive Scale." *Arch Gen Psychiatry*, vol. 48, November 1989.

Assessment

The nurse should have a clear understanding of the difference between obsessions and compulsions as well as common behaviors associated with each. Table 7-3 presents the Yale-Brown Obsessive-Compulsive Scale. The nurse can use this tool along with detailed discussion to guide the assessment of the client with OCD.

History

Gather history of the patient's obsessions and compulsions, and the extent to which it is interfering with his or her daily life. Treatment is usually done in an outpatient setting, but patients may be hospitalized when they have become completely unable to carry out their daily routines.

General Appearance and Behavior

The nurse will assess the patient's appearance and behavior. Expected behaviors include anxiety, tenseness, and a worried look. Patient's overall appearance is often unremarkable.

Mood and Affect

The patient may report an overwhelming feeling of anxiety in response to his or her obsessive thoughts, urges, or images.

Judgment and Insight

The patient recognizes that his or her obsessions are irrational, but he or she is unable to stop them. The patient will continue to engage in ritualistic behavior when the anxiety becomes overwhelming.

Self-Care Considerations

Like other anxiety disorders, the OCD patient often has difficulty sleeping. Performing rituals may take time away from sleep, or the anxiety may interfere with a good night's sleep and the feeling of waking refreshed. Loss of appetite and weight may also be evident. In severe cases, poor personal hygiene is observed due to the patient's inability to complete tasks.

Predisposing Factors to Obsessive-Compulsive Disorder

Psychoanalytical Theory

Psychoanalytical theorists suggest that individuals with OCD have weak, underdeveloped egos for reasons such as poor parent-child relationship or conditional love. This concept views patients with OCD as having regressed to earlier developmental stages of the infantile superego (harsh, punitive characteristics) that have now reappeared as part of their psychopathology.

Learning Theory

Learning theorists explain that OCD behavior as a conditioned response to a traumatic event. This event produces anxiety and discomfort, and the individual learns to prevent this anxiety and discomfort by avoiding this situation with which they are associated. This is called passive avoidance. When passive avoidance is not possible, this individual learns to enlist in behaviors that relieve the anxiety and discomfort associated with the traumatic situation. This is called active avoidance and describes the behaviors associated with OCD.

Diagnosis

An analysis of the assessment data with background knowledge regarding predisposing factors to the disorder will assist in determining the priority of problems and help formulate the plan of care. Common nursing diagnosis for the patient with OCD includes the following NANDA nursing diagnoses:

- Anxiety
- Ineffective coping
- Ineffective role performance

Planning/Implementation:

Appropriate nursing interventions are to be selected to address specific problems identified for the patient experiencing OCD. These priority interventions include the following:

- Offer support, encouragement, and compassion.
- Explore with patient the types of situations that increase anxiety and result in ritualistic behaviors.
- Encourage the patient to talk about feelings, obsessions, and rituals in detail.
- Encourage independence and give positive feedback for independent behaviors.
- Encourage techniques to manage and tolerate anxiety responses.
- Emphasize the importance of medication compliance as an important part of treatment.

Evaluation

In evaluating the outcomes of the nursing interventions in the care of the patient with OCD, the following questions should be asked:

- Is the patient able to refrain from rituals when anxiety increases?
- Does the patient recognize the relationship between increasing anxiety and their dependence on ritualistic behaviors for relief?
- Can the patient verbalize a plan of action for dealing with stressful situations in the future?
- Can the patient perform activities of daily living independently?
- Is the patient compliant with his or her prescribed medications and does he or she understand that this is an important part of the treatment?

7.6 Post-Traumatic Stress Disorder

Diagnostic Criteria for Post-Traumatic Stress Disorder

(cautionary statement)

A. The person has been exposed to a traumatic event in which both of the following were present:

(1) The person experienced, witnessed, or was confronted with an event or events that involved actual or threatened death or serious injury, or a threat to the physical integrity of self or others.

(2) The person's response involved intense fear, helplessness, or horror. *Note:* In children, this may be expressed instead by disorganized or agitated behavior.

B. The traumatic event is persistently reexperienced in one (or more) of the following ways:

(1) Recurrent and intrusive distressing recollections of the event, including images, thoughts, or perceptions. *Note:* In young children, repetitive play may occur in which themes or aspects of the trauma are expressed.

(2) Recurrent distressing dreams of the event. *Note:* In children, there may be frightening dreams without recognizable content.

(3) Acting or feeling as if the traumatic event were recurring (includes a sense of reliving the experience, illusions, hallucinations, and dissociative flashback episodes, including those that occur on awakening or when intoxicated). *Note:* In young children, trauma-specific reenactment may occur.

(4) Intense psychological distress at exposure to internal or external cues that symbolize or resemble an aspect of the traumatic event.

(5) Physiological reactivity on exposure to internal or external cues that symbolize or resemble an aspect of the traumatic event.

C. Persistent avoidance of stimuli associated with the trauma and numbing of general responsiveness (not present before the trauma), as indicated by three (or more) of the following:

(1) Efforts to avoid thoughts, feelings, or conversations associated with the trauma

(2) Efforts to avoid activities, places, or people that arouse recollections of the trauma

(3) Inability to recall an important aspect of the trauma

(4) Markedly diminished interest or participation in significant activities

(5) Feeling of detachment or estrangement from others

(6) Restricted range of affect (i.e., unable to have loving feelings)

(7) Sense of a foreshortened future (i.e., does not expect to have a career, marriage, children, or a normal life span)

D. Persistent symptoms of increased arousal (not present before the trauma), as indicated by two (or more) of the following:

(1) Difficulty falling or staying asleep

(2) Irritability or outbursts of anger

(3) Difficulty concentrating

(4) Hypervigilance

(5) Exaggerated startle response

E. Duration of the disturbance (symptoms in Criteria B, C, and D) is more than one month.

F. The disturbance causes clinically significant distress or impairment in social, occupational, or other important areas of functioning.

Traumatic events that are experienced directly include, but are not limited to, military combat, violent personal assault (sexual assault, robbery), being kidnapped, being taken hostage, terrorist attack, torture, incarceration as a prisoner of war or in a concentration camp, severe auto accidents, natural or manmade disasters, or being diagnosed with a life-threatening illness. For children, sexually traumatic events may include developmentally inappropriate sexual experiences without threatened or actual violence or injury. Witnessed events include, but are not limited to, observing the serious injury or unnatural death of another person due to violent assault, accident, war, or disaster, or unexpectedly witnessing a dead body or body parts.

Assessment

During the assessment process, the nurse should show support and compassion for the individual with PTSD. Reassure the patient that he or she is in a safe environment. An awareness of characteristic symptoms which include a reexperiencing of the traumatic event, a sustained high level of anxiety or arousal, or generalized numbing of responsiveness are to be expected. Symptoms of depression are common as well as "survival guilt" when others perished during the traumatic event, but the patient survived.

History

The health history will reveal that there is a history of trauma or abuse. It is not necessary or encouraged to prompt the patient to detail specific events of the trauma or abuse. This is usually done during individual psychotherapy sessions.

Thought Process and Content

These patients often report reliving the trauma through flashbacks or nightmares. Patients also report intrusive, persistent thoughts that often interfere with their ability to focus and concentrate and to perform their daily tasks.

Intellectual Processes

The patient is usually oriented to reality except when experiencing a flashback or dissociative episode. During this time, the patient may not respond to the nurse or may not be able to communicate at all. The nurse may note that those patients who have been abused or traumatized may have memory gaps in which there are periods for which they have no clear memories.

Physiologic Considerations

Most of these patients report difficulty sleeping due to nightmares or anxiety over the anticipation of nightmares. Overeating or lack of appetite is also common. Quite often, these patients use alcohol or other drugs to sleep or block out intrusive thoughts or memories.

Diagnosis

An analysis of the assessment data with background knowledge regarding predisposing factors to the disorder will assist in determining the priority of problems and help formulate the plan of care. Common nursing diagnosis for the patient with PTSD includes the following NANDA nursing diagnoses:

- Ineffective coping
- Risk for self-mutilation
- Post-trauma response
- Chronic low self-esteem
- Powerlessness
- Disturbed sleep pattern
- Sexual dysfunction
- Spiritual distress
- Social isolation

Planning/Implementation

- Stay with patient during periods of flashbacks or nightmares.
- Obtain an accurate history from significant others about the trauma and the patient's specific response.
- Encourage patient to talk about trauma at his or her own pace.
- Discuss coping strategies in response to the trauma.
- Assist the patient to try to comprehend the trauma if possible.
- Acknowledge feelings of guilt or self-blame that the patient may express.
- Assess for self-destructive ideation or behavior.
- Identify community resources from which the patient can seek out assistance and support.

Evaluation

In evaluating the outcomes of the nursing interventions in the care of the patient with PTSD, the following questions should be asked:

- Is the patient able to discuss the traumatic event without experiencing panic anxiety?
- Does the client experience flashbacks?
- Can the client sleep without medication?
- Has the patient learned new coping strategies for assistance with recovery and is he or she able to utilize them in times of stress?
- Has the patient maintained or reestablished relationships with significant others?
- Is the patient able to look to the future with optimism?
- Is the patient involved with any support groups of victims of similar traumatic experiences?

7.7 Substance-Induced Anxiety Disorder

The *DSM-IV-TR* describes the essential features of this disorder as prominent anxiety symptoms that are judged to be due to the direct physiological effects of a substance (i.e., drug of abuse, a medication, or toxin exposure). The symptoms may occur during substance intoxication or withdrawal, and may involve prominent anxiety, panic attacks, phobias, or obsessions or compulsions.

Diagnosis of this disorder is made only if the anxiety symptoms are in excess of those usually associated with the intoxication or withdrawal syndrome and warrant independent clinical attention.

Nursing care of the patient with substance-induced anxiety disorder is directly related to the substance and the context in which the symptoms occurred: intoxication or withdrawal. Nursing interventions utilized for anxiety symptoms were discussed earlier in this chapter.

Treatment Modalities

Individual Psychotherapy

When patients are given an opportunity to express and discuss their personal difficulties with a sympathetic therapist, there is a marked decrease in anxiety. The psychotherapist can use logical explanations to assist the patient in understanding the circumstances that create anxiety in their personal lives.

Behavior Therapy

Systematic desensitization and implosion therapy (flooding) are two common forms of behavior therapy used to treat patients with phobic disorders and to reform stereotyped behavior of patients with PTSD.

Systematic desensitization is a type of Pavlovian therapy developed by South African psychiatrist Joseph Wolpe. The patient is taught relaxation skills in order to extinguish fear and anxiety responses to specific phobias. Once taught these skills, the patient must use them to react toward and overcome situations in an established hierarchy of fears.

Implosion therapy involves the patient imagining situations or participation in real-life situations that he or she finds extremely frightening for a prolonged period of time. The therapist "floods" the patient with a vivid description of an anxiety, provoking the situation to arouse anxiety. The therapy continues until the topic no longer produces inappropriate anxiety.

Group Therapy

This type of therapy is strongly recommended for patients with PTSD. It has especially proven effective with Vietnam veterans. The group is able to share their experiences with fellow veterans, talk about their problems in a social setting, and have an opportunity to discuss options to manage their aggression toward others.

Psychopharmacology

Antidepressants, anxiolytics, and antihypertensives are the medications of choice to treat antianxiety disorders. They are discussed in detail in Chapter 3. Figure 7-3 lists the antianxiety medication, classification, and the type of anxiety disorder the medication is used to treat.

DRUG NAME GENERIC (TRADE)	CLASSIFICATION	ANXIETY DISORDER IT TREATS
Aprazolam (Xanax)	Benzodiazepine	Anxiety, panic disorder, OCD, social phobia, agoraphobia
Buspirone (Buspar)	Nonbenzodiazepine anxiolytic	Anxiety, OCD, social phobia, GAD
Chlorazepate (Tranxene)	Benzodiazepine	Anxiety
Chlordiazepoxide (Librium)	Benzodiazepine	Anxiety
Clomipramine (Anafranil)	Tricyclic antidepressant	OCD
Clonazepam (Klonopin)	Benzodiazepine	Anxiety, panic disorder, OCD
Clonidine (Catapres)	Beta-blocker	Anxiety, panic disorder
Diazepam	Benzodiazepine	Anxiety, panic disorder
Fluoxetine (Prozac)	SSRI antidepressant	Panic disorder, OCD, GAD
Hydroxyzine (Vistaril, Atarax)	Antihistamine	
Imipramine (Tofranil)	Tricyclic antidepressant	Anxiety
Paroxetine (Paxil)	SSRI antidepressant	Anxiety, panic disorder, agoraphobia Social phobia, GAD
Propanolol (Inderal)	Alpha-adrenergic agonist	Anxiety, panic disorder, GAD
Sertraline (Zoloft)	SSRI antidepressant	Panic disorder, OCD, social phobia, GAD

OCD: obsessive compulsive disorder, GAD: generalized anxiety disorder, SSRI: selective serotonin reuptake inhibitor

Figure 7-3 Drugs used to treat anxiety disorders.

Chapter 7 Questions

Matching

1. Anxiety
2. Moderate anxiety
3. Neurosis
4. Fear
5. Panic
6. Mild anxiety
7. Agoraphobia
8. Obsessions
9. Regression
10. Neurosis
11. Repression
12. PTSD
13. Severe anxiety
14. Compulsions
15. Psychosis

A. A reaction to a specific danger.

B. The person focuses on a specific detail and ignores everything else. Cognitive skills decrease and behavior is automatic.

C. Illogical, intense, persistent fear of a specific object or social situation that causes extreme distress and interferes with normal functioning.

D. Unwanted repetitive behaviors or mental acts that the person feels driven to perform in response to an obsession.

E. Cluster of symptoms including hallucinations, delusions, and disorganized thinking and behavior.

F. Excluding emotionally painful or anxiety-provoking thoughts and feelings from conscious awareness.

G. Feelings of dread or apprehension.

H. Moving back to a previous developmental stage to have needs met or feel safe.

I. Involves disorganization of personality and disturbed behavior. May lose touch with reality.

J. Focus is only on immediate concerns, with narrowing perceptual field.

K. A disturbing pattern of behavior demonstrated by someone who has experienced a traumatic event.

L. A feeling that something is different and the person is more alert with an increase in his or her perceptual field.

M. Disturbances characterized by excessive anxiety that is expressed directly or altered through defense mechanisms.

N. Intense, excessive anxiety or fear about being in places or situations from which escape may prove difficult or embarrassing.

O. Anxiety that involves no distortion of reality.

P. Unwanted, intrusive, and persistent thoughts, impulses, or images that are experienced and cause great anxiety or distress.

Fill in the Blank

17. The three major biological systems believed to contribute to the development of anxiety responses are the
_____, _____, and _____.

18. The two main classifications of medications to treat anxiety disorders are the
_____ and _____.

19. This type of anxiety disorder is characterized by obsessions (thoughts, images, impulses) that cause marked anxiety and/or compulsions that attempt to offset anxiety. This disorder is called

_____.

20. This type of phobia involves the individual becoming severely anxious to the point of panic when attending social engagements alone, interacting with the opposite sex, eating in public, or being the center of attention. These are examples of _____ phobia.

Multiple Choice

21. When assessing a patient with anxiety, the nurse's questions should be
    A. Open-ended
    B. Specific and direct
    C. After breakfast
    D. After the anxiety has diminished

22. During an assessment, a patient tells the nurse that before going to bed at night, she checks the locks to her front door 20 times. The nurse recognizes that this type of behavior is indicative of:
    A. Generalized anxiety disorder
    B. Panic disorder
    C. Obsessive-compulsive disorder
    D. Post-traumatic stress disorder

23. Which of the following interventions would be best for a patient experiencing a panic attack?
    A. Stay with the patient
    B. Place the patient in physical restraints
    C. Attempt to teach the patient relaxation techniques
    D. Offer a diversional activity such as playing cards

24. A patient is prescribed lorazepam (Ativan) to treat his anxiety. It is most important that the nurse assess the patient's:
    A. Family support
    B. Alcohol or illegal drug use
    C. Motivation for treatment
    D. Sleep habits

25. One possible reason for panic disorder may be
    A. Poor bonding
    B. Dopamine deficiency
    C. Lorazepam (Ativan) excess
    D. Inhibition of GABA

Chapter 7 Answers

Matching

1. G		9. H	
2. J		10. M	
3. O		11. F	
4. A		12. K	
5. I		13. B	
6. L		14. D	
7. N		15. E	
8. P		16. C	

Fill in the Blank

17. GABA system, norepinephrine system, serotonin system

18. benzodiazepines and antidepressants

19. obsessive compulsive disorder (OCD)

20. social

Multiple Choice

21. **B.** This type of questioning helps the patient to focus and can also assist in decreasing his or her anxiety.

22. **C.** Obsessive compulsive disorder includes repetitive behaviors.

23. **A.** The patient's safety is the priority. A very anxious patient should not be left alone, which could cause his or her anxiety to escalate.

24. **B.** Drinking alcoholic beverages (a CNS depressant) or using illegal drugs when taking a benzodiazepine will potentiate the depressant effects.

25. **D.** Gamma-aminobutyric acid (GABA) is the amino acid neurotransmitter believed to be dysfunctional in anxiety disorders.

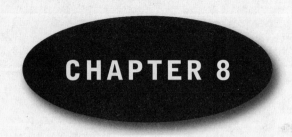

CHAPTER 8

Somatoform and Dissociative Disorders

8.1 Somatoform Disorders

It was in the 1800s that medical professionals first began considering the influence of psychosocial determinants on illnesses. *Psychosomatic* is a term used to relate the connection between the psyche and body. *Somatization* is the transference of emotional experiences and states into physical symptoms. It is the process in which anxiety is transformed into physical symptoms, illness, or complaints. Somatoform disorders are characterized by these physical symptoms, which suggest a medical disorder but do not show a demonstrable organic pathology or a known pathophysiological explanation. In somatoform disorders, individuals do not voluntarily control the symptoms or deficits; the presentations are not willful.

There are five specific somatoform disorders that are described by the American Psychiatric Association:

1. *Somatization disorder*— Characterized by the presence of multiple physical symptoms. Begins by the age of 30 and lasts for several years. This disorder includes a combination of pain, gastrointestinal, sexual, and pseudoneurological symptomology. See Box 8-1.

Box 8-1: Diagnostic Criteria for Somatization Disorder

A. A history of many physical complaints beginning before age 30 that occur over a period of several years and result in treatment being sought or significant impairment in social, occupational, or other important areas of functioning.

B. Each of the following criteria must have been met, with individual symptoms occurring at any time during the course of the disturbance:

 1. *Four pain symptoms*: A history of pain related to at least four different sites or functions (e.g., head, abdomen, back, joints, extremities, chest, rectum, during menstruation, during sexual intercourse, or during urination).

 2. *Two gastrointestinal symptoms*: A history of at least two gastrointestinal symptoms other than pain (e.g., nausea, bloating, vomiting other than during pregnancy, diarrhea, or intolerance of several different foods).

 3. *One sexual symptom*: A history of at least one sexual or reproductive symptom other than pain (e.g., sexual indifference, erectile or ejaculatory dysfunction, irregular menses, excessive menstrual bleeding, vomiting throughout pregnancy).

---

4. *Other pseudoneurological symptoms*: A history of at last one symptom of deficit suggesting a neurological condition not limited to pain (e.g., conversion symptoms such as impaired coordination or balance, paralysis or located weakness, difficulty swallowing or lump in the throat, aphonia, urinary retention, hallucinations, loss of touch or pain sensation.

C. Either 1 or 2:

1. After appropriate investigation, each of the symptoms in Criterion B cannot be fully explained by a known general medical condition or the direct effects of a substance (e.g., a drug of abuse or a medication).

2. When there is a related general medical condition, the physical complaints or resulting social or occupational impairment are in excess of what would be expected from the history, physical examination, or laboratory findings.

D. The symptoms are not intentionally produced or feigned (as in factitious disorder or malingering).

American Psychiatric Association (2000), with permission.

2. *Conversion disorder*—Also referred to as conversion reaction, this disorder involves unexplained and sudden deficits in sensory or motor functioning (e.g., blindness, paralysis). There is a suggestion of a neurological disorder, but it is related to psychological influences. A key feature is the exhibition of an attitude of *la belle indifference* (lack of concern or distress). See Box 8-2.

Box 8-2: Diagnostic Criteria for Conversion Disorder

A. One or more symptoms or deficits affecting voluntary motor or sensory function that suggests a neurological or other general medical condition.

B. Psychological factors are judged to be associated with the symptom or deficit because the initiation or exacerbations of the symptom or deficit is preceded by conflicts or other stressors.

C. The symptom or deficit is not intentionally produced or feigned (as in factitious disorder or malingering).

D. The symptom or deficit cannot, after appropriate investigation, be fully explained by a general medical condition, by the direct effects of a substance, or as a culturally sanctioned behavior or experience.

E. The symptom or deficit causes clinically significant distress or impairment in social, occupational, or other important area of functioning or warrants medical evaluation.

F. The symptom or deficit is not limited to pain or sexual dysfunction, does not occur exclusively during the course of somatization disorder, and is not better accounted for by another mental disorder.

Specify type of symptom or deficit:

With motor symptom or deficit

With sensory symptom or deficit

With seizures or convulsions

With mixed presentation

American Psychiatric Association (2000), with permission.

---

3. *Pain disorder*—Has a primary complaint of physical pain which is not relieved by analgesics and is significantly influenced by psychological factors regarding onset, severity, exacerbation, and maintenance. See Box 8-3.

Box 8-3: Diagnostic Criteria for Pain Disorder

A. Pain in one or more anatomical sites is the predominate focus of the clinical presentation and is of sufficient severity to warrant clinic attention.

B. The pain causes clinically significant distress or impairment in social, occupations, or other important areas of functioning.

C. Psychological factors are judged to have an important role in the onset, severity, exacerbation, or maintenance of the pain.

D. The symptom or deficit is not intentionally produced or feigned (as in factitious disorder or malingering).

E. The pain is not better accounted for by a mood, anxiety, or psychotic disorder and does not meet criteria for dyspareunia.

May be coded as:

Pain Disorder Associated with Psychological Factors:

Psychological factors are judged to have the major role in the onset, severity, exacerbation, or maintenance of the pain.

> **Acute**: Duration of less than 6 months
> **Chronic**: Duration of 6 months or longer

Pain Disorder Associated with Both Psychological Factors and a General Medical Condition:

Both psychological factors and a general medical condition are judged to have important roles in the onset, severity, exacerbation, or maintenance of the pain.

> **Acute**: Duration of less than 6 months
> **Chronic**: Duration of 6 months or longer

Pain Disorder Associated with a General Medical Condition:

A general medical condition has a major role in the onset, severity, exacerbation, or maintenance of the pain.

American Psychiatric Association (2000), with permission.

---

4. *Hypochondriasis*—Characterized by the fear of having a serious disease (disease conviction) or the likelihood of suffering from a serious disease (disease phobia). Individuals experiencing this disorder are considered to be misinterpreting physical sensations or functions. See Box 8-4.

Box 8-4: Diagnostic Criteria for Hypochondriasis

A. Preoccupation with fears of having, or the idea that one has, a serious disease, based on the person's misinterpretation of bodily symptoms.

B. The preoccupation persists despite appropriate medical evaluation and reassurance.

C. The belief in Criterion A is not of delusional intensity (as in delusional disorder, somatic type) and is not restricted to a circumscribed concern about appearance (as in body dysmorphic disorder).

D. The preoccupation causes clinically significant distress or impairment in social, occupational, or other important areas of functioning.

E. The duration of the disturbance is at least 6 months.

F. The preoccupation is not better accounted for by generalized anxiety disorder, obsessive-compulsive disorder, panic disorder, a major depressive episode, separation anxiety, or another somatoform disorder.

American Psychiatric Association (2000), with permission.

---

5. *Body dysmorphic disorder*—Characterized by a preoccupation with an imagined or exaggerated defect in physical appearance. See Box 8-5.

Box 8-5: Diagnostic Criteria for Body Dysmorphic Disorder

A. Preoccupation with an imagined defect in appearance. If a slight physical anomaly is present, the person's concern is markedly excessive.

B. The preoccupation causes clinically significant distress or impairment in social, occupational, or other important areas of functioning.

C. The preoccupation is not better accounted for by another mental disorder (e.g., dissatisfaction with body shape and size in anorexia nervosa).

American Psychiatric Association (2000), with permission.

Two other disorders, *malingering* and *factitious disorders* are distinguished from somatoform disorders in that individuals intentionally produce or feign symptoms for ulterior motives. Malingering is the intentional production of false or grossly exaggerated physical or emotional symptoms. There is a motive for the presence of these symptoms or deficits such as avoiding work or school, evading criminal repercussions, securing financial retribution, or securing drugs. As there are no real symptoms, or simply a gross exaggeration of minor symptoms or deficits, the individual is able to cease complaints upon achievement of his or her goal.

A factitious disorder evidences itself when an individual willfully produces or fabricates physical or emotional symptoms or deficits exclusively for attention. These individuals may even inflict an injury to themselves to receive this attention.

A. *Munchausen's syndrome*—A common term used to describe factitious disorder, this is when an individual produces or feigns symptoms or causes harm to self in an attention-seeking manner

B. *Munchausen's by proxy*—When an individual inflicts illness or injury on someone else in an attempt to seek attention from medical professionals or to have him- or herself identified as hero when he or she then acts in a way to save the victim.

Prevalence

Somatization disorder occurs in 0.2 percent to 2 percent of the general population. Conversion disorder occurs in less than 1 percent of the population. Pain complaints are frequent in medical practices, and more likely to occur in women to men, at a ratio of 2:1. Though it presents at any age, the most typical ages are the 40s and 50s. Most individuals associated with pain disorder are those classified as "blue collar workers." Pain disorder is commonly seen in medical practice, with 10 percent to 15 percent of people in the United States reporting work disabilities related to back pain. Hypochondriasis is reported to occur in 1 percent to 5 percent of the general population, equally common between men and women. Common age of onset for this disorder is early adulthood. The occurrence of body dysmorphic disorder is rare, and occurs more often in practices of dermatology and plastic surgery. The age is typically late teens to 20s and unmarried.

Pathophysiology

Many theorists believe that individuals who experience somatoform disorders internalize stress, anxiety, or frustrations. Subsequently, these feelings are expressed through physical symptoms. The individual experiencing somatoform disorders is not producing or feigning the symptoms or deficits. This internalization is an ego defense mechanism. Biological theory suggests that individuals experiencing these disorders misinterpret usual and normal physical sensations, unintentionally exaggerating the sensations and attributing the experience to a disease-process or illness. There may be a genetic predisposition for the development of somatization disorder, as demonstrated by a familiar tendency for occurrence (studies of twins, frequency within families).

8.2 Application of the Nursing Process for Somatoform Disorders

Assessment

- It is essential that the physical health status of the individual be investigated to establish that there is no underlying illness or disease-process requiring medical interventions. Awareness of the individual's culture and ethnic background allows discerning the presence of a culture-bound syndrome. It is also important that patients that have been diagnosed with somatoform disorders not be prejudged if they do offer somatic (physical) complaints. Evaluation of the physical symptoms should be performed in a respectful, thorough, and objective manner.

- A complete health assessment, including laboratory studies, is necessary to rule out physical illness. Assessment of the nature, location, onset, characteristics, and duration of the symptoms/deficits and the patient's ability to meet basic needs is basic. Determination of volition in regards to symptoms/deficits is required.

- Nursing history data is collected from the individual, family, significant others, prior treatment documentation, and others involved in the care of the person. Onset of symptoms/deficits will be dependent upon the disorder. Typically the individual will provide a detailed history of past physical problems and numerous diagnostic tests and procedures. Ascertain a pattern of seeking care from different health-care providers. Assess the type and amount of medication (prescribed and over-the-counter). Attention to verbalized complaints regarding the quality of care received may offer some insight into the patient's perception (an exception is the individual experiencing conversion disorder).

- A mental status assessment (as discussed in Chapter 4) is conducted to ascertain general appearance and motor behavior, mood/affect, sensorium and intellectual processes, judgment and insight (insight is typically impaired—denies life stressors or minimizes response to stressors), self-concept, roles/relationships (employment status, family/significant other support system), and physiologic and self-care concerns. Determination should be made of the individual's primary gain (the illness allows for delay of responsibilities) and secondary gain (sick role allows for dependency needs to be met). This information is conveyed to the treatment team.

- Assessed symptoms include affective (lability, exaggerated emotions, minimal distress regarding crisis related to personal health, mood may be depressed or anxious, etc.), behavioral (psychomotor retardation, ambulating slowly and rigidly, poor hygiene and grooming, social isolation), cognitive (content of thinking is focused on exaggeration of physical concerns, responds to questions about emotional status with comments related to physical health or experiences, preoccupation with illness or disease process, etc.), and physiological (overall appearance is not greatly influenced, psychomotor retardation may be evidenced, facial expression indicating pain/discomfort, relief of symptoms evidenced with attention of health-care provider, often offer complaints of disturbed sleep patterns, decrease in mobility and activity tolerance, possible physiologic responses to pain medications (side effects or withdrawal symptoms, etc.).

- It is essential to assess the individual's culture with regard to influence on the type and frequency of physical complaints. Some cultures and religions disapprove of expressing emotions, which can result in the use of somatic behaviors to process life stressors and anxiety. It should also be noted that those individuals in a lower socioeconomic, educational, and/or occupational status use somatic complaints more regularly.

Diagnosis

An analysis of the data will assist in determining the priority problems and help formulate the plan of care. Common nursing diagnoses for the patient with major depressive disorder include the following:

- Ineffective individual coping related to severe level of anxiety/low self-esteem.
- Ineffective coping related to repressed anxiety and unmet dependency needs.
- Ineffective denial related to threat to self-concept.
- Impaired social interaction related to fear of physical symptoms/disability.
- Disturbed body image related to low self-esteem.
- Chronic pain related to severe level of anxiety.

Planning/Implementation

Appropriate nursing interventions are to be selected to address specific problems identified for the patient experiencing major depressive disorder. The establishment of a therapeutic relationship is core in all clinical nursing situations. It is important that the approach to care be in a nonjudgmental, caring, and supportive manner. Awareness of one's own feelings regarding the dependency issues experienced with the patient's experiencing somatoform disorders should be evaluated. Patients who cope with their anxieties through somatization can prove to be frustrating for health clinicians. Typically, patients have employed these maladaptive coping skills for years, and these responses are not readily changed. Progress is slow and painstaking; many times the patients experience a slip back into their maladaptive coping on the road to wellness. Though clinicians are accepting of the symptoms as presented by the patient and avoid debate regarding the significance of the symptoms/illness, nurses must ensure that a positive reward is not provided for negative behaviors.

An essential component of nursing interventions is patient education. Core approaches for each disorder discussed include: education of symptoms on a physiologic level, offering information related to the mind-body interaction with focus on the influence of anxiety/stress on an individual, and education to assist the patient in the development and utilization of adaptive coping skills. See Figure 8-1 for appropriate plan of care for the patient with somatoform disorders.

NURSING DIAGNOSIS	NURSING INTERVENTION
Ineffective coping	1. Monitor ongoing assessment of the patient—lab reports and other data to ensure no pathology of complaints 2. Recognize and accept that the patient's complaints are their reality 3. Identify primary and secondary gains for the individual 4. Initially meet the patient's dependency needs, but focus on minimizing gains for somatic complaints 5. Encourage appropriate expression of fears and concerns/anxieties. Set limits on rumination of physical complaints 6. Teach adaptive coping skills to manage anxiety (relaxation, distraction, assertiveness, etc.) 7. Assist the patient to identify and use appropriate methods for getting recognition from others
Chronic pain	1. Assess physical symptoms of pain, physical complaints, and daily activities 2. Monitor ongoing assessments and recognize/accept that the patient's pain is real to them 3. Administer pain medication as prescribed, provide comfort measures without reinforcing pain behavior 4. Provide 1:1 at times other than expressing of presence of pain 5. Encourage the patient to express feelings and increase recognition that anxiety promotes exacerbation of symptoms 6. Patient education of alternative methods to decrease anxiety (relaxation, distraction, etc.)
Social isolation	1. Establish therapeutic relationship with the patient through use of effective communication techniques and limit-setting for maladaptive behaviors 2. Discuss with the patient reasons for social isolation. Help the patient to identify own wants and needs 3. Assess the patient's willingness to alter behavior to facilitate increase in socialization 4. Assist the patient to increase understanding on how the focus on pain/illness discourages others from wanting to spend time with him/her 5. Provide positive feedback for appropriate responses and attempts to improve socialization with others
Fear	1. Ongoing assessment to ensure organic pathology is ruled out 2. Determine primary and secondary gains of illness/disease for patient 3. Assist the patient to identify episodes of increased anxiety/symptoms. Help to establish a pattern of increased physical complaints with increased anxiety 4. Initially allow the patient timed intervals for expressing physical complaints/concerns with a planned decrease in occurrence 5. Patient education to assist the patient in the development and utilization of effective coping skills to manage anxiety more effectively
Disturbed body image	1. Assess the patient's self-perception. Acknowledge and accept that the patient's view of self is their reality 2. Assist the patient to understand that their self-view is exaggerated in relation to significance of an actual physical anomaly 3. Encourage the patient to participate in activities that build esteem through attributes other than appearance 4. During 1:1 focus on strengths and abilities. Encourage patient to identify these attributes 5. Encourage expression of fears and anxieties 6. Patient education related to alternative adaptive coping skills

Figure 8-1 Nursing diagnosis and intervention.

Evaluation

The fifth phase of the nursing process is evaluation. In this stage, a reassessment is done to determine if the nursing interventions selected were effective in assisting the patient to meet the objectives of care. Some of the outcomes that should be revisited include the following:

- Is the individual able to cope with life stressors with alternative methods than somatic problems?
- Is the individual able to verbalize their anxieties and fears/concerns?
- Is the individual able to verbalize an understanding of the connection between anxiety and physical symptoms/deficits? Is he or she able to verbalize irrationality of fear and interpret bodily sensations accurately?
- Does the individual report relief from pain while demonstrating more adaptive coping techniques?
- Is the patient able to increase socialization through voluntary participation in activities?
- Is the patient able to identify individual strengths and positive attitudes?
- Is there a decrease in rumination about physical symptoms/deficits?

8.3   Dissociative Disorders

The *DSM-IV-TR* describes the essential feature of dissociative disorders as a disruption in the usually integrated functions of consciousness, memory, identity, or perception. Individuals with anxiety disorders experience distress with regard to their feelings and thoughts, but do not encounter any alterations in perception of bodily sensations. Those individuals experiencing somatoform disorders have distress with regard to physicality, but do not evidence alteration in thought processes. Individuals with dissociative disorder experience a disruption in consciousness, memory, identity, or environmental perception.

There are four types of dissociative disorders described: dissociative amnesia, dissociative fugue, dissociative identity disorder, and depersonalization disorder. These disorders are the result of experiences of severe anxiety that has been repressed and exacerbates via dissociative behaviors. The ego is protected from the painful anxiety through detachment from the exposure.

1. *Dissociative amnesia*—Inability to recall important personal information, typically of a traumatic or stressful nature. See Box 8-6.

Box 8-6: Diagnostic Criteria for Dissociative Amnesia

A. The predominant disturbance of one or more episodes of inability to recall important personal information, usually of a traumatic or stressful nature, that is too extensive to be explained by ordinary forgetfulness.

B. The disturbance does not occur exclusively during the course of dissociative identity disorder, dissociative fugue, post-traumatic stress disorder, acute stress disorder, or somatization disorder and is not due to the direct physiological effect of a substance (e.g., a drug of abuse, a medication) or a neurological or other general medical condition (e.g., amnestic disorder due to head trauma).

C. The symptoms cause clinically significant distress or impairment in social, occupational, or other important areas of functioning.

American Psychiatric Association (2000), with permission.

---

2. *Dissociative fugue*—The individual experiences episodes of suddenly leaving home or work, being unable to recall identity and perhaps even assuming a new identity. See Box 8-7.

Box 8-7: Diagnostic Criteria for Dissociative Fugue

A. The predominant disturbance is sudden, unexpected travel away from home or one's customary place of work, with inability to recall one's past.

B. Confusion about personal identity or assumption of a new identity (partial or complex).

C. The disturbance does not occur exclusively during the course of a dissociative identity disorder and is not due to the direct physiological effects of a substance (e.g., drug abuse, a medication) or a general medical condition (e.g., temporal lobe epilepsy).

D. The symptoms cause clinically significant distress or impairment in social, occupational, or other important areas of functioning.

American Psychiatric Association (2000), with permission.

---

3. *Dissociative identity disorder*—In the past, this disorder was referred to as multiple personality disorder (MPD). The individual manifests two or more distinct identities that repeatedly take control of his or her behavior. See Box 8-8.

Box 8-8: Diagnostic Criteria for Dissociative Identity Disorder

A. The presence of two or more distinct personality states (each with its own relatively enduring pattern of perceiving, relating to, and thinking about the environment and self).

B. At least two of these identities or personality states recurrently take control of the person's behavior.

C. Inability to recall important personal information that is too extensive to be explained by ordinary forgetfulness.

D. The disturbance is not due to the direct physiological effects of a substance (e.g., blackouts or chaotic behavior during alcohol intoxication) or a general medical condition (e.g., complex partial seizures).

Note: In children, the symptoms are not attributable to imaginary playmates or other fantasy play.

American Psychiatric Association (2000), with permission.

---

4. *Depersonalization disorder*—The individual experiences an incessant or recurrent feeling of being disaffiliated from their mental processes or body/reality testing is intact; there is no evidence of psychosis. See Box 8-9.

Box 8-9: Diagnostic Criteria for Depersonalization Disorder

A. Persistent or recurrent experiences of feeling detached from, and as if one is an observer of, one's mental processes or body (e.g., feeling like one is in a dream).

B. During the depersonalization experience, reality testing remains intact.

C. The depersonalization causes clinically significant distress or impairment in social, occupational, or other important areas of functioning.

D. The depersonalization experience does not occur exclusively during the course of another mental disorder, such as schizophrenia, panic disorder, acute stress disorder, or other dissociative disorder, and is not due to the direct physiological effects of a substance (e.g., drug abuse, a medication) or a general medical condition (e.g., temporal lobe epilepsy).

American Psychiatric Association (2000), with permission.

Prevalence

These disorders are rare in occurrence; however, when experienced, they present as a dramatic and severe disturbance in personality functioning. Dissociative disorders are more prevalent in individuals that experience childhood physical or sexual abuse. Dissociative amnesia occurs most frequently in younger women, and typically under conditions such as natural disasters or war. Dissociative fugue is also a rare condition, occurring during times of great psychological stress. Dissociative identity disorder occurs three to nine times more often in females than males, with onset generally in childhood, despite characteristics remaining hidden until later years.

Pathophysiology

There are no known causes of dissociative disorders. As discussed in Chapter 3, the limbic system is a complex set of structures that lies on both sides of the thalamus, just under the cerebrum. This system appears to be primarily responsible for our emotional life and has a lot to do with the formation of memories. Current research suggests that the limbic system is involved in the development of dissociative disorders. Early trauma affecting the development of the limbic system may lead to the occurrence of dissociation.

8.4   Application of the Nursing Process for Dissociative Disorders

Assessment

- The diagnosis of dissociative disorder requires that medical and neurological illness, substance abuse, and other psychiatric illnesses be eliminated. It is essential that the physical health status of the individual be investigated to establish that there is no underlying illness or disease-process requiring medical interventions.

- The focus of the assessment will be on identity, memory, and consciousness. Exploring the occurrence of childhood, recent, or current trauma and abuse (physical, sexual, or emotional). Detailed events need not be examined during the assessment, as this will be reviewed during psychotherapy sessions.

- Nursing history data is collected from the individual, family, significant others, prior treatment documentation, and others involved in the care of the person. In assessing the patient's ability to identify self, attention is focused on terms the individual uses to describe him- or herself (referencing in the third person, calling self by another name, using the pronoun "we" instead of "I").

- A mental status assessment (as discussed in Chapter 4) is conducted, ensuring assessment to ascertain general appearance and motor behavior (often evidences hypervigilence, attention to personal boundary/spacing, can exhibit increased psychomotor agitation), mood/affect (lability is likely related to dissociation, potential flashbacks, etc.), sensorium and intellectual processes (patient will be oriented if not experiencing dissociation or a flashback, may be reports of memory gaps, presence of intrusive thoughts), judgment and insight (typically insight is aligned with the duration of patient's disorder and treatment progress, problem-solving skills may be impaired), self-concept (typically evidence low self-esteem), roles/relationships (generally report relationship problems—socially, occupationally, and interpersonally), and physiologic and self-care concerns (many experience disturbed sleep patterns, comorbid substance abuse issues). This information is conveyed to the treatment team.

- Assessed symptoms include affective (lability, depression, anxiety), behavioral (hypervigilence, psychomotor agitation), cognitive (memory impairments, confusion, disconnection), and physiological (overall appearance is not greatly influenced, often offer complaints of disturbed sleep patterns, decrease in mobility and activity tolerance, possible physiologic responses to pain medications (side effects or withdrawal symptoms, etc.).

- Assessment of the presence of a culture-bound syndrome (combination of psychiatric and somatic symptoms that are evidenced only in one specific culture (geographical location). The concept of culture specific illnesses is controversial, however, it is included in the *DSM-IV-TR*.

  - *Pibloktoq (Arctic hysteria)*—Occurring exclusively in the Eskimo population living in the Arctic Circle, usually during the winter. Symptoms include intense hysteria, depression, insensitivity to extreme cold temperatures. May be related to Vitamin A toxicity.

- *Amok*—Malaysian culture term used to describe occurrence of individual, who has never demonstrated violence previously, who suddenly and without provocation attempts to kill or seriously injure someone.
  - *Dromomani (traveling fugue)*—French. An uncontrollable urge to wander—spontaneously depart from normal routine and travel long distances, taking up another identity and occupation.
  - *Kundalini syndrome*—Hindu. A complex pattern of sensory, motor, mental, and affective symptoms (spontaneous body movement, depersonalization, spontaneous trancelike states).
- Core symptoms
  - Amnesia or fugue related to traumatic event
  - Symptoms of depersonalization
  - Alterations in consciousness, memory, identity
  - Abuse of substances
  - Disorganization or dysfunction in usual patterns of behavior
  - Feelings of being out of control (memories, behaviors, awareness)
  - Inability to explain actions or behaviors when in altered state

Diagnosis

An analysis of the data will assist in determining the priority problems and help formulate the plan of care. Common nursing diagnoses for the patient with major depressive disorder includes the following:

- Risk for self-mutilation
- Ineffective coping
- Post-trauma response
- Powerlessness
- Disturbed personal identity
- Ineffective role performance
- Spiritual distress

Planning/Implementation

Appropriate nursing interventions are to be selected to address specific problems identified for the patient experiencing major depressive disorder. See Figure 8-2 for the appropriate plan of care for the patient with dissociative disorder.

- Maintaining the patient's safety is always a priority nursing intervention. The nurse must continually assess potential for self-harm or suicidal tendencies and take appropriate actions.
- Assisting the patient to use grounding techniques during episodes of dissociating or flashbacks will help the patient remain in the here and now. Validation of feelings while reinforcing the current safe environment are essential actions to help maintain reality and diminish the dissociative experience.
- Encouraging the use of journaling provides patients to document their feelings as they occur and reflect on precipitating stimulus. This initial step will allow access to problem-solving to identify triggers and more effective coping strategies.
- Promotion of self-esteem is essential in the care of a patient experiencing dissociative disorders. Assisting an increase in self-worth and encouraging identification of personal strengths allows for patients to use their inner fortitude to alter self-perception from victim to survivor.
- Facilitating the formation of social and community supports allows for the patient to have available connections to help when feelings of loneliness, depression, or increasing anxiety. Establishment of relationships in the community encourages decreasing dependency on health care providers.
- Patient education is a basic nursing intervention. Stress reduction education to provide appropriate alternatives for anxiety relief is essential.

NURSING DIAGNOSIS	NURSING INTERVENTIONS
Post-trauma syndrome	1. Provide care for any physical injuries present 2. Provide psychological support through establishment of a therapeutic relationship, attentive listening, nonjudgmental acceptance, offer reassurance of personal safety 3. Observe for changes in behavior and mood, assess for potential for self-harming behaviors 4. Allow individual to verbalize feelings as tolerated 5. Provide a safe and nonthreatening environment 6. Explore and enhance support systems/resources
Powerlessness	1. Assess the individual's locus of control related to health situation 2. Assess potential for self-injurious behaviors 3. Establish a therapeutic relationship using therapeutic communication techniques, active listening behaviors, and offering of self 4. Assist the individual to identify goals to achieve, participate in the planning of their care, and efforts to regain control through education of illness and treatment regimen 5. Encourage verbalization of feelings related to incident, identifying feelings of powerlessness and circumstances that precipitate these feelings
Spiritual distress	1. Establish a therapeutic relationship with the patient 2. Assess patient's spiritual, religious and cultural beliefs, and health care practices 3. Acknowledge the patient's spiritual concerns and encourage ventilation of feelings 4. Provide patient education related to stages of grieving process and expected symptoms to decrease anxiety, promote an understanding, and encourage feelings of normalcy 5. Monitor and promote supportive social contacts, encourage visits with spiritual/religious advisors 6. Assist the patient in identifying and creating own experiences and develop skills to deal with life situation
Disturbed personal identity	1. Assess the patient for history of abuse 2. Assess for any history of seizure disorders, conduct a structured clinical interview adhering to criteria for dissociative disorders 3. Avoid use of labeling (such as "multiple personality disorder") 4. Establish a therapeutic relationship, allow permission for patient to share experiences, focus on assisting the patient to decrease problem behaviors 5. Encourage verbalization of feelings related to self, identifying strengths 6. Integrate personal identity issues into decisions and choices to assist patient to develop problem-solving skills
Ineffective role performance	1. Assess patients perception of role, discuss factors that may increase difficulty in managing current responsibilities 2. Encourage verbalization of feelings related to changes in role performance. 3. Assess for influences of cultural, religious beliefs, and health care practices and expectations of role 4. Encourage involvement of family members/ significant others in discussions regarding feelings and perceptions of role changes for the patient 5. Reinforce the patient's strengths and internalized beliefs

Figure 8-2 Nursing care plan for dissociative disorders.

Evaluation

The fifth phase of the nursing process is evaluation. In this stage, a reassessment is done to determine if the nursing interventions selected were effective in assisting the patient to meet the objectives of care. Some of the outcomes that should be revisited include the following:

- Has the patient's safety been maintained?
- Has the patient's anxiety been decreased? Is he or she able to employ alternative stress reduction behaviors?
- Is the patient able to identify and express fears and anxieties with staff?
- Is the patient able to verbalize the presence of multiple personalities and reasons why these personalities exist?

- Is the patient able to demonstrate the ability to perceive stimuli correctly?
- Can the patient maintain a sense of reality during stressful situations?
- Can the patient verbalize a correlation between stressful situations and dissociative symptoms experienced?
- Is the patient able to identify community resources?

Chapter 8 Questions

Multiple Choice

1. The most appropriate goal of care for a client who has experienced a dissociative fugue is
   A. The patient will remember what occurred during the fugue state by discharge.
   B. The patient will development and utilize adaptive coping skills to manage life stressors by discharge.
   C. The patient will report no feelings of dissociation by discharge.
   D. The patient will verbalize two strengths by discharge.

Scenario: Eileen is a 26-year-old female, admitted to your unit with a diagnosis of dissociative identity disorder (DID). The psychiatrist reports that she has been involved in treatment since the age of 11 and has been a victim of childhood sexual abuse. During her outpatient treatment, nine personalities have been identified. During the physical assessment, you note that Eileen has several burn marks on her ankles and wrists. As you describe the expectation of her hospitalization, Eileen states, "I'm not going to any groups."

Questions 2 to 4 are based on the above scenario. Select the answer that is most appropriate.

2. Which of the following is the priority nursing diagnosis?
   A. Self-care deficit
   B. Impaired sensory perception
   C. Risk for self-mutilation
   D. Noncompliance

3. In establishing trust with Eileen, you must
   A. Relate to her as though she does not have multiple personalities.
   B. Establish a relationship with each of the individual personalities.
   C. Ignore behaviors of personalities other than "Eileen."
   D. Explain to Eileen that you will only work with her when she presents as the primary personality (Eileen).

4. The ultimate goal of treatment with Eileen is
   A. Integration of all the personalities into one.
   B. To have control over changing personalities to fit appropriate social forums.
   C. To identify which of the personalities Eileen wants to become.
   D. To recognize the existence of the various personalities.

5. Which of the following nursing strategies is the most appropriate for the patient experiencing dissociative amnesia?
   A. Use of abreaction—encouraging remembering the events in detail in order to reexperience abusive memories.
   B. Use of antidepressant and anxiolytics.
   C. Introduction of known stressors to initiate amnesic episode for further assessment.
   D. Expose the patient to stimuli that represents pleasant past memories.

6. You are assigned to care for John this evening. During your one-on-one, he tells you that he has had a depersonalization experience that has been frightening. Which is the best response to this admission?

   A. "Don't worry about that. You always come back as John."

   B. "Let's talk about the stressors you have."

   C. "It must be scary being here in the hospital."

   D. "That sounds like it was very frightening. Tell me more about your experiences."

7. A patient experiencing amnesia is brought into the emergency room by his family. You are performing an initial nursing assessment. Which of the following symptoms would you expect to find?

   A. Disheveled appearance.

   B. The patient has been experiencing a gradual loss of memory of the past six months.

   C. The family reports the patient has been under severe stress.

   D. Confabulation of history data.

8. A 48-year-old male presented to the emergency room with complaints of muscle aches, breathlessness, sleeping problems, and loss of appetite. After a comprehensive physical assessment, there is no pathology related to his current symptoms. While gathering data for your nursing history, you find out that he recently lost his job and is fearful of how he will support his family. Which of the following nursing diagnoses is the most appropriate?

   A. Powerlessness-related ineffective coping as evidenced by physical symptoms

   B. Post-trauma response related to loss of economic status as evidenced by reported loss of employment

   C. Parental role conflict related to inability to meet financial and physical needs of family as evidenced by loss of employment

   D. Ineffective individual coping related to ineffective role performance as evidenced by physical manifestations of anxiety

9. A young woman is found wandering the campus of a local community college. She is not able to identify herself, presents as confused and disoriented. During the nursing assessment, she is unable to recount the events of the evening. After medical clearance, she is evaluated by the psychiatrist in the emergency room. She is diagnosed with dissociative amnesia. The most appropriate nursing diagnosis for this patient is

   A. Disturbed personal identity

   B. Spiritual distress

   C. Risk for violence; self-directed

   D. Anxiety related to altered thought process

10. A 22-year-old female is admitted to your unit. During your initial assessment, she tells you that she is a dancer. This evening she suddenly experiences paralysis of her right leg; she is now not even able to ambulate independently. Encouraging her to verbalize her feelings about this current situation and her career as a dancer, you are surprised when she indicates that she is not concerned about the possible impact. This is known as:

    A. Primary gain

    B. Secondary gain

    C. *La belle indifference*

    D. Malingering

Scenario: Georgia frequently comes into the clinic where you work. She complains of various physical symptoms, yet none of the work-ups has evidenced any pathology. She has been diagnosed with somatization disorder.

Questions 11 to 13 are based on the above scenario. Select the answer that is most appropriate.

11. In assessing Georgia, you would expect to find

    A. Complaints of symptoms deficits involving multiple body systems

    B. Georgia confiding that she is terrified she has a terminal illness

    C. Loss or deficit in sensoruium functioning

    D. Uncovering that Georgia feels that she has a bodily deformation or defect

12. The defense mechanism associated with somatization disorder is

    A. Denial

    B. Repression

    C. Suppression

    D. Displacement

13. One day Georgia comes into the clinic and complains about a pain in her back that she never experienced before. She tells you that she is supposed to be seeing her psychiatrist in 30 minutes. The most appropriate response would be

    A. "Listen Georgia, I told you that I don't have time for all your complaints. You know it's all in your head."

    B. "Well, it's OK if you are late for you appointment. Tell me more about the pain."

    C. "I'll tell Dr. Jones about this pain, but you should go to your appointment. It is important to be on time."

    D. "I'll call the doctor. It seems that your pain medication is not working well. Maybe she would like to order another medication."

14. You notice that a young mother has been frequently bringing her two-year-old child into the emergency room. She has reported sleep problems, decreased appetite, spiking temperatures, incessant crying, and generalized discomfort. Each time the child has been treated and discharged home for follow-up with the pediatrician. Tonight the mother brings in the baby, who is unconscious. The emergency room doctor suspects that the mother has a factitious disorder. What is the common term for this specific presentation?

    A. Munchausen's syndrome

    B. Munchausen's by proxy

    C. Malingering

    D. Hypochondriasis

15. Psychosocial theorists believe that people with somatoform disorders keep stress, anxiety, or frustrations inside rather than expressing them outwardly. The term used to describe this is

    A. Primary gain

    B. Secondary gain

    C. Internalization

    D. Hysteria

16. Providing care for a patient diagnosed with somatoform disorder can be challenging. An important consideration for the nurse includes

    A. Self-awareness issues

    B. Understanding of pathophysiology

    C. Knowledge of pain medications and side effects

    D. Awareness that the patient chooses to experience the symptoms/deficits rather than deal with the anxiety

17. Paroxetine (Paxil) has been prescribed for your patient, who is diagnosed with a somatoform disorder. Patient education would include the following:

    A. Take the medication with a full glass of water.

    B. Possible side effect of nausea.

    C. Patient may experience increased flatulence or constipation.

    D. The patient may experience increased appetite.

18. The following statement is correct about individuals with hypochondriasis:

    A. They typically exaggerate or fabricate physical symptoms for attention.

    B. They misinterpret normal bodily sensations as symptoms of disease.

    C. They do not evidence increased stress related to their physical symptoms.

    D. All of the above.

19. A patient who was scheduled for a piano recital experienced severe numbness to the right hand and was unable to participate in the recital. Not having to play at the recital is best described as:

    A. Primary gain

    B. Internalization

    C. Emotion-centered coping

    D. Secondary gain

20. Your patient asks you during a one-on-one, "The doctor says I have a body dysmorphic disorder. What is that?" The best response you could offer is

    A. "That is an illness not explained by a medical condition."

    B. "What happens over time due to excessive worrying about a disease."

    C. "A disorder where there is a defect in the appearance of a body or part."

    D. "When someone has a preoccupation with an imagined or exaggerated defective body part."

Matching

21. Hysteria

22. Malingering

23. Psychosomatic

24. Repressed memories

25. Somatization

26. Pain disorder

A. A stimulus, as fear or pain, that disturbs or interferes with the normal physiological equilibrium of an organism.

B. A period during which a person suffers from loss of memory, often begins a new life, and, upon recovery, remembers nothing of the amnesic phase.

C. The organization of the constituent elements of the personality into a coordinated, harmonious whole.

D. A conversion symptom of false pregnancy.

E. A polysymptomatic disorder characterized by recurrent multiple somatic complaints unexplained by organic pathology, violent emotional outbursts, and disturbances in sensory and motor function.

F. A theoretical concept used to describe a significant memory, usually of a traumatic nature, that has become unavailable for recall; also called motivated forgetting in which a subject blocks out painful or traumatic times in one's life.

27.	Amnesia	G.	The expression of psychological stress through physical symptoms.
28.	Fugue	H.	A conscious process of intentionally producing symptoms for an obvious environmental goal.
29.	Pseudocyesis	I.	Diagnosis used once medical evaluation rules out organic cause for physical distress.
30.	Aphonia	J.	Release of emotional tension achieved through recalling a repressed traumatic experience.
31.	Abreaction	K.	Pertaining to a physical disorder that is caused by or notably influenced by emotional factors.
32.	Hypnosis	L.	Intervention used to remind the individual that they are in the present, and safe.
33.	Integration	M.	Used in psychoanalysis, the uncensored expression of ideas, impressions and thoughts passing through the mind.
34.	Dissociation	N.	The splitting off of a group of mental processes from the main body of consciousness, as in amnesia or certain forms of hysteria.
35.	Derealization	O.	An unconscious process that protects an individual from unacceptable or painful ideas or impulses.
36.	Free association	P.	Inability to speak.
37.	Conversion disorder	Q.	Loss of a large block of interrelated memories; complete or partial loss of memory.
38.	Grounding techniques	R.	A disorder in which physical symptoms occur without apparent physical cause and instead appear to result from psychological conflict or need.
39.	Defensive mechanisms	S.	An artificially induced altered state of consciousness, characterized by heightened suggestibility and receptivity to direction, used to access the unconscious.
40.	Stressor	T.	An alteration in perception leading to the feeling that the reality of the world has been changed or lost.

Chapter 8 Answers

Multiple Choice

1. **B.** An expected outcome of care is that the patient gains effective coping skills. This will help to reduce anxiety to a level where dissociation is unlikely to occur. Individuals do not recall events that occur during a fugue state, nor are they aware of depersonalization.

2. **C.** Self-mutilation is not an uncommon occurrence in patients diagnosed with DID. Noted during your nursing assessment in observance of the injuries to her wrist and ankles, this patient remains at risk for further self-injurious behaviors. Priority care is determined according to Maslow's hierarchy of needs— physical, safety, social, esteem, and self-actualization.

3. **B.** The nurse must develop a trusting relationship with the original personality and with each of the subpersonalities. Each of the personalities envision him- or herself as a separate entity and must be initially treated as such.

4. **A.** The goal of therapy for a patient diagnosed with DID is to gain optimal functioning and to integrate the existing personalities into one personality.

5. **D.** Many cases of dissociative amnesia resolve spontaneously when the patient is removed from the stressful stimulation. Patients exposed to painful information that the amnesia is protecting them from remembering may decompensate. Exposure to stimuli of pleasant experiences in the past may assist the patient in recovering less pleasant memories.

6. **D.** This response conveys empathy and encourages the patient to further describe his experiences. A and C dismiss the affective component of the verbalization and dismiss his feelings. B is an appropriate response by making a connection between stress and the event, but is not the most appropriate compared with D.

7. **C.** Amnesia is typically precipitated by stress resulting from conflict or trauma. It occurs spontaneously and is not volitional. Loss of memory related to dementia may evidence symptoms of confabulation, self-care deficits, and gradual loss of memory.

8. **C.** Parental role conflict is when a parent experiences role confusion and conflict in response to a crisis. This patient's crisis involves the recent loss of employment and subsequent financial problems.

9. **A.** The patient's symptoms are indicative of personal identity disturbance related to a traumatic event. Her symptoms include inability to recall identity, inability to integrate consciousness, memory, identity, or motor behavior.

10. **C.** In conversion disorder, the symptom usually occurs suddenly and often the patient expresses a lack of concern (*la belle indifference*). This behavior is often a clue that the problem is psychological rather than physical.

11. **A.** Somatization disorder is a syndrome of multiple somatic complaints that cannot be explained medically and are associated with psychosocial distress.

12. **B.** Repression is the unconscious hiding of uncomfortable thoughts. In the case of somatization disorder, repression of anxiety exacerbates through somatic complaints.

13. **C.** Informing the patient that this new symptom will be referred to her doctor will address the importance that the possibility of organic pathology must always be considered; however, it is equally important not to give positive reinforcement for negative behaviors.

14. **B.** Factitious disorder occurs when a person intentionally produces or feigns physical or psychological symptoms to solely gain attention (Munchausen's syndrome). Munchausen's by proxy is the term used when a person inflicts illness or injury on someone else to gain this attention.

15. **C.** Internalization is the term used to describe keeping stress and feelings inside and expressing them through somatization.

16. **A.** The nurse must be able to provide care for the patient with somatoform disorders without responding in anger or frustration. Typically, patient progress is slow and many times there are stalls in movement toward goals. The nurse must be able to accept the patient and his or her continuing complaints and criticisms without judgment. It is important to remember that the somatic complaints are not under the patient's control.

17. **B.** Paxil is an SSRI, and common side effects include nausea, vomiting, diarrhea, and loss of appetite.

18. **B.** Individuals with hypochondriasis misinterpret routine physical sensations as evidence of a serious illness. They are not reassured by normal diagnostic findings. Answer A would indicate somatization disorder, and C would indicate conversion disorder.

19. **A.** Primary gains are the direct external benefits that the symptom provides (relief from anxiety, conflict, or distress). Secondary gains are internal or personal benefits (attention due to presence of symptoms).

20. **D.** Body dysmorphic disorder is when an individual becomes excessively concerned over a perceived defect in physical appearance or body part.

Matching

21. E	**31.** J
22. H	**32.** S
23. K	**33.** C
24. F	**34.** N
25. G	**35.** T
26. I	**36.** M
27. Q	**37.** R
28. B	**38.** L
29. D	**39.** O
30. P	**40.** A

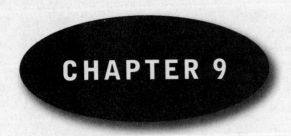

CHAPTER 9

The Schizophrenias

9.1 Schizophrenia

The term *schizophrenia* was introduced by the Swiss psychiatrist Eugen Bleuler in 1908. The word is a combination of two Greek words, *schizein,* "to split," and *phren*, "mind." Bleuler did not believe that there was a "split" personality, but a split between the cognitive and emotional aspects of the personality. Schizophrenia is a devastating brain disease that affects the person's emotions, thinking, language, social behavior, occupational functioning, and the ability to perceive reality accurately.

Of all the mental illnesses, schizophrenia accounts for more lengthy hospitalizations, causes more discord in family life, and is responsible for an exorbitant financial cost to individuals and their governments. Schizophrenia carries with it a stigma not only by society but also by the medical community. The following are types of schizophrenia. The diagnosis is made according to the patient's predominant symptoms.

Schizophrenia, paranoid type: Characterized by the presence of delusions of persecution or grandeur and auditory hallucinations related to a single theme. The person is usually guarded and suspicious, and may be hostile and aggressive. Onset of symptoms is usually in the late 20s or 30s. There is less regression of mental faculties, emotional responses, and behavior as compared to other types of schizophrenia. There is usually minimal social impairment, and a good prognosis when it comes to occupational functioning and independent living.

Schizophrenia, disorganized type: Once called hebephrenic schizophrenia, the onset of symptoms is usually before age 25, and its course is usually chronic. There is poor contact with reality, and behavior is more regressed and primitive. Speech is disorganized and may be accompanied by silliness and incongruous laughter. Bizarre mannerisms and facial grimaces are common, and personal appearance is poor and neglected. There is also extreme social impairment.

Schizophrenia, catatonic type: Characterized by marked abnormalities in motor behavior and may be manifested in the form of stupor or excitement.

Catatonic stupor: Characterized by extreme psychomotor retardation. The individual exhibits a pronounced decrease in spontaneous activity and movements. Mutism (absence of speech) is common, and negativism (a motiveless resistance to all directions or attempts to be moved) may also be evident. A waxy flexibility (posturing) may be exhibited.

Catatonic excitement: Manifested by a state of extreme psychomotor agitation. These movements are frenzied and purposeless, and often accompanied by continuous incoherent verbalizations and shouting. Patients in this state are often destructive and violent toward others, and require physical and medical control to protect them from injuring themselves as well as others. Their excitement can also cause them collapse from complete exhaustion.

Schizophrenia, undifferentiated type: This diagnosis is given when the individual with schizophrenic symptoms does not meet the criteria for any of the subtypes, or they may meet the criteria for more than one subtype. Their behavior is psychotic, but the symptoms cannot be easily classified into any of the subtype diagnostic categories.

Schizophrenia, residual type: This diagnosis is made when the individual has a history of at least one previous episode of schizophrenia with prominent psychotic symptoms. Residual schizophrenia occurs in the individual who has a chronic form of the disease, and is the stage that follows an acute episode (hallucinations, delusions, bizarre behavior). In this stage, there is continuing evidence of the illness, but no prominent psychotic symptoms. Residual symptoms may include poor personal hygiene, social isolation, inappropriate or blunted affect, illogical thinking, poverty of or elaborate speech, or apathy.

Signs/Symptoms

The symptoms of schizophrenia are divided into two major categories: positive and negative symptoms. Positive symptoms are often seen early in the onset of the illness and often precipitate hospitalization. These symptoms usually respond to antipsychotic medications. Negative symptoms develop over a long period of time, and most interfere with the client's ability to initiate and maintain relationships, conversations, make decisions, maintain a job, and attend to their own personal grooming and hygiene. Below are examples of both positive and negative symptoms.

Positive Signs/Symptoms

Delusions—False fixed beliefs that cannot be corrected by reasoning.

Hallucinations—False sensory perceptions or perceptual experiences that do not exist in reality.

Concrete thinking—An overemphasis on specific details and impairment in the ability to use abstract concepts.

Perseveration—Persistent adherence to a single idea or topic. May include verbal repetition of a word, phrase, or sentence.

Ambivalence—Refers to simultaneously holding two opposing emotions, attitudes, ideas, or wishes toward the same person, situation, or object.

Echopraxia—Imitating the movements and gestures of another person that the client is observing.

Flight of ideas—Continuous flow of verbalization in which the client rapidly jumps from one subject to another.

Ideas of reference—The client misinterprets the messages and external events of others, thinking they have special meaning to just them.

Associative looseness—Fragmented or poorly related thoughts and ideas. Thinking becomes haphazard, confused, and illogical.

Negative Signs/Symptoms

Anhedonia—Inability to feel joy or pleasure from life, relationships, or activities.

Apathy—Indifferent feelings towards people, events, and activities.

Avolition—Lack of motivation or ambition, inability to initiate tasks, or drive to take action.

Blunted affect—Restricted range of emotional feelings, mood, or tone.

Catatonia—Abnormal motor behavior exhibited by either extreme motor agitation or extreme psychomotor retardation.

Flat affect—Immobile or absence of facial expression or a blank look.

Poverty of speech—Restriction in the amount of speech in which answers can range from brief to monosyllabic answers.

Diagnostic Criteria for Schizophrenia

A. *Characteristic symptoms*—Two (or more) of the following, each present for a significant portion of time during a one-month period (or less if successfully treated):

    (1) Delusions

    (2) Hallucinations

(3) Disorganized speech (i.e., frequent derailment or incoherence)

(4) Grossly disorganized or catatonic behavior

(5) Negative symptoms (i.e., affective flattening, alogia, or avolition)

Note: Only one Criterion A symptom is required if delusions are bizarre or hallucinations consist of a voice keeping up a running commentary on the person's behavior or thoughts, or two or more voices conversing with each other.

B. *Social/occupational dysfunction*—For a significant portion of the time since the onset of the disturbance, one or more major areas of functioning such as work, interpersonal relations, or self-care are markedly below the level achieved prior to the onset (or when the onset is in childhood or adolescence, failure to achieve expected level of interpersonal, academic, or occupational achievement).

C. *Duration*—Continuous signs of the disturbance persist for at least six months. This six-month period must include at least one month of symptoms (or less if successfully treated) that meet Criterion A (i.e., active-phase symptoms) and may include periods of prodromal or residual symptoms. During these prodromal or residual periods, the signs of the disturbance may be manifested by only negative symptoms or two or more symptoms listed in Criterion A present in an attenuated form (i.e., odd beliefs, unusual perceptual experiences).

D. *Schizoaffective and mood disorder exclusion*—Schizoaffective Disorder and Mood Disorder with Psychotic Features have been ruled out because either (1) no major depressive, manic, or mixed episodes have occurred concurrently with the active-phase symptoms or (2) if mood episodes have occurred during active-phase symptoms, their total duration has been brief relative to the duration of the active and residual periods.

E. *Substance/general medical condition exclusion*—The disturbance is not due to the direct physiological effects of a substance (i.e., a drug of abuse, a medication) or a general medical condition.

F. *Relationship to a pervasive developmental disorder*—If there is a history of autistic disorder or another pervasive developmental disorder, the additional diagnosis of schizophrenia is made only if prominent delusions or hallucinations are also present for at least a month (or less if successfully treated).

9.2 Psychotic Disorders

Schizophrenia is a psychotic disorder. The term *psychotic* refers to delusions, any prominent hallucinations, disorganized speech, or disorganized catatonic behavior. Other psychotic disorders include the following:

Schizophreniform disorder. The essential features of this disorder are identical to those of schizophrenia, with the exception that the duration, including prodromal, active, and residual phases, is at least one month but less than six months. If the diagnosis is made while the individual is still symptomatic but has been so for less than six months, it is qualified as provisional. The diagnosis is changed to schizophrenia if the clinical picture persists beyond six months.

Schizophreniform disorder is thought to have a good prognosis if at least two of the following features are present:

1. Onset of prominent psychotic symptoms within four weeks of first noticeable change in usual behavior or functioning
2. Confusion or perplexity at the height of the psychotic episode
3. Good premorbid social and occupational functioning
4. Absence of blunted or flat affect

Brief psychotic disorder. The essential feature of this disorder is the sudden onset of psychotic symptoms that may or may not be preceded by a severe psychosocial stressor. The episode lasts at least one day but less than one month, and the individual returns to his or her premorbid level of functioning.

Schizoaffective disorder. This disorder is characterized by an uninterrupted period of illness during which time there is a strong element of symptomatology associated with the mood disorders (depressive, manic, or mixed episode) concurrent with symptoms that meet the criteria for schizophrenia. The symptoms must not be due to any substance use or abuse or to a general medical condition.

Delusional disorder. The essential feature of this disorder is the presence of one or more nonbizarre delusions that persist for at least one month. The subtype of delusional disorder is based on the predominant delusional theme.

- *Erotomanic type*—The individual believes that someone, usually of a higher status, is in love with him or her. Famous people are often the subject of erotomanic delusions.
- *Grandiose type*—Delusions of inflated worth, talent, knowledge, power, or a special relationship to a deity or famous person.
- *Jealous type*—Delusions that the individual's sexual partner is unfaithful.
- *Persecutory type*—Delusions that the person (or someone to whom the person is close) is being malevolently treated in some way. Frequent themes include being spied on, cheated, conspired against, followed, harassed, or prevented from pursuing long-term goals.
- *Somatic type*—Delusions that the person has some physical defect or general medical condition. Some common somatic delusions include the individual believing he or she has an infestation of insects in or on their skin or a foul odor emitting from his or her mouth, skin, rectum, or vagina. The individual may also believe he or she has dysfunctional body parts.
- *Mixed type*—Delusions characterized by more than one of the above types, but no one theme predominates.

Shared psychotic disorder. The essential feature of this disorder, also called *folie à deux*, is a delusional system that develops in the second person as a result of a close relationship with another person who already has a psychotic disorder with prominent delusions. The person with the primary delusional disorder is usually the dominant person in the relationship, and the delusional thinking is gradually imposed on the more passive partner. This occurs over a long-term relationship, particularly when the couple had been socially isolative.

Psychotic disorder due to a medical condition. The essential features of this disorder are prominent hallucinations and delusions that can be directly attributed to a general medical condition. The diagnosis is not made if the symptoms occur during the course of a delirium or chronic, progressing dementia. Figure 9-1 shows a number of medical conditions that can cause psychotic symptoms.

Substance-induced psychotic disorder. The essential features of this disorder are the presence of prominent hallucinations and delusions that are determined to be directly attributable to the physiological effects of a

Neurological conditions	Neoplasms Cerebrovascular disease Huntington's disease Epilepsy Auditory nerve injury Deafness Migraine headache CNS infections
Endocrine conditions	Hyperthyroidism Hypothyroidism Hyperparathyroidism Hypoparathyroidism Hypoadrenocorticism
Metabolic conditions	Hypoxia Hypercarbia Hypoglycemia
Autoimmune disorders	Systemic lupus erythematosus
Others	Fluid or electrolyte imbalance Hepatic or renal diseases

Figure 9-1 Medical conditions that can cause psychotic symptoms.

substance (i.e., a drug of abuse, a medication, or toxin exposure). The diagnosis is made in the absence of reality testing and when history, physical examination, and laboratory findings indicate use of substances. Substances identified by the *DSM-IV-TR* that are believed to induce psychotic disorders are listed in Figure 9-2.

Drugs of abuse	Alcohol
	Amphetamines and related substances
	Cannabis
	Cocaine
	Hallucinogens
	Inhalants
	Opioids
	Phencyclidine and related substances
	Sedatives, hypnotics, and anxiolytics
Medications	Anesthetics and analgesics
	Anticholinergic agents
	Anticonvulsants
	Antidepressant medication
	Antihistamines
	Antihypertensive agents
	Antimicrobial medications
	Antiparksonian agents
	Cardiovascular medications
	Chemotherapeutic agents
	Corticosteroids
	Disulfiram
	Gastrointestinal medications
	Muscle relaxants
	Nonsteroidal anti-inflammatory agents
Toxins	Anticholinesterase
	Carbon dioxide
	Carbon monoxide
	Nerve gases
	Organophosphate insecticides
	Volatile substances (e.g., fuel or paint)

Figure 9-2 Substances that may cause psychotic disorders.

Psychotic disorder not otherwise specified. This disorder is characterized by psychotic symptoms (i.e., delusions, hallucinations, disorganized speech, grossly disorganized or catatonic behavior) about which there is inadequate information to make a specific diagnosis or about which there is contradictory information, or disorders with psychotic symptoms that do not meet the criteria for any specific psychotic disorder.

9.3   Trends of Schizophrenia

Epidemiology

The lifetime prevalence of schizophrenia worldwide is 1 percent, with no differences in how it affects race, social status, environment, or culture. The most typical age of onset is late adolescence or early adulthood. Men and women are equally affected, although there are some differences. Those with an early onset (18 to 25 years) are more often male, have poorer premorbid adjustment, have more evidence of structural brain abnormalities, and have more prominent negative symptoms. Individuals with a later onset are likely to be females, have less structural brain abnormalities, and have better outcomes. Childhood schizophrenia does exist, although rare, and occurs in 1 out of 40,000 children compared to 1 out of 100 adults.

Comorbidity

Substance abuse disorders occur in approximately 40 percent to 50 percent of individuals with schizophrenia. Substance abuse is associated with multiple negative outcomes, including homelessness, incarceration, violence, suicide, and HIV. Substance abuse in schizophrenia occurs more with men and exhibits more pronounced psychotic symptoms, greater noncompliance with medication regimen, and a poorer prognosis. Nicotine dependence is also very common among schizophrenics and may be as high as 80 percent to 90 percent.

Etiology

The cause of schizophrenia still remains uncertain. There seems to be no single factor that can be implicated in the etiology. Results from many studies seem to suggest that the disease probably results from a combination of influences that include psychological, biological, and environmental factors.

Biologic Influences

Refer to Chapter 3 for a more thorough review of the biological implications of mental illness.

Genetics

How schizophrenia is inherited is still uncertain. No reliable biological marker has been found. Studies do show that relatives of individuals with schizophrenia have a much higher probability of developing the disease than does the general population. It is still unknown as to which genes are important in the vulnerability to schizophrenia, or whether one or multiple genes are involved.

Twin studies. The rate of schizophrenia among identical twins is 4 times that of fraternal twins and approximately 50 times that of the general population. Interestingly, identical twins raised apart have the same rate of developing the illness as do those who were raised together. Due to the fact that in about 50 percent of the cases only one of a pair of identical twins develops schizophrenia, some scientists believe that environmental factors interact with genetic factors.

Biochemical Influences

The oldest biological theory in explaining schizophrenia attributes a pathogenic role to abnormal brain biochemistry.

The Dopamine Hypothesis

This theory suggests that schizophrenia may be caused by an excess of dopamine-dependent neuronal activity in the brain. There is pharmacological support, as a result of studies have demonstrated the action of antipsychotic drugs (i.e., Thorazine or Haldol) blocking the activity of dopamine, thereby reducing some of the symptoms of schizophrenia. Amphetamines, cocaine, levodopa, and Ritalin are drugs that increase the activity of dopamine in the brain. These drugs can actually exacerbate the symptoms of schizophrenia in a psychotic individual.

Postmortem studies of schizophrenic brains have shown a significant increase in the average number of dopamine receptors in about two thirds of the brains that were studied. This suggests that an increased dopamine response may not be important in all schizophrenic clients. The current position of the dopamine hypothesis is that manifestations of acute schizophrenia may be related to increased numbers of dopamine receptors in the brain and respond to neuroleptic drugs that block these receptors. Manifestations of chronic schizophrenia are probably unrelated to numbers of dopamine receptor, and neuroleptic drugs are unlikely to be as effective in treating these chronic symptoms.

Alternative Biochemical Hypothesis

There have been other biochemical abnormalities implicated in the predisposition to schizophrenia including the neurotransmitters norepinephrine, serotonin, acetylcholine, and aminobutyric acid, as well as neuroregulators.

Anatomical Abnormalities

Brain imaging techniques such as computed tomography (CT), positron emission tomography (PET), and magnetic resonance imaging (MRI) have provided evidence that some people with schizophrenia have structural brain abnormalities, such as:

- Ventricular enlargement
- Cerebellar atrophy
- Sulci (fissures) enlargement on the surface of the brain
- Frontal lobe atrophy

Postmortem studies of people who have had schizophrenia also revealed a reduction in gray matter in the temporal and frontal lobes. Those individuals with the most tissue loss also had the most severe symptoms (hallucinations, delusions, depression).

9.4 Application of the Nursing Process

Assessment

In this first step of the nursing process, the nurse must not make assumptions about the patient's abilities or limitations based solely on the medical diagnosis of schizophrenia. Without an accurate assessment, problem identification, objectives of care, and outcome criteria, the patient's plan of care will be inaccurate.

- Patients in an acute episode of their illness can rarely make an accurate contribution to their history, so data will need to be obtained from family members if possible, old medical records, or other individuals who know the patient well and can report on the progression of the patient's behavior.
- Questions that should be asked regarding history include the following:
  - Have you ever been hospitalized in a psychiatric setting?
  - When and where was the patient's last hospitalization?
  - What was the age of onset?
  - What medications are you currently taking, and what have you taken in the past?
  - Have you ever harmed yourself or tried to harm yourself or others?
  - Do you currently have thoughts to harm yourself or others?
  - Are you hearing voices or sounds that others cannot hear now or in the past?
  - Have you ever participated in outpatient treatment or programs?
  - What makes you angry, frustrated, or scared?
  - Do you have anyone who provides emotional support?
- The nurse must be knowledgeable with behaviors common to schizophrenia to be able to obtain an adequate assessment. This includes behavioral disturbances in eight areas of functioning as presented in previous editions of the *Diagnostic and Statistical Manual of Mental Disorders*. They include the following:
  - Content of thought (i.e., delusions, religiosity, paranoia)
  - Form of thought (i.e., associative looseness, circumstantiality, mutism)
  - Perception (i.e., hallucinations, illusions)
  - Affect (i.e., inappropriate or flat, apathy)
  - Sense of self (i.e., echolalia, echopraxia, depersonalization)
  - Volition (i.e., emotional ambivalence)
  - Impaired interpersonal functioning and relationship to the external world (i.e., autism, poor personal grooming, and ADLs)
  - Psychomotor behavior (i.e., waxy flexibility, posturing, pacing, or rocking)
- The nurse should assess for positive and negative symptoms, as discussed earlier in this chapter.
- The patient's judgment or lack thereof will need to be assessed. Judgment is often impaired in patients with schizophrenia. Because judgment is directly based on one's ability to interpret the environment correctly, the individual with impaired thought processes and environmental misinterpretations will have great difficulty with judgment. This patient may not recognize the need to wear warm clothes in cold weather or to eat on a regular basis.
- Safety for both the nurse and patient is a priority when assessing and caring for a patient with schizophrenia. The patient may be paranoid or suspicious of the nurse and the environment. It is extremely important that the nurse be aware of the patient's body language, history (if possible), escalating agitation, verbalizations, and tone. The nurse must approach the patient in a nonthreatening manner, give the patient ample space, and know when to end the interview. The nurse should also conduct the interview in a safe area where there are other personnel nearby. The nurse must institute interventions that will keep the patient, nurse, and others safe. This may include the administration of medication, escorting the patient to a less stimulating environment, or, as a last resort, using restraints.
- Cultural differences are very important when assessing a patient with schizophrenia. Thoughts or beliefs such as witchcraft that may be considered delusional in one culture are commonly accepted in other cultures. Also seeing a saint or the Virgin Mary, or hearing God's voice, may be a normal part of one's religious experience but considered auditory/visual hallucinations in others.

Diagnosis

An analysis of the assessment data will assist in determining the priority of problems and help formulate the plan of care. Common nursing diagnosis for the patient with schizophrenia/psychotic disorders includes the following:

- Disturbed thought processes
- Disturbed sensory perception
- Social isolation
- Risk for violence
- Impaired verbal communication
- Self-care deficit
- Disabled family coping
- Ineffective health maintenance
- Interrupted family process

Planning Implementation

Appropriate nursing interventions are to be selected to address specific problems identified for the patient diagnosed with schizophrenia. See Figure 9-3 for appropriate plan of care for the patient diagnosed with schizophrenia.

NURSING DIAGNOSIS	NURSING INTERVENTIONS
Disturbed thought process	• Convey acceptance of patient need for false belief, but indicate that you do not share belief. • Do not argue or deny the belief • Reinforce focus on reality
Disturbed sensory perception	• Observe patient for signs of hallucinations (listening pose, laughing or talking to self) • Avoid touching patient without warning • Convey an attitude of acceptance to encourage patient to share content of hallucination with you. • Do not reinforce the hallucination. • Assist the patient in understanding the connection between anxiety and hallucinations. • Try to distract the patient from the hallucination.
Social isolation	• Convey an accepting attitude by making brief, frequent contacts. • Offer to be with patient during group activities that he/she may find difficult. • Give recognition and positive feedback for patient voluntarily interacting with others.
Risk for violence	• Maintain low level of stimuli in patient's environment. • Observe patient behavior frequently. • Remove all dangerous objects from patient's environment. • Redirect violent behavior with physical outlets for anxiety. • Staff should maintain a calm attitude toward patient. • Have sufficient staff available to indicate a show of strength to patient if it becomes necessary. • Administer medications as ordered by M.D. If patient is not calmed by medication or verbal intervention, mechanical restraints may be necessary
Impaired verbal communication	• Attempt to decode incomprehensible communicating patterns. Seek validation and clarification. • Facilitate trust and understanding by maintaining staff assignments as consistently as possible. • Orient patient to reality consistently.
Disabled family coping	• Identify level of family functioning. • Provide information for the family about patient illness, treatment required, and long-term prognosis. • Teach family members how to respond to bizarre behavior and communication patterns, in the event that the patient becomes violent.

Figure 9-3 Schizophrenia care plan.

Pharmacological Interventions for Schizophrenia and Other Psychotic Disorders

Drugs used to treat psychotic disorders are called *antipsychotic medications or neuroleptics.* Although this group of medications does not cure schizophrenia, they alleviate many of its psychotic symptoms.

There are two groups of antipsychotic medications. The older or conventional (traditional) antipsychotic agents are dopamine antagonist (see Chapter 3). These medications target the positive signs, such as hallucinations, delusions, and disorganized thinking. These conventional antipsychotics are becoming obsolete and less often prescribed due to their significant side effects, which can range from mild discomfort to permanent movement disorders. Because many of these side effects are so uncomfortable and frightening, many patients become noncompliant, which leads to relapse. These troubling side effects are called *extrapyramidal side effects (EPS).* They include the following:

- *Akathisia*—Characterized by restless movement, pacing, an inability to remain still, and a description of inner restlessness. Patients have described it as "feeling like jumping out of their skin."

- *Dystonia*—Characterized by spasms of the head and neck, or eye muscles (oculogyric crisis). These spasms may also be accompanied by protrusion of the tongue, dysphagia, and laryngeal/pharyngeal spasms, which can lead to a constricted airway, causing a medical emergency. These spasms can be both frightening and painful for the patient.

- *Pseudoparkinsonism*—Characterized by a shuffling gait, muscle stiffness, mask-like face, cogwheeling rigidity, drooling, and akinesia (slowness and difficulty initiating movement).

- *Tardive dyskinesia (TD)*—A late-appearing side effect of antipsychotic medications, characterized by abnormal, involuntary movements such as tongue protrusion, lip smacking, blinking, and grimacing, with involuntary tonic muscular spasms of the fingers, toes, neck, trunk, or pelvis. TD can be disfiguring and incapacitating. Early symptoms, which consist of the oral movements, often disappear with the discontinuation of the antipsychotic medication. There is no proven cure for the advanced symptoms. *The Abnormal Involuntary Movement Scale (AIMS)* was developed by the National Institute of Mental Health (NIMH) to screen patients for late-appearing movement disorders. As described in Chapter 5, the patient is observed in several positions, and the severity of symptoms is rated 0 to 4. The AIMS can be administered every three to six months. If the nurse observes an increase in the AIMS score, she or he should notify the physician immediately so the dosage or medication can be changed in order to prevent further advancement of tardive dyskinesia.

Most patients will develop a tolerance to EPS after months of therapy.

A group of medications called *antiparkinsonian agents,* which include benztropine (Cogentin), trihexyphenidyl (Artane), amantadine (Symmetrel), and diphenhydramine (Benadryl), an antihistamine, are cholinergic blockers that counteract the extrapyramidal symptoms and are often prescribed along with the antipsychotic medication.

Other common side effects include anticholinergic manifestations which can include blurred vision, dry mouth, constipation, and urinary retention. Sedation and weight gain as well as photosensitivity are also potential side effects of neuroleptic therapy.

- *Neuroleptic Malignant Syndrome (NMS)*—This is a rare but potentially fatal side effect of antipsychotic drugs. It is characterized by high fever, muscle rigidity, tachycardia, incontinence, stupor, increased muscle enzymes (particularly creatine phosphokinase), and leukocytosis. The patient's medications would be discontinued, and supportive symptomatic care would be given. Eventually, antipsychotic drugs can be carefully reintroduced.

- *Agranulocytosis*—This is a medical emergency that develops abruptly and is characterized by fever, ulcerative sore throat, and leucopenia. Medication should be immediately discontinued, and the patient may need reverse isolation and antibiotic therapy.

The second group of antipsychotics is called *atypical antipsychotics*. They are both dopamine and serotonin antagonists. They are considered the new generation and first emerged in 1990s with the medication clozapine (Clozaril). This medication produces agranulocytosis in a small number of patients and also increases the risk for seizures. Patients who are being treated with clozapine must have a baseline WBC as well as a differential before therapy can begin. A WBC must be done biweekly for the next six months and then monthly thereafter if blood counts have been acceptable. WBC should be monitored for four weeks after the discontinuation of clozapine. Another common side effect of clozapine that is often embarrassing for the patient is excessive drooling. The atypical antipsychotics, which also include risperidone, olanzapine, quetiapine, ziprasidone, and aripiprazole, also target the positive symptoms but diminish the negative symptoms (poor social interaction, blunted or inappropriate affect, lack of motivation). This group causes very few if any extrapyramidal symptoms

See Figures 9-4 and 9-5 for typical and atypical medications used to treat schizophrenia.

Adjuncts to Antipsychotic Drug Therapy

Antimanic Medications

Lithium has been beneficial in suppressing episodic violence in schizophrenia as well as addressing many of the more distressing symptoms when this medication is given along with an antipsychotic.

Benzodiazepines

The addition of these agents can improve positive and negative symptoms by approximately 50 percent.

GENERIC NAME (TRADE NAME)	ROUTE	DOSAGE (mg.)	SPECIAL CONSIDERATIONS/ SIDE EFFECTS
Chlopromazine (Thorazine)	PO, IM, L	75-400	Anticholonergic side effects, photosensitivity, orthostatic hypotension, decreased libido, weight gain, sedation, EPS, tardive dyskinesia, NMS
Fluphenazine (Prolixin)	PO, IM, L	2.5-10	Anticholonergic side effects, photosensitivity, orthostatic hypotension, decreased libido, weight gain, sedation, EPS, tardive dyskinesia, NMS
Haloperidol (Haldol)	PO, IM	1-100	Anticholonergic side effects, photosensitivity, orthostatic hypotension, decreased libido, weight gain, sedation, EPS, tardive dyskinesia, NMS
Loxapine (Loxitane)	PO, IM	20-250	Anticholonergic side effects, photosensitivity, orthostatic hypotension, decreased libido, weight gain, sedation, EPS, tardive dyskinesia, NMS
Molindone (Moban)	PO	15-225	Anticholonergic side effects, photosensitivity, orthostatic hypotension, decreased libido, weight gain, sedation, EPS, tardive dyskinesia, NMS
Perphenazine (Trilafon)	PO, IM, IV	8-48	Anticholonergic side effects, photosensitivity, orthostatic hypotension, decreased libido, weight gain, sedation, EPS, tardive dyskinesia, NMS
Thioridazine (Mellaril)	PO	150-800	Anticholonergic side effects, photosensitivity, orthostatic hypotension, decreased libido, weight gain, sedation, EPS, tardive dyskinesia, NMS
Trifluoperazine (Stelazine)	PO, IM	4-40	Anticholonergic side effects, photosensitivity, orthostatic hypotension, decreased libido, weight gain, sedation, EPS, tardive dyskinesia, NMS
Thiothixene (Navane)	PO, IM	6-30	Anticholonergic side effects, photosensitivity, orthostatic hypotension, decreased libido, weight gain, sedation, EPS, tardive dyskinesia, NMS
Haloperidol decanoate (Haldol)	IM	50-250	Given deep muscle Z-track Given every 2-4 weeks
Fluphenazine decanoate (Prolixin)	IM	6.25-50	Given deep muscle Z-track Given every 2-4 weeks

PO = oral; IM = intramuscular; L = liquid
EPS = extrapyramidal symptoms; NMS = neuroleptic malignant syndrome

Figure 9-4 Typical antipsychotic drugs.

GENERIC NAME (TRADE NAME)	ROUTE	DOSAGE (mg.)	SPECIAL CONSIDERATIONS/ SIDE EFFECTS
Aripiprazole (Abilify)	PO, L	10-30	Nausea, vomiting, headaches, constipation, insomnia, weight gain, blurred vision, increased salivation, hyperglycemia, EPS
Clozapine (Clozaril)	PO	1-6	Agranulocytosis, seizures, sedation, hypersalivation, tachycardia, weight gain, orthostatic hypotension, hyperglycemia, NMS
Olanzapine (Zyprexa)	PO, zyprexa injectable	5-20	Weight gain, headache, fever, dizziness, dry mouth, orthostatic hypotension, tachycardia, hyperglycemia, EPS
Quetiapine (Seroquel)	PO	150-750	Dizziness, headache, constipation, dry mouth, dyspepsia, weight gain, orthostatic hypotension, hyperglycemia, NMS, EPS, TD
Risperidone (Risperdal)	PO, risperdal consta injectable	1-6	Agitation, anxiety, sedation, insomnia, dizziness, headache, constipation, rhinitis, rash, hyperglycemia, tachycardia, EPS
Ziprasidone (Geodon)	PO, geodon injectable	40-160	Headache, nausea, dyspepsia, diarrhea, constipation, prolonged QT interval, orthostatic hypotension, rash, hyperglycemia, EPS

PO = oral; IM = intramuscular; L = liquid
EPS = extrapyramidal symptoms; NMS = neuroleptic malignant syndrome; TD = tardive dyskinesia

Figure 9-5 Atypical antipsychotic drugs.

Antidepressants
Depression, which is very common among schizophrenics, can improve with the administration of antidepressants in conjunction with antipsychotics.

Advanced Practice Interventions
Medication is the single most important factor in preventing relapse in a patient with the diagnosis of schizophrenia. When psychosocial interventions are coupled with medication therapy, the chances of relapse are further decreased.

Milieu Therapy
Many patients need the structure of inpatient hospitalization. Patients in the acute phase of schizophrenia improve more in a structured milieu than on an open unit that allows greater freedom. A therapeutic milieu provides safety, activities, opportunities for learning how to resolve conflicts, and opportunities for learning vocational and social skills.

Individual Therapy
Reality-oriented individual therapy is the most appropriate approach to psychotherapy for schizophrenia. The main focus of this type of therapy is to reduce anxiety and establish trust through truthfulness and a demonstration of respect toward the individual. Individual psychotherapy for schizophrenics is long term and takes patience and perseverance on the part of the therapist. It may take years before the individual is able to demonstrate some degree of independent functioning.

Group Therapy
Group therapy has been shown to be especially effective in the outpatient setting and most useful over the long-term course of the illness. The social interaction, cohesiveness, and reality testing achieved in the group have been proven to be highly therapeutic for these individuals.

Behavior Therapy

Behavior modification has been known to reduce bizarre, disturbing, and aggressive behaviors and increase more appropriate behaviors. This is done by

- Setting clearly defined goals
- Using simple concrete instructions to encourage appropriate behavior
- Attaching positive, negative, and apathetic reinforcements to adaptive and maladaptive behavior.

This type of therapy can be a very powerful tool in helping patients change their undesirable behaviors.

Social Skills Training

Considerable attention is given to the improvement of social skills. This is done by role play with immediate feedback from the therapist. Emphasis is placed on functional skills that are relevant to activities of daily living.

Family Therapy

Family therapy usually consists of pychoeducational programs that treat the family as a resource, focusing on problem solving and helping behaviors for coping with stress. Family therapy also teaches families to reshape patterns of communication and problem solving.

Evaluation

The fifth phase of the nursing process is evaluation. In this stage, a reassessment is done to determine if the nursing interventions selected were effective in assisting the patient to meet the objective of care. Following are some questions that should be considered:

- Have the patient's psychotic symptoms decreased or disappeared?
- Does the patient have a clear understanding of his or her medication regimen and understand the importance of compliance?
- Has the patient established trust with at least one staff member?
- Is the patient's anxiety level under control?
- Is the patient able to utilize appropriate coping mechanisms in response to stress and anxiety?
- Is the patient depressed or does he or she have any suicidal thoughts or plans?
- Is the patient able to interact with others in an appropriate manner?
- Does the patient voluntarily attend therapy activities?
- Is the patient self-isolating?
- Does the patient exhibit the necessary functional abilities for community living?
- Does the patient and his or her family have an adequate understanding of schizophrenia?
- Is the patient knowledgeable of resources from which he or she can seek assistance outside the hospital setting?
- Does the family have information regarding support groups that they can participate in, and from which they can seek assistance in dealing with their ill family member?

Schizophrenia is a lifelong illness, and therefore individuals with this disorder will need the help and support of their family as well as the community. The patient may be referred to a social worker or directly to case management services after discharge from inpatient hospitalization. Although the support of professionals in the community is important, the nurse must be aware of the patient's need for autonomy and potential abilities to manage his or her own health.

Chapter 9 Questions

Self-Learning Exercise

Scenario: Keisha is a 28-year-old married homemaker, and mother of two children, ages seven and four. Her husband Tyrone has noticed that his wife has become increasingly withdrawn and isolated, and no longer takes the children out to the park or on play dates. She has become more argumentative, and both he and the children have observed Keisha muttering to herself and sometimes cocking her head to the side and listening as if someone is talking to her. Today, Tyrone called the crisis team when his wife locked the door announcing no one could leave because there is "someone out there trying to harm them." Keisha arrives in the emergency department in an agitated state, exhibiting psychotic symptoms. The nurse notes that her affect is flat and she is guarded upon approach, and continuously scans the environment. Keisha is admitted to the psychiatric unit with a diagnosis of schizophreniform disorder.

Questions 1 to 8 are based on the above scenario. Select the answer that is most appropriate.

1. The initial nursing intervention for Keisha is to

    A. Provide a safe environment.

    B. Give an injection of risperdal consta Q 2 hours.

    C. Place in four-point restraints.

    D. Invite patient into an ongoing therapy group.

2. The psychiatrist orders haloperidol (Haldol) 5 mg. PO STAT and then 2 mg. PO BID and benztropine (Cogentin) 1 mg. PO BID. Why is haloperidol ordered?

    A. To promote rest.

    B. To prevent neuroleptic malignant syndrome.

    C. To decrease psychotic symptoms.

    D. To increase the patient's appetite.

3. Why is benztropine ordered?

    A. To promote rest.

    B. To increase the patient's appetite.

    C. To counteract the extrapyramidal symptoms.

    D. To decrease psychotic symptoms.

4. The primary goal of the clinical team working with Keisha is to

    A. Decrease her anxiety and begin to establish a trusting relationship.

    B. Improve her relationship with her husband and children.

    C. Encourage participation in therapy groups.

    D. Encourage interaction with her peers.

5. Keisha's belief that "someone" is trying to harm her and her family is an example of

    A. Delusion of reference

    B. Delusion of grandeur

    C. Somatic delusion

    D. Delusion of persecution

6. Keisha is observed by the nurse tilting her head to the side and listening intensely. The nurse recognizes that Keisha is probably experiencing

    A. A religious delusion

    B. Auditory hallucinations

    C. Extrapyramidal symptoms

    D. Catatonia

7. What would be the most appropriate intervention for the symptom just described in the previous question?

    A. Call the M.D.

    B. Give benztropine (Cogentin) 2 mg. IM STAT.

    C. Ask Keisha to describe what she is hearing.

    D. Ask if she is experiencing stiffness.

8. Keisha and her husband Tyrone will be attending a weekly family therapy group. What is the primary focus of this type of group?

    A. To increase family understanding of the illness and improve their interactions with one another.

    B. To introduce the couple to other families with similar challenges.

    C. To increase their social skills.

    D. To discuss ADLs.

9. A nursing intervention that is helpful when caring for a person diagnosed with schizophrenia is

    A. Limiting your contact with the patient to one to two brief interactions daily.

    B. Directly ask the patient about the hallucination or delusion he or she is experiencing.

    C. Ignore the patient's bizarre behavior.

    D. Assume understanding of what the patient means by "we" or "they."

10. In which of the following situations, is the nurse aware that the patient is experiencing auditory hallucinations?

    A. Ms. Smith yells out, " I'm not a bad person! Stop saying those horrible things about me!"

    B. Ms. Smith shares, "I see aliens every afternoon at 1 p.m. in the Day Room."

    C. Ms. Smith shouts to the nurse, "There are caterpillars and worms crawling on my skin!"

    D. Ms. Smith informs the nurse, "I'm not taking my medication. I know that it is poisoned!"

11. Which of the following are considered *positive signs* of schizophrenia?

    A. Delusions, hallucinations, ambivalence

    B. Blunted affect, apathy, catatonia

    C. Hallucinations, alogia, flat affect

    D. Delusions, hallucinations, disorganized thinking

12. The nurse is taking care of a patient who has been taking haloperidol (Haldol) for three days. The patient suddenly cries out, and the nurse observes the patient's eyes appearing to roll back in their sockets, as well as his neck being twisted uncomfortably to one side. Which of the following PRN medications ordered will the nurse administer?

    A. Haloperidol (Haldol) 5 mg. PO prn

    B. Chlorpromazine (Thorazine) 25 mg. PO prn

    C. Diphenhydramine (Benadryl) 25 mg. IM prn

    D. Benztropine (Cogentin) 2 mg. PO prn

13. During discharge teaching of a patient who is taking clozapine (Clozaril), it is essential that the nurse include which of the following information?

    A. Remind the patient of the importance of following through with blood work for his or her WBC.

    B. Inform the patient about the importance of fiber in his or her daily diet.

    C. Remind patient to take daily multivitamins.

    D. Caution the patient to wear protective clothing when out in the bright sunlight.

14. A patient with a known diagnosis of schizophrenia presents in the emergency department verbalizing a series of jumbled words and phrases that make no sense to the listener. The nurse realizes that this is an example of what unusual speech pattern?

    A. Echolalia

    B. Word salad

    C. Neologisms

    D. Clang associations

15. The overall objective of psychiatric rehabilitation is for the patient to achieve

    A. An improvement in social skills

    B. Control of anxiety

    C. Recovery from the illness with improved functioning

    D. Control of symptoms

Matching

16. Abnormal Involuntary Movement Scale (AIMS)

17. Akathisia

18. Ambivalence

19. Anhedonia

20. Apathy

21. Avolition

22. Blunted affect

23. Catatonia

24. Command hallucinations

25. Delusions

26. Dystonia

A. False beliefs with no basis in reality.

B. Simultaneously holding two attitudes, emotions, or ideas toward the same person.

C. The brief test developed by the NIMH to detect tardive dyskinesia.

D. Gives private meaning to the communication of others, or misinterprets the messages of others.

E. Serious and often fatal condition seen in patients who are treated with antipsychotics. Symptoms include muscle rigidity, high fever, increased muscle enzymes, and leukocytosis.

F. Late-appearing side effect of antipsychotic therapy, characterized by involuntary movements such as lip smacking, blinking, tongue protrusion, and grimacing.

G. Imitation of movements and gestures of another person.

H. Muscle cramps of the head and neck.

I. Lack of motivation or ambition.

J. Absence of any facial expression that would exhibit mood or emotions.

K. False sensory perceptions or perceptual experiences.

27. Echopraxia
28. Extrapyramidal side effects
29. Flat affect
30. Hallucination
31. Ideas of reference
32. Neuroleptic malignant syndrome
33. Perseverance
34. Pseudoparkinsonism
35. Tardive dyskinesia

L. Restless movement, inability to remain still.

M. Voices demanding that the person take action, often to harm themselves or others.

N. Reversible movement disorders caused by neuroleptic medication.

O. Neuroleptic induced Parkinson-like symptoms such as shuffling gait, masklike faces, and cogwheeling.

P. Persistently repeats the same word or idea in response to different questions.

Q. Inability to experience pleasure.

R. Abnormalities in motor behavior and may manifest in the form of stupor or excitement.

S. Demonstration of disinterest or indifference in the environment.

T. Restricted range of emotional feeling, tone, or mood.

Chapter 9 Answers

Multiple Choice

1. **A.** Providing a safe environment is the main priority on any inpatient psychiatric unit.
2. **C.** Antipsychotics are prescribed to decrease psychotic symptoms.
3. **C.** To counteract the extrapyramidal effects.
4. **A.** Primary goal of treatment team with a newly admitted patient is to begin establishing a trusting relationship.
5. **D.** The belief that others intend to harm or persecute them.
6. **B.** Auditory hallucinations.
7. **C.** Asking the patient what he or she is experiencing will help the nurse to determine interventions that will help the patient, as well as keep the patient safe.
8. **A.** The goal is to help patients and their families better understand the illness and how to deal with it on a daily basis.
9. **B.** It is key to know and understand what the patient is experiencing.
10. **A.** An example of an auditory hallucination.
11. **D.** Delusions, hallucinations, and disorganized thinking are all examples of positive symptoms of schizophrenia.
12. **C.** Diphenhydramine (Benadryl) is a antihistamine/antiparksonian that is fast acting when given IM to reduce extrapyramidal side effects.
13. **A.** It is essential that patients receiving clozapine (Clozaril) therapy have their WBC monitored.
14. **B.** Word salad.
15. **C.** Recovery from the illness and improved functioning is the primary goal of rehabilitation.

Matching

16. C
17. L
18. B
19. Q
20. S
21. I
22. T
23. R
24. M
25. A

26. H
27. G
28. N
29. J
30. K
31. D
32. E
33. P
34. O
35. F

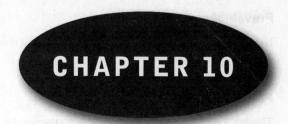

CHAPTER 10

Personality Disorders

10.1   Personality Disorders

An individual's personality is consistent characteristics evidenced through behaviors and connectiveness with self, others, and his or her environment. Regardless of varying situations, people typically respond in an unchanging way, maintaining basic traits and responses. The personality is influenced by many factors: biologic, genetic, and developmental (experience). Personality disorders, which include borderline personality disorder, antisocial personality disorder, and other similar illnesses, were first defined by the DSM as diagnosable illnesses in 1980. The diagnosis of a personality disorder occurs when these traits become immaleable, and maladaptive and interfere with daily functioning. The ineffective behavioral patterns are typically evident in childhood or adolescence, and many times diagnosis and treatment does not occur unless the individual experiences a crisis or comorbid illness. Characteristics that are present in all personality disorders include the following:

- Maladaptive responses to stress
- Impairments in occupational and interpersonal relationships
- Ability to create interpersonal conflict
- Ability to provoke others through enmeshing boundaries

The individual diagnosed with a personality disorder does not typically acknowledge that there is a problem with his or her behavior, frequently becoming distressed by the response to his or her behaviors by others.

This chapter discussed various theories related to the development of the personality discussed previously in this book. It is important for the nurse to understand the development of the personality prior to learning about maladaptive personality development, and that personality disorders are long-term issues that are not treatable by medications. The individual diagnosed with a personality disorder does not generally seek out psychiatric treatment, and is hospitalized only when a coexisting Axis I diagnosis is present. When pharmacological approaches are used in his or her treatment, the goal is targeted to symptoms of the subtype. The goals of individual and group therapy are as follows:

- Assist the individuals to build trusting relationships.
- Educate regarding basic activities of daily living.
- Provide support.
- Diminish anxiety.
- Enhance interpersonal relationships.

Prevalence

NIMH-funded researchers recently reported that roughly 9 percent of U.S. adults have a personality disorder as defined by the *DSM-IV*.

Pathophysiology

The etiology of personality disorders appears to be the combination of various environmental, biological, and psychological factors. Negative experiences in childhood, such as abuse (physical and sexual), genetic components (temperament), experiential learning, socialization experiences, and learning are a few components in the development of personality disorders. The cluster B disorders—that is, antisocial and borderline personality disorders—have garnered most of the attention in research. Psychoanalytical and developmental theories suggest that unsuccessful mastery of tasks in the early developmental levels in conjunction with negative childhood experiences result in personality disorders. Borderline personality disorder has been associated with failure to navigate the separation-individualization process which occurs during toddlerhood. From a sociocultural perspective, it is also believed that borderline personality disorder results from the experience of childhood sexual abuse.

10.2   Categories of Personality Disorders

- **Cluster A:** Individuals are described as odd, eccentric.

  A. *Paranoid personality disorder*—"A pervasive distrust and suspiciousness of others such that their motives are interpreted as malevolent, beginning by early adulthood and present in a variety of contexts" (APA, 2000).

  B. *Schizoid personality disorder*—"A pervasive pattern of detachment from social relationships and a restricted range of expression in interpersonal settings, beginning by early adulthood and present in a variety of contexts" (APA, 2000).

  C. *Schizotypal personality disorder*—"A pervasive pattern of social and interpersonal deficits marked by acute discomfort with, and reduced capacity for, close relationships as well as by cognitive or perceptual distortions and eccentricities of behavior, beginning in early adulthood and present in a variety of contexts" (APA, 2000).

- **Cluster B:** Individuals are described as dramatic, emotional, and erratic.

  A. *Antisocial personality disorder*—"A pervasive pattern of disregard for a violation of the rights of others occurring since the age 15" (APA, 2000).

  B. *Borderline personality disorder*—"A pervasive pattern of instability of interpersonal relationships, self-image, and affects, and marked impulsivity beginning in early adulthood and present in a variety of contexts" (APA, 2000).

  C. *Histrionic personality disorder*—"A pervasive pattern of excessive emotionality and attention-seeking, beginning in early adulthood and present in a variety of contexts" (APA, 2000).

  D. *Narcissistic personality disorder*—"A pervasive pattern of grandiosity (in fantasy and behavior), need for admiration, and lack of empathy, beginning in early adulthood and present in a variety of contexts" (APA, 2000).

- **Cluster C:** Individuals are described as anxious, fearful.

  A. *Avoidant personality disorder*—"A pervasive pattern of social inhibition, feelings of inadequacy, and hypersensitivity to negative evaluation, beginning in early adulthood and present in a variety of contexts" (APA, 2000).

  B. *Dependent personality disorder*—"A pervasive and excessive need to be taken care of that leads to submissive and clinging behavior and fear of separation, beginning by early adulthood and present in a variety of contexts" (APA, 2000).

  C. *Obsessive-compulsive personality disorder*—"A pervasive pattern of preoccupation and orderliness, perfectionism, and mental and interpersonal control at the expense of flexibility, openness, and efficiency, beginning by early adulthood and present in a variety of contexts" (APA, 2000).

- **Other Related Disorders:**
  A. *Depressive personality disorder*—"A pervasive pattern of depressive cognitions and behaviors present in a variety of contexts" (APA, 2000).
  B. *Passive-aggressive personality disorder*—"A negative attitude and pervasive pattern of passive resistance to demands for adequate social and occupational performance, present in a variety of contexts" (APA, 2000).

10.3　Application of the Nursing Process

Assessment

- There are several structured assessment tools that can be used in the diagnosis of personality disorders. The length of the clinical interview needed to adequately employ these is not always available. The most common standardized testing for evaluation of the personality is the Minnesota Multiphasic Personality Inventory (MMPI).
- Nursing history data is collected from the individual, family, significant others, prior treatment documentation, and others involved in the care of the person. Included in this is a full medical history. Attention to the occurrence of past or present physical, sexual or emotional abuse, history of suicidal or aggressive ideations or behaviors, current use of medications (prescription and OTC), and substance use/abuse.
- Note objective and subjective symptoms related to the specific diagnosis:
  ○ Appears suspicious, distrustful.
  ○ Uses defense mechanisms (especially projection).
  ○ Appears socially withdrawn, emotionally aloof, with odd mannerisms, or extroverted and superficial, flamboyant.
  ○ Responds with indifference to approval or criticism from others, or hypersensitivity.
  ○ Exhibits unstable mood, impulsivity, manipulation.
  ○ Exhibits poor self-concept, low self-esteem.
  ○ Exhibits dramatic behaviors, frequent outbursts of anger, increased frustration and intolerance, and attention-seeking behaviors.
  ○ Expresses rigid, moralistic, and judgmental opinions; acts in a controlling and demanding manner in relationships.
  ○ Idealizes organization, order, and perfection.
  ○ Demonstrates anger through passive-aggressive behaviors.
  ○ Has difficulty in interpersonal relationships, occupational issues, involvement with the legal system.
- A mental status assessment (as discussed in Chapter 4) is conducted, ensuring assessment to ascertain presence of suicidal ideations; if present, the nurse assesses further regarding the intent and plan. This information is conveyed to the treatment team.
- Use of self-care techniques is an important consideration for those administering care to the individual with a personality disorder. Self-awareness of responses toward the patient is essential to evaluate frequently due to the intense feelings that can be evoked in caring for this population. Open communication within the multidisciplinary treatment team, sufficient clinical supervision and support, and reinforcement of characteristics of the personality disorders among the team will help to minimize the negative influences (splitting, countertransference, manipulation, etc.).
- Cultural considerations: Judgments about personality functioning must involve a consideration of the individual's ethnic, cultural, and social background. Determination of the influence of one's background must be evaluated before exhibited behaviors are attributed to a personality disorder.

Diagnosis

An analysis of the data will assist in determining the priority problems and help formulate the plan of care. Common nursing diagnoses for the patient with personality disorder include the following:

Cluster A

- Social isolation
- Disturbed thought process
- Chronic low self-esteem
- Fear

Cluster B

- Ineffective coping
- Risk for violence; other directed
- Role performance, ineffective
- Self-mutilation, risk for
- Self-esteem, chronic low

Cluster C

- Anxiety
- Denial, ineffective individual
- Decisional conflict
- Social interaction, impaired

Planning/Implementation

Appropriate nursing interventions are to be selected to address specific problems identified for the patient experiencing personality disorder. It is important to have the individual and family involved in setting realistic goals of treatment.

See Figure 10-1 for an overview of the characteristics of the subtypes and appropriate nursing interventions.

- Structure is provided through the establishment of a therapeutic relationship. This professional interaction allows for the identification of acceptable and desired behaviors, provides opportunities for role modeling, and encourages a consistent approach to care. A therapeutic relationship assists the nurse in establishing clear and firm boundaries of the relationship.
- Limit-setting is an intervention frequently used in the nursing care of the patient diagnosed with a personality disorder. This intervention must be done with a matter-of-fact, nonjudgmental approach. This action is a three step process:
  1. Identification of the behavioral limit, or rule. It is essential that the specific unacceptable behavior or rule is identified.
  2. The expected, acceptable behavior or rule is identified.
  3. The consequence(s) of not adhering to the identified behavior or rule is outlined. This consequence must have meaning for the individual to be effective.
- Confrontation is a technique used to assist in managing manipulative or deceptive behavior. The nurse identifies a specific concerning behavior in a nonjudgmental and clinically neutral manner.
- Cognitive restructuring is an intervention helpful in altering an individual's pattern of thinking. It focuses the patient on recognition of negative thoughts and feelings and encourages restoring those with more positive thinking.
- Treatment modalities:
  - *Interpersonal psychotherapy*—IPT is a time-limited psychotherapy that focuses on the relations between the individual and others and on building interpersonal skills. IPT is based on the belief

	CLINICAL PRESENTATION	NURSING INTERVENTIONS
CLUSTER A		
Paranoid personality disorder	Hypervigilence, pervasive mistrust, suspiciousness, oversensitive, and misinterpret environmental cues. Maintain esteem through projection, do not accept personal responsibility or accountability. Appear aloof and withdrawn, conflicts with authority figures are common	Establish a trusting, therapeutic relationship, maintain a consistent professional demeanor due individuals, heightened sense of paranoia, facilitate the individuals sense of control through active involvement in planning of care, assist them to be able to validate concepts before taking action
Schizoid personality disorder	Constricted affect, emotionally cold and uninvolved, difficulty experiencing and expressing emotion, aloof and indifferent, inappropriately serious about most everything. Typically isolative in work situations, can appear shy, anxious, and uneasy in social situation	Nursing actions focus on increasing socialization skills to facilitate functioning in the community
Schizotypal personality disorder	Eccentric appearance, may demonstrate magical thinking or sensory distortions not clearly psychotic in origin	Focus of nursing interventions is development of self-care and social skills, and improving overall activities in daily functioning
CLUSTER B		
Antisocial personality disorder	Low tolerance for frustration, require immediate, gratification, impetuous, exploitative, ignore conventional authority and rules cold and callous—can be intimidating and belligerent. Poor; insight and judgment, present as confident and self-assured, but are quite shallow and emotionally empty, manipulative, difficulty maintaining long-term commitments	Establish a trusting and therapeutic relationship to help promote responsible behavior, use of limit-setting and confrontation assist the individual to learn effective problem-solving skills, management of emotions (anger and frustration) using concepts such as time-out. Assisting enhancement of role performance
Borderline personality disorder	Instability in affect, identity, and relationships. Desperate in seeking relationships, however, push others away due to clinging and distancing behaviors, splitting manipulation, self-destructive behaviors, and impulsivity. Pervasive mood is dysphoria, expressing feelings of boredom, restlessness, frustration, and "emptiness," repetitive and self-mutilative behaviors (cutting, scratching, burning)	Nursing interventions will most probably occur during times of crisis. Providing a safe and nonthreatening environment, safety from self-injurious behaviors, limit-setting techniques, establishing and maintaining boundaries
Histrionic personality disorder	Self-dramatizing, attention-seeking, overly gregarious, and seductive. All-consuming need for approval, failure to achieve this results in dejection and anxiety. Distractible and tangential, relationships are superficial and short-lived, discomfort when not the center of attention	Use of feedback to advise the individual about their socialization skills, offering appropriate alternatives, role modeling of appropriate social skills and communication behaviors, assisting the individual to identify strengths, increase assertiveness
Narcissistic personality disorder	Self-centeredness, unrealistic self-image, superiority to others, entitlement, mood is typically optimistic, relaxed, and cheerful, can become hostile, rageful, shame, and humility if needs not met. Unable to recognize expressing or empathize others feelings, insight is limited, underlying poor self-esteem, difficulty working with others	Use of self-awareness skills to avoid anger and frustration as a result of the individuals presentation, goal is to gain cooperation of the individual. Limit-setting, improving coping skills and helping the patient develop alternative behaviors to deal with perceived threats to self
CLUSTER C		
Avoidant personality disorder	As a child often overly inhibited, uncomfortable in new environments, shy, fearful, poor eye contact, anxious, awkward, appear as devastated by real or imagined criticism, occupational difficulties due to shyness and awkwardness prohibiting challenging positions. Very low self-esteem.	Supportive and reassuring approach, exploration of positive self-aspects, discern positive contacts with others and investigate etiology of self-criticism. Education to employ self-affirmations, and improve self-esteem, social skills, and improve interpersonal relationships.
Dependent personality disorder	Notable lack of self-confidence, passive, acquiescence, overly generous, thoughtful and minimize their own attributes. Pollyannaish to others, but when alone pessimistic, dejected, and negative. Frequently anxious, self-critical, preccupied with fear of being left alone, loss of support from another. Difficulty in decision-making. Feel unable to function independently.	Establish a therapeutic relationship to encourage expression of feelings related to loss of any relationships while promoting independence and autonomy. Assist in identifying personal strengths and attributes, assistance in activities of daily living to promote independence in functioning, education related to effective problem-solving and decision-making. Use of effective communication techniques to avoid continuance of a dependent position in a relationship.
Obsessive-compulsive personality disorder	Formal and serious demeanor, expresses need to be perfect from childhood. Inability to express emotions or exhibit independent behavior, preoccupation with orderliness in most (if not all) areas, poor listening skills, poor judgment and decision-making skills, literal interpretation of social situations, low self-esteem, self-deprecating, difficulty with interpersonal relationships-few friends, unemotional with others. Marital and relationships with offspring difficulty due to inflexibility and unemotionality. Occupationally can have difficulty due to need for perfection.	Establish a trusting, therapeutic relationship. Assist the individual in refocusing goals from perfection of product to timeliness of completion. Assist them to tolerate less-than-perfect work. Use of cognitive restructuring techniques. Assist the individual to allow others to take control of projects or planning's to decrease need for total control.
OTHER RELATED DISORDERS		
Depressive personality disorder	Behaviors exhibited are similar to those of an individual with depression, the personality disorder is less severe. Sad, gloomy, dejected affect. Report persistent unhappiness, hopelessness. Anhedonia, worrisome, negative thinking, judgment, and decision-making intact, but influenced by pessimism. Low self-esteem.	Establish a safe, therapeutic relationship. Suicidal assessment, offer specific, factual feedback to minimize negative thoughts of self, cognitive restructuring techniques, patient education to improve social skills, provide opportunities to practice new skills, effective communication skills.
Passive-aggressive personality disorder	Superficially cooperative, angry and self-assertive, or dependent and submissive, pervasive negative attitude, affect may be sad or angry, judgment and decision-making are typically inpaired, ambivalent and indecisive. Opposition, resistance, obstructiveness.	Establish therapeutic relationship, self-awareness to help manage resistance. Assist individual to recognize the presence of anger and exhibition through behaviors, patient education to assist in effective communication skills, recognition of feelings.

Figure 10-1 Personality disorder characteristics.

that interpersonal factors may contribute heavily to psychological problems. It is commonly distinguished from other forms of therapy in its emphasis on the interpersonal experiences rather than biological etiologies. The goal of IPT is to alter the individual's relations with others by fostering adaptation to current interpersonal roles and situations.

- *Psychoanalytical psychotherapy*—The focus of this long-term therapy is to increase awareness of the unconscious factors that negatively influence relationships and behaviors, to identify the patterns of behavior, and, ultimately, to change them.

- *Milieu or group therapy*—This approach is most common when the individual is involved in inpatient treatment, partial hospitalization, or day treatment settings. The primary goal is management in group situations. This approach is helpful in increasing awareness and responsiveness to the needs and rights of others, and in decreasing social anxieties.

- *Cognitive behavioral therapy*—This intervention is a combination of cognitive and behavioral approaches to rectify situations involving dysfunctional emotions, behaviors, and cognitions. It can be used in individual or group settings.

- *Case management*—This approach is appropriate for those individuals diagnosed with personality disorder that are persistently and severely impaired and would benefit from increased social support, crisis management, and organized and structured care.

- *Psychopharmacology*—Though this approach has no direct influence on the diagnosis itself, it can be helpful in the management of symptoms. Most of these classifications of medications are discussed in other areas of this book. The nurse is expected to understand the indications of the medications, the potential adverse effects for both continuing assessments of the individual, and the provision of patient education.

- Antipsychotic medications can be useful in the treatment of psychotic symptoms.

- Antidepressants will help those individuals experiencing depressive symptoms (social isolation, low self-esteem, etc.). SSRIs are useful in addressing the symptoms of impulsivity, mood instability, and self-injurious behaviors.

- Mood stabilizers are useful in targeting impulsive behaviors.

- Anxiolytics help to reduce symptoms of anxiety.

Evaluation

The fifth phase of the nursing process is evaluation. In this stage, a reassessment is done to determine if the nursing interventions selected were effective in assisting the patient to meet the objectives of care. Some of the outcomes that should be revisited include the following:

- Is the individual able to relate comfortably with the nurse on a one-to-one basis?
- Does the individual participate in group situations with support?
- Is the patient able to minimize unusual mannerisms?
- Has the patient demonstrated a decrease in impulsivity?
- Has there been a decrease in manipulative behaviors, and has the patient shown an increase in ability to verbalize needs directly?
- Has the patient exhibited improvement in respecting the rights and needs of others? Adherence to rules and policies of the unit?
- Has the patient been able to express positive statements of self-evidencing improvement in self-esteem?
- Does the patient interact with peers in social situations?
- Does the patient demonstrate decreased anxiety and the use of adaptive coping skills in daily activities?
- Is the patient able to independently make decisions?
- Can the family and significant others maintain general boundaries? Set appropriate limits?

Chapter 10 Questions

1. You are working in the health clinic when June comes to the reception area stating, "I don't feel good; I need to see the doctor. I have an appointment at 1 p.m. and it's now 1:15 p.m." In a very dramatic and highly emotional manner, she goes on, "Can't you see I'm on death's door? I can't possibly wait another moment. I might just die." Which of the following is the best way for you to respond?

   A. Immediately call for a stretcher, telling the staff that June's behavior is so disruptive she needs to be seen first.

   B. Confront June about her unreasonable behavior and emphasize that many other people are waiting to be seen as well.

   C. Ignore June's behavior and do not confront her, as it may lead to an escalation of behaviors.

   D. In a calm, controlled, and nonthreatening manner, inform June of the reason for the delay and offer to reschedule her appointment for another time, if she would like.

2. You are the charge nurse on an inpatient psychiatric unit. Mr. Frank comes to you and reports, "Jim stole $10.00 from me." Jim is a 46-year-old male with an Axis II diagnosis of antisocial personality disorder. What is the most appropriate statement for you to make to Jim?

   A. "Jim, Mr. Frank said you took his money. Why did you do that?"

   B. "Mr. Frank is an old man. He can't stand up for himself."

   C. "Jim, tell me how you felt when you took Mr. Frank's money."

   D. "Jim, you have not followed the unit policies. The consequence of stealing is the loss of privileges. You will not be able to attend the recreation group this evening to see the movie."

3. You attend an in-service that discusses strategies useful when working with patients diagnosed with personality disorders. Which of the following recommendations would be helpful in assisting you with self-awareness?

   A. Therapeutic communication techniques

   B. Discussing your feelings with the patient and asking how they see the situation

   C. Seeking direction from your peers and nurse manager

   D. Wait until a problem is identified by someone

Scenario: This evening, you are assigned to care for Eileen, who has a diagnosis of borderline personality disorder. During your one-on-one with Eileen, she confides in you that she has cut herself, using a razor that the day staff "forgot to get back."

Questions 4 to 6 are based on the above scenario. Select the answer that is most appropriate.

4. The priority nursing diagnosis is

   A. Violence, risk for: self-directed

   B. Self-mutilation

   C. Ineffective coping

   D. Low self-esteem

5. What is the first thing you would do?

   A. Explore with Eileen what she was feeling prior to cutting.

   B. Place Eileen on a special status ensuring one-on-one supervision.

   C. Assess the injury and provide first aid.

   D. Notify the doctor.

6. Eileen tells you, "The evening staff is the best; you would have never forgotten to take the razor back." Which defense mechanism is being used by Eileen?

   A. Projection

   B. Displacement

   C. Splitting

   D. Undoing

7. As the nurse involved in the treatment of a patient with antisocial personality disorder, it is important when establishing the plan of care that you remember

   A. The psychiatrist must provide an accurate diagnosis and establish the treatment plan to maintain the most appropriate care.

   B. The patient will respond more quickly to an unstructured plan of care.

   C. Only the nursing staff needs to be involved in the development of the nursing care plan.

   D. All members of the multidisciplinary treatment team must agree on the diagnosis, goals, and plan of care.

Scenario: During your shift in the psychiatric emergency room, John is brought in for an evaluation after he was arrested for burglary and sent to the county jail. During his initial assessment at the jail, the nurse practitioner noted that John was hostile, verbally threatening, and showed no remorse for his actions. She reports that he stated, "I wasn't doing anything, just minding my business when those jokers stopped me. I don't know how all that stuff got in my car. I think someone put it there." John stated that, "If you put me in a cell, I'm busting some faces before I go in."

Questions 8 to 11 are based on the above scenario. Select the answer that is most appropriate.

8. Which of the following diagnoses is the most appropriate for John?

   A. Schizotypal personality disorder

   B. Borderline personality disorder

   C. Antisocial personality disorder

   D. Passive-aggressive personality disorder

9. During your nursing assessment of John, which would you expect to experience?

   A. Compliance with facility rules

   B. Expression of good insight into his behaviors

   C. Long-standing employment history

   D. Disregard for the court system and laws

10. John is to be admitted for further evaluation and initiation of treatment. You establish the following nursing diagnosis: Risk for violence, other directed, related to inability to tolerate frustrations. Which nursing interventions would be appropriate?

   A. Establish a trusting relationship, conveying acceptance.

   B. Place John on a special monitoring status, search him and his room, removing all contraband.

   C. Encourage John to verbalize feelings gradually, exploring alterative ways of handling his frustrations.

   D. A and B

   E. A, B, and C

11. The most appropriate treatment modality for John would include

   A. Interpersonal psychotherapy

   B. Individual counseling

   C. Milieu therapy

   D. Psychoanalytical psychotherapy

12. You are reassigned to another unit in the hospital after restructuring has occurred. During the staff meeting, you suggest that the schedule be done like it was on the floor you came from—a blank schedule is posted and everyone works together to fill it out. Tess, your nurse manager, responds,: "What? You just come over and already you are trying to run the unit? The schedule gets done the way it gets done, by me. No one else has a say." This is an example of which personality disorder?

    A. Passive-aggressive personality disorder

    B. Obsessive-compulsive personality disorder

    C. Antisocial personality disorder

    D. Paranoid personality disorder

13. The unit holiday party is next week. Anne works on your unit as the secretary. She does not usually go to any of the unit parties or functions, but you specifically tell her where the party will be and what time it is. She replies, "Oh, I don't know' I would really like to. Do you really think they want me there? I didn't think anyone really liked me." This is an example of which personality characteristics?

    A. Histrionic personality disorder

    B. Avoidant personality disorder

    C. Dependent personality disorder

    D. Asocial personality disorder

14. Which characteristics would you expect to find in the patient diagnosed with narcissistic personality disorder?

    A. Exaggerated sense of self-worth, entitlement, presents with an optimistic mood

    B. Presents as aloof, socially isolative, can experience magical thinking

    C. Mistrustful of others, suspicious and tense/irritable

    D. Sensitive to rejection, very socially withdrawn

15. Which of the following statements best describes a patient with personality disorder?

    A. They are able to recognize individual strengths and weaknesses.

    B. They can establish long lasting, healthy relationships.

    C. They are not able to see themselves objectively.

    D. They exhibit adaptive coping skills.

16. Which of the following personality disorders will require strategies to minimize or decrease manipulative behaviors?

    A. Schizoid personality disorder

    B. Borderline personality disorder

    C. Paranoid personality disorder

    D. Obsessive-compulsive personality disorder

17. Patients diagnosed with antisocial personality disorder typically use which of these defense mechanisms?

    A. Projection

    B. Compensation

    C. Regression

    D. Suppression

18. Personality disorders are diagnosed on which axis of the multiaxial diagnostic system used by the APA?

    A. Axis I

    B. Axis II

    C. Axis III

    D. Axis IV

19. Personality disorders are caused by

    A. Biological and psychological influences

    B. Contaminants

    C. Heredity

    D. Social interactions

20. The nurse should have an understanding of what theories before studying about and treating individuals with personality disorders?

    A. Personality development

    B. Nursing

    C. Advanced psychotherapy

    D. Pharmacology

Matching

21. Personality

22. Histrionic

23. Narcissistic

24. Schizoid

25. Schizotypal

26. Manipulative

27. Splitting

28. Character

29. Cognitive restructuring

30. Dysphoric

31. Limit-setting

32. Confrontation

33. Decatastrophizing

34. Temperament

35. Time-out

A. Leaving the area to a neutral place to regain internal control

B. Establishing parameters of acceptable and desirable patient behaviors

C. The aggregate of features and traits that form the individual nature of an individual

D. Natural predisposition

E. State of dissatisfaction, anxiety, restlessness

F. An outgoing and gregarious individual

G. Defense mechanism used by individuals with borderline personality disorder

H. Actions that are abrupt, unplanned, and directed towards immediate gratification

I. Technique used in cognitive therapy to assist the patient to examine validity of negative autonomic thoughts

J. Exaggerated belief in one's importance

K. Inordinate preoccupation with oneself

L. Technique used to manage manipulative or deceptive behavior by pointing out the problematic behavior

M. "Latent schizophrenic"—behavior is odd but does not reach level of schizophrenia

N. Learning to refute negative thinking with more positive and reality-based thoughts

O. Technique used to alter the process of negative, self-deprecating thoughts and feelings and change them to more positive ones; the patient develops skills to cease the process.

36. Thought-stopping

37. Positive self-talk

38. Impulsivity

39. Grandiose

40. Extroverted

P. Excessive emotionality, attention-seeking, and overly dramatic behavioral responses

Q. Technique where the patient rewords negative thoughts into positive ones

R. Personality disorder marked by dissociation, passivity, withdrawal, inability to form relationships, and indifference to praise or criticism

S. Sum of an individual's relatively fixed personality traits and typical responses to events

T. Purposeful behavior directed at meeting one's desires/needs with regard for the rights, needs, and desires of another

Chapter 10 Answers

1. D. The correct response involves role-modeling appropriate behavior by communicating in a calm, nonthreatening manner. Offering to reschedule the appointment allows the patient to choose the disposition in a nonjudgmental manner. Facilitating an immediate response to her acting-out behaviors reinforces her inappropriate behaviors. If the behavior were ignored, most probably June would continue to escalate.

2. D. The most appropriate statement is to reinforce the limit-setting strategies by identifying the inappropriate behavior and consequences of that behavior. The other choices are incorrect because the patient with an antisocial personality disorder is unlikely to have compassion for another, and you should avoid allowing the patient to excuse his or her behaviors.

3. C. It is important to recognize that proactive measures be taken for those providing care for patients with personality disorders. These individuals can be challenging and overwhelming for caregivers to manage. Open communication with your peers and clinical supervision by your nurse manager are recommended aspects of self-care for the nurse working with personality disorders to assist in maintaining boundaries and objectivity. Therapeutic communication is an appropriate technique that will benefit the patient. Discussing your feelings with the patient is not appropriate, nor therapeutic.

4. B. The patient is not at risk for self-injuring behaviors; she has actually harmed herself. Though ineffective coping skills and social isolation are appropriate nursing diagnoses for borderline personality disorder patients, neither is a priority when a patient has harmed herself.

5. C. All of the mentioned interventions are appropriate, but the first thing that needs to be done is to assess the patient's physical needs.

6. C. Splitting is a primitive defense mechanism commonly used by individuals diagnosed with borderline personality disorder, who see self and others as "all good, or all bad." Projection is the putting of one's unacceptable feelings on another, displacement is transferring feelings from one target to another considered less threatening, and undoing symbolically negates an experience that an individual cannot tolerate.

7. D. Individuals diagnosed with antisocial personality disorder frequently use manipulation to attempt to control their environment. To accomplish this, they will play staff against each other. The treatment team must be united in their approach to care. The other responses are incorrect in that they do not foster team cohesiveness, which is essential in the treatment of this patient.

8. C. Antisocial personality disorder is a pattern of socially irresponsible, exploitative, guiltless behavior. Individuals diagnosed with this disorder have a very low frustration tolerance, are easily provoked to attack, and typically are quick to demean or degrade. Schizotypal personality disorders present as aloof, isolative, and bland, and may exhibit psychotic symptoms. Borderline personality disorders are characterized by a pattern of intense and chaotic relationships, affective instability, and impulsivity. Passive-aggressive personality disorder individuals are considered to passively exhibit covert aggression.

9. **D.** Antisocial personality disorder individuals generally have a disregard for the law. They typically see themselves as victims and do not accept nor acknowledge responsibility for the consequences of their behaviors. They have difficulty sustaining employment and in developing any long-term relationships, and one of the more distinct characteristics is their tendency to ignore authority and rules.

10. **E.** All of the listed interventions are appropriate for a nursing care plan for risk for other-directed violence. An accepting attitude promotes feelings of self-worth, close observation allows for immediate intervention to ensure safety, and removal of dangerous objects ensures the priority of safety.

11. **C.** Milieu therapy is especially appropriate for patients diagnosed with antisocial personality disorder because feedback from peers is most effective. The therapist can be seen as an authority figure, with whom these patients have a difficult time accepting and responding appropriately to.

12. **B.** Individuals with obsessive-compulsive personality disorder are overly disciplined, rigid, and preoccupied with rules. They are typically inflexible when it comes to changing routines. Individuals with paranoid personality disorder appear as tense and hypervigilant. They avoid interactions with others and feel that others try to take advantage of them. Antisocial personality disorder individuals typically are exploitative and manipulative. Passive-aggressive personality disorder characteristics include passively expressing covert aggression.

13. **B.** Avoidant personality disorder characteristics include being extremely sensitive to rejection. While they may certainly desire social relationships, this fear is overpowering and leads to a very withdrawn social life. There is no personality disorder identified as "asocial." Dependent personality disorder characteristics include submissiveness and toleration of mistreatment by others to ensure the continuance of a relationship. Histrionic personality disorder is often characterized by flamboyant, colorful, and dramatic behaviors. There is a need for constant affirmation of approval by others.

14. **A.** Individuals diagnosed with narcissistic personality disorder have a self-inflated ego and believe that they have a right for special considerations. B describes schizotypal personality disorder, C describes paranoid personality disorder, and D describes avoidant personality disorder.

15. **C.** The only statement that appropriately describes an individual diagnosed with personality disorder is the one that says these individuals are not able to see themselves objectively. They typically are not able to accept personal responsibility for their behaviors and frequently create negative responses in others.

16. **B.** Individuals diagnosed with borderline personality disorder typically use manipulation to allay fears of separation.

17. **A.** Patients diagnosed with antisocial personality disorder typically envision themselves as victims. Projection is the primary defense mechanism they use. Compensation is covering up a real or perceived weakness by emphasizing an attribute one considers more desirable, regression is retreating in response to an earlier level of development, and suppression is the voluntary blocking of unpleasant feelings and experiences.

18. **B.** Personality disorders are coded on Axis II. Clinical disorders are located on Axis I, medical illnesses on Axis III, and environmental/psychosocial stressors on Axis IV.

19. **A.** It is believed that personality disorders are in response to various biological (hereditary, temperament) and psychological (experiential learning, social interactions) influences. They are not contagious, and it is felt that all individuals exhibit behaviors associated with various personality disorders at some point.

20. **A.** The nurse should be familiar with theories related to the normal development of the personality to provide a knowledgeable foundation before learning about what is identified as maladaptive personality development. Medications are not indicated in the treatment of personality disorders. While certain medications are appropriate for the treatment of symptoms associated with the disorder, medications will not affect the presence of the disorder.

Matching

21. C	**31.** B
22. P	**32.** L
23. K	**33.** I
24. R	**34.** D
25. M	**35.** A
26. T	**36.** O
27. G	**37.** Q
28. S	**38.** H
29. N	**39.** J
30. E	**40.** F

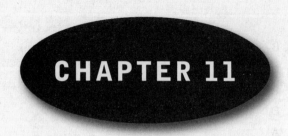

CHAPTER 11

Mood Disorders and Suicide

Many mentally healthy individuals experience occasional episodes of feeling sad or "down," or feelings of great joy and happiness. This can be a typical response to disappointments and happy events faced in everyday life. These intermittent periods occur as we struggle to effectively cope with real or perceived losses or failures, or respond to elated moods in response to positive experiences. It is not unusual when we feel down that we describe ourselves as "depressed" and experience feelings of decreased energy (anergia), or that when we are experiencing great joy, we have boundless energy and an elated mood. In both examples, disturbances can occur in sleep patterns and appetite.

Despite these feelings of wanting to retreat from the world, or remain involved in the experiences bringing us happiness, our everyday responsibilities spur us on to participate in work, family, and other activities. When unable to function adaptively, the individual is considered to be experiencing a mood disorder. There are accounts of mood disturbances dating back over the years to various ancient cultures (Babylonian, Hebrew, and Egyptian).

It was not until the 1950s that treatment became available for those individuals with severe depression or mania. This chapter reviews major depressive disorder, bipolar disorder, and suicide.

11.1   Mood Disorders

Major depressive disorder is characterized by one or more major depressive episodes without a history of mania, mixed, or hypomanic episodes. A major depressive episode is a period of two weeks of depressed mood, or anhedonia. Major depressive disorder is categorized as:

- *Single episode or recurrent*—First diagnosis or experiences of two or more episodes.
- *Mild, moderate, or severe*—These are determined by the severity of the symptoms.
- *With psychotic features*—Presence of disturbances in sensory perception or thought processes.
- *With catatonic features*—Psychomotor impairments, for example, psychomotor retardation (with or without waxy flexibility, stupor, excessive motor activity), negativism, mutism, echolalia, echopraxia.
- *With melancholic features*—A severe form of major depressive episode where symptoms are exaggerated with regard to depression of spirits and gloomy forebodings.
- *Chronic*—When episode of depressed mood has been continuous for two years.
- *With seasonal pattern*—Occurs typically in the fall and winter months. Was previously referred to as Seasonal Affective Disorder (SAD).
- *With postpartum onset*—Depressive symptoms occurring within four weeks postpartum

See Box 11-1 for *DSM-IV-TR* diagnostic criteria for major depressive disorder.

Box 11-1: Criteria for Major Depressive Episode

A. Five (or more) of the following symptoms have been present during the same 2-week period and represent a change from previous functioning; at least one of the symptoms is either (1) depressed mood or (2) loss of interest or pleasure.

Note: Do not include symptoms that are clearly due to a general medical condition, or mood-incongruent delusions or hallucinations.

1. Depressed mood most of the day, nearly every day, as indicated by either subjective report (e.g., feels sad or empty) or observation made by others (e.g., appears tearful).

Note: In children and adolescents, can be an irritable mood.

2. Markedly diminished interest or pleasure in all, or almost all, activities most of the day, nearly every day (as indicated by either subjective account or observation made by others).

3. Significant weight loss when not dieting or weight gain (e.g., a change of more than 5% of body weight in a month), or decrease or increase in appetite nearly every day.

Note: In children, consider failure to make expected weight gains.

4. Insomnia or hypersomnia nearly every day.

5. Psychomotor retardation or agitation nearly every day (observable by others, not merely subjective feelings of restlessness or being slowed down).

6. Fatigue or loss of energy nearly every day.

7. Feelings of worthlessness or excessive or inappropriate guilt (which may be delusional) nearly every day (not merely self-reproach or guilt about being sick).

8. Diminished ability to think or concentrate, or indecisiveness, nearly every day (either by subjective account or as observed by others).

9. Recurrent thoughts of death (not just a fear of dying), recurrent suicidal ideation without a specific plan, or a suicide attempt or a specific plan for committing suicide.

B. The symptoms do not meet criteria for a Mixed Episode.

C. The symptoms cause clinically significant distress or impairment in social, occupational, or other important areas of functioning.

D. The symptoms are not due to the direct physiological effects of a substance (e.g., a drug of abuse, a medication) or a general medical condition (e.g., hypothyroidism).

E. The symptoms are not better accounted for by Bereavement, i.e., after the loss of a loved one, the symptoms persist for longer than 2 months or are characterized by marked functional impairment, morbid preoccupation with worthlessness, suicidal ideation, psychotic symptoms, or psychomotor retardation.

DSM-IV-TR with permission.

Prevalence

Major depressive disorder occurs twice as often in women than men.

Pathophysiology

Neurotransmitters indicated in the pathophysiology of major depressive disorders include the following:

- Norepinephrine
- Acetylcholine
- Dopamine

- Serotonin
- Gamma-aminobutyric acid

Application of the Nursing Process

Assessment

- While there are no specific lab values that will diagnose the presence of major depressive disorder, sleep EEG abnormalities are evident in greater than half of outpatients and in 90 percent of inpatients.
- Symptoms develop over days to weeks. A prodromal period may include anxiety symptoms. Mild depressive symptoms may last weeks to months before the onset of a full major depressive episode.
- Nursing history data is collected from the individual, family, significant others, prior treatment documentation, and others involved in the care of the person.
- A mental status assessment (as discussed in Chapter 4) is conducted, ensuring assessment to ascertain presence of suicidal ideation. If present, the nurse assesses further regarding the intent and plan. This information is conveyed to the treatment team.
- Assessed symptoms include affective (despair, hopelessness, worthlessness, blunted affect, apathy, etc.), behavioral (psychomotor retardation, ambulating slowly and rigidly, poor hygiene and grooming, social isolation), cognitive (delusional thinking, confusion, indecisiveness, impaired concentration and attention, alterations in sensory perceptions, self-deprecation, etc.), and physiological (general physical retardation, diminished libido, trouble getting to sleep or staying asleep, anorexia, etc.)
- Core symptoms of major depressive episode are the same for children and adolescents:
  - Somatic complaints
  - Irritability
  - Social withdrawal
- Culture can influence the experience and communication of symptoms of depression. Following are cultural aspects to consider:
  - *Latino/Mediterranean*—Somatic complaints offered versus feelings of sadness/guilt
  - *Chinese/Asian*—Reports of weakness, tiredness, or "imbalance"
  - *Middle Eastern*—"Heart" problems
  - *Hopi*—Reports of being "heartbroken"

  Additionally, during times of crisis, cultural consideration must be given before considering the reports of the individual as an alteration in thinking (delusion).
- Completion of depression rating scales can assist in creating a diagnostic picture.

Diagnosis

An analysis of the data will assist in determining the priority problems and help formulate the plan of care. Common nursing diagnoses for the patient with major depressive disorder include the following:

- Risk for suicide
- Imbalanced nutrition: Less than body requirement
- Imbalanced nutrition: More than body requirement
- Anxiety
- Hopelessness
- Ineffective role performance
- Self-care deficit
- Chronic low self-esteem

- Disturbed sleep pattern
- Impaired social interaction
- Powerlessness
- Dysfunctional grieving
- Disturbed thought processes
- Disturbed sensory perceptions

Planning/Implementation

Appropriate nursing interventions are to be selected to address specific problems identified for the patient experiencing major depressive disorder. See Figure 11-1 for appropriate plan of care for the patient with major depressive disorder.

- A first priority is to ensure the safety of the patient. Staff are directed to follow established procedures and protocols for suicidal precautions as warranted. Formulating a contract for safety with the client, when the time frame has elapsed, another is initiated. This chapter will discuss the suicidal patient in a later section.

- Establishing a therapeutic relationship is essential in facilitating the expression of the patient's feelings. As noted in the diagnostic section, impaired social interaction can be experienced by the depressed patient. Short, frequent intervals of connectiveness will assist in building a trusting and therapeutic relationship. During these short interactions, the nurse continues to assess the patient and monitor for dangerousness.

- Be nonjudgmental in acceptance of the patient. Despite verbalization of negativism and pessimism related to self-esteem issues, assist the patient to identify strengths and positive self-value.

- Encourage the patient to express feelings in an honest and reflective manner. Anger is often present in depression; if needed, provide measures for the patient to release feelings of hostility

- Depressed patients can experience psychomotor retardation. The nurse may experience feelings of frustration related to the patient impairment in communication. However, use of the therapeutic techniques of offering self and silence will benefit the patient through demonstration of genuineness, concern, and caring.

- Promotion of activities of daily living and basic physical care are important interventions for the client experiencing depression. Lethargy and lack of energy is a common experience in depression. Assessment of the patient's ability to perform self-care activities directs when greater assistance is required. Continual assessment of these activities is essential in determining the changes in the patient's psychomotor abilities.

- Monitor and encourage appropriate nutritional and fluid intake. Many patients with depression experience a significant decrease in appetite. Offer frequent, small amounts of food so that they may not be as overwhelming. Ensure that the foods are energy-dense and protein-enriched until the patient is able to ingest adequate amounts. Consultation with the dietician to address the patient's individual needs is encouraged.

- Assessment and monitoring of sleep patterns is important. Patients with depression can experience both hypersomnia and insomnia. Interventions will be specific to the presenting symptom. Use of sleep agents, environmental manipulation, and patient education related to relaxation techniques are appropriate actions to promote sleep. Ensuring attention to maintaining the proper sleep-wake pattern may necessitate encouraging the patient to remain out of bed during the day hours to promote sleep at night. It is important to assess if the patient feels refreshed upon awakening to determine effectiveness of sleep.

- Encourage the patient to attend and participate in available unit activities to promote physical activity and socialization.

NURSING DIAGNOSIS	NURSING INTERVENTIONS
Risk for suicide	1. Assess for suicidal ideation. Ask the patient directly and if suicidal ideation is present, further assess for intent or plan.
	2. Provide a safe and nonthreatening environment. Ensure all potentially dangerous objects are removed from the direct area, provide close supervision of the patient during meals and medication times. Conduct room searches as dictated by facility policy and procedure.
	3. Encourage the patient to formulate a contract for safety.
	4. Upon assessment of dangerousness, ensure adequate level of monitoring the patient. Consider the use of 1 : 1 supervision, frequent checks (every 15 minutes). Consider placing the patient in a room in close proximity to the nurse's station. If the patient is deemed to be a high risk to harm self—constant 1 : 1 may be necessary, even during bathroom/shower use.
	5. Observation of the patient not placed on a 1 : 1 should be done at frequent and **irregular** times. Most especially do not establish patterns of rounds during change of shift, night hours, and ensure observations are done when the unit acuity is elevated.
	6. Use therapeutic communication techniques to facilitate honest communication regarding feelings of the patient. Anger, many times, is present in the depressed patient. Allow opportunity for the patient to vent these feelings without fear of retribution or punishment.
Low self-esteem	1. Employ therapeutic communication techniques to establish a relationship with the patient to convey respect and acceptance of the patient.
	2. Encourage the patient to identify indiviual strenghts, resources, and prior effective coping skills (identify use of ineffective coping skills)
	3. Allow the patient to establish the pace for working through their issues/problem
	4. Identify the defense mechanisms used by the patient in managing their situation, initiate patient education as appropriate to assist in addressing maladaptive defense mechanism.
	5. Provide psychoeducation for the patient and significant others
	6. Encourage participation in group activities which will offer methods of accomplishment for the patient. Encourage independence as able.
	7. Provide patient education related to improving assertiveness and communication skills
Imbalanced nutrition: less than body requirement	1. Assess the patient 's nutritional status per facilities screening tool
	2. Monitor for signs and symptoms of malnutrition (hair, skin, conjunctiva).
	3. Review laboratory findings (serum albumin, prealbumin, serum total protein, serum ferritin, transferring, Hgb, Hct, and electrolytes.
	4. Monitor food intake at meals, including fluids. Note if the patient partakes in snacks or eats during visiting with significant others
	5. Provide energy-dense and protein-rich nutrients as tolerated, until intake improves. Allow the patient to eat in small amounts at frequent intervals
	6. The patient's appetite may not coincide with the unit routine. Allowance for this variance will increase opportunity to encourage consumption.
Disturbed sleep pattern	1. Assess the patients sleep pattern, noting any recent changes
	2. Encourage the patient to express concerns or issues that may be interfering in their sleep
	3. Plan nursing care to facilitate appropriate number of uninterrupted sleep hours
	4. Ensure an environment conducive for sleep, administer medication as prescribed to promote a normal sleep pattern.
	5. Encourage the patient to actively participate in unit groups or exercise during the day hours to enhance ability to achieve adequate sleep at night. Patient education related to the relationship of activity and rest, and in relaxation techniques should be provided.
	6. Assess the patient, in the morning, encouraging a description of sleep experience.
Self-care deficit	1. Assess and monitor the patient for ability to perform ADL's. Monitor the patient's ability to complete the tasks, reminding what needs to be done. Provide positive reinforcement for achieving the goals.
	2. Ensure privacy and encourage the patient to perform self-care activities in an unrushed manner
	3. Provide assistance as needed
	4. Set realistic goals (brush hair, brush teeth) that may be accomplished within a shift to increase esteem.
	5. If the patient is unable to accomplish basic ADL needs, provide daily hygiene to prevent alteration in skin integrity or infectious process from occurring.

Figure 11-1 Depressive disorder care plan.

Related Mood Disorders:

Following are some other mood disorders classified in the *DSM-IV-TR*:

- *Dysthymic disorder* is characterized by at least two years of depressed mood for more days than not with some additional less severe symptoms that do not meet the criteria for a major depressive episode.

- *Premenstrual dysphoric disorder* is not an official diagnosis in the *DSM-IV-TR*; however, it does provide a set of research criteria that encourages further study of the incidence. Characteristics include a significantly depressed mood, anxiety, mood swings, and decreased interest in activities in the time frame prior to menses, subsiding shortly after the onset of menstruation.

- *Cyclothymic disorder* is characterized by two years of numerous episodes of hypomanic symptoms that do not meet the criteria for bipolar disorder.

- *Substance-induced mood disorder* is characterized by prominent and persistent disturbance in mood assessed to be directly and physiologically a consequence of substances (alcohol, drugs, toxins).

- *Mood disorder* due to a general medical condition characterized by a prominent and persistent mood disturbance assessed to be directly related to a medical condition (neurological, metabolic, endocrine, autoimmune, chronic disorder).

- *Seasonal affective disorder* (SAD)

  1. *Fall-onset*—Also referred to as winter depression. Characteristics include hypersomnia, increased appetite with weight gain, irritability.

  2. *Spring-onset*—Less common occurrence, characterized by insomnia, decreased appetite with weight loss.

- *Postpartum depression* meets all the requirements of a major depressive episode with the onset occurring within four weeks after delivery.

11.2 Bipolar Disorder

Bipolar disorder, previously referred to as manic-depressive disorder, results in a significant and severe shift in an individual's mood, energy, and ability to function. Mood swings experienced by those diagnosed with bipolar disorder can involve episodes of mania (extreme "highs") to episodes of severe depression.

During episodes of mania, the individuals experience euphoria, grandiosity, increased physical energy, and insomnia. There is a noticeable impairment in judgment—rapid thoughts ("racing thoughts"), impulsivity, pressured and rapid speech, and expansive mood. There can be psychosis present during a manic episode. Hypomania is a milder form, typically not severe enough to result in a noticeable disruption in social or occupational functioning. Refer to Box 11-2 for the criteria for a manic episode.

Box 11-2: Diagnostic Criteria for a Manic Episode

A. A distinct period of abnormally and persistently elevated, expansive, or irritable mood, lasting one week (or any duration if hospitalization is necessary).

B. During the period of mood disturbance, 3 (or more) of the following symptoms have persisted (4 if the mood is only irritable) and have been present to a significant degree:

  1. Inflated self-esteem or grandiosity

  2. Decreased need for sleep

  3. More talkative than usual or pressured to keep talking

  4. Flight of ideas or subjective experiences that thoughts are racing

  5. Distractibility

(Continued)

6. Increase in goal-directed activity or psychomotor agitation

7. Excessive involvement in pleasurable activities that have a high potential for painful consequences

C. The mood disturbance is sufficiently severe to cause marked impairment in occupational functioning or in usual social activities or relationships with others, or to necessitate hospitalization to prevent harm to self or others, or there are psychotic features.

D. The symptoms are not due to the direct physiological effects of a substance (e.g., a drug of abuse, a medication, or other treatment) or a general medical condition (e.g., hypothyroidism).

American Psychiatric Association, with permission.

The classic form of bipolar disorder is referred to as bipolar I disorder. This involves recurrent episodes of mania and depression. Those individuals who experience only a hypomania, where the depressive episodes are more frequent and intense than the mania, are characterized as bipolar II disorder.

Prevalence

Bipolar disorder occurs almost equally among men and women. The average age for a first manic episode is in the early 20s; however, it should be noted that the spectrum ranges from adolescence to 50-plus years of age. Though diagnosed in children and adolescents, it is a difficult process due to the unique differences in how children respond to illness than adults (presentation of symptoms). Adolescents are more likely to have psychotic symptoms (disturbances in sensory perception and/or disturbed thought processes). There are likely to be incidences of school truancy, antisocial behaviors, school failure, and substance abuse.

Pathophysiology

There are many factors that together produce the disorder. There is a genetic component (familiar predisposition), as well as environmental. While many incidences of bipolar disorder occur without an identifiable causation, trauma, or stressful life experiences have precipitated episodes of bipolar disorder in individuals who are genetically predisposed. Certain medications have been known to trigger a manic episode. Steroids, used to treat somatic illnesses, are the most common. Additionally, other medications such as antidepressants, amphetamines, and narcotics have the potential for mania.

Application of the Nursing Process
Assessment

- There are no specific blood tests, X-rays, or scans that will diagnose bipolar disorder.
- Obtaining a history from patients may prove to be challenging. If they are experiencing a manic state, they may exhibit flight of ideas, rapid and pressured speech, racing thoughts, and so on. If they are experiencing a depressive episode, they may evidence lethargy, refuse to be motivated to participate, or experience impaired social interaction.
- The nursing history data is collected from the individual, from family or significant others, from prior treatment documentation, and from others involved in the care of the person.
- A mental status assessment (discussed in Chapter 4) is conducted, ensuring assessment related to mania, as impulsive behaviors may result in harm to self or others.
- Mania symptoms are described in three stages: hypomania, acute mania, and delirious mania. Assessed symptoms include affective (euphoria, grandiosity, lability, or evidence of depression as previously discussed), behavioral (increased psychomotor agitation, continual movement, rapid and pressured speech, impulsivity, poor boundaries, or behaviors related to depression as discussed previously), cognitive (delusional thinking, impaired concentration and attention, confusion, flight of ideas, etc.), and physiological (individuals experiencing mania can ignore the need for food or sleep

for several days. Personal hygiene is often ignored. They may discard needed items and place themselves at risk for harm to self or others.

- Core symptoms of hypomania include the following:
  - ○ Cheerful and expansive mood with underlying irritability which is quickly revealed when the individual's self-perceived needs are unmet.
  - ○ Elevated self-worth; thought processes are rapid. Goal-directed activities are negatively influenced due to increased distractibility.
  - ○ Increased psychomotor activity, present as "social" and "outgoing," though the individual experiences difficulty forming interpersonal relationships due to lack of connectiveness. Generally are very gregarious, talking and laughing inappropriately and loudly.
- Core symptoms of acute mania include symptoms of hypomania and the following:
  - ○ Grandiose, heightened, or agitated mood, easily irritable or angered.
  - ○ Insomnia, ADLs neglected, dress is bizarre and inappropriate.
  - ○ Rapid and pressured speech, flight of ideas, rapid and pressured speech, highly distractible.
  - ○ Exaggerated self-esteem, presence of delusional thinking and hallucinations.
  - ○ Poor judgment in situations with severe consequences, impulsivity, sexual acting out, excessive spending.
  - ○ Substance abuse.
- Core symptoms of delirious mania involve the symptoms associated with acute mania and are a rare critical form of mania. They include the following:
  - ○ Severe lability of mood, experience of panic level of anxiety.
  - ○ Cognition and perception are significantly impaired with confusion, severe disorganization, and extreme distractibility, and the individual can be incoherent.
  - ○ Physical activity reaches frantic level, with severe agitation, intense impulsivity, and potential for death due to exhaustion or injury.
- Core symptoms in children and adolescents are similar to those exhibited by adults; however, younger children may demonstrate more intermittent or erratic changes in their mood, energy level, and behaviors. They may also present with accelerated mood swings, belligerence, agitation, irritability, and explosiveness.
- Cultural considerations that were discussed under major depressive episodes are relevant to manic episodes.
- Assessment tools are available to screen for signs and symptoms of bipolar disorder (mania and depression). These tools may be used by the individual, or in the case of a child/adolescent, his or her parent or guardian.

Diagnosis

An analysis of the data will assist in determining the priority problems and help to formulate the plan of care. Common nursing diagnoses for the individual with bipolar disorder include the following:

- Imbalanced nutrition: less than body requirements
- Disturbed sleep pattern
- Self-care deficit
- Fatigue
- Disturbed thought process
- Disturbed sensory perception
- Risk for injury
- Risk for violence; other directed
- Social isolation
- Chronic low self-esteem
- Sexual dysfunction
- Impaired verbal communication

Planning/Implementation

Appropriate nursing interventions are to be selected to address specific problems identified for the patient experiencing bipolar disorder. See Figure 11-2 for an example of a plan of care. Priority interventions include the following:

- Safety plays an important and primary role in the nursing care of a patient experiencing mania. A safe environment and assessment of the presence of suicidal ideations or thoughts/plans to harm others is essential.
- Special monitoring of the individual on the unit is prudent due to impulsive behaviors. Patients typically have poor insight and poor personal boundaries, and frequently present as aggressive toward others. These behaviors may evoke retaliation from others on the unit.
- It is a priority to meet the physiologic needs of the patient diagnosed with bipolar disorder. Disturbed sleep pattern and decreased nutritional intake must be monitored and addressed.
- Mania results in impaired concentration and attention. The use of therapeutic communication will facilitate effective communication and allow opportunities for patients to appropriately express themselves.
- The promotion of appropriate behaviors is necessary due to the occurrence of socially unacceptable and risky behavior typically exhibited by patients experiencing mania.
- The administration of medications requires an understanding of the indications, desired effects, and possible side effects. Additionally, the nurse needs to be aware of the special considerations of neuroleptic and mood stabilizers. Incorporating this information into patient education will increase the patient's understanding of the importance of medication, which may influence compliance.

11.3　Pharmacologic Interventions

Pharmacological Interventions for Depressive Disorders

Antidepressant medications are believed to work by slowing the removal of certain neurotransmitters (serotonin and norepinephrine) from the brain. As discussed earlier in this book, neurotransmitters are essential for normal brain function and are involved in the control of the mood and other responses and functions. Antidepressants increase the availability of these chemicals, restoring the imbalance and relieving the symptoms of depression. Several kinds of antidepressants are prescribed:

Selective Serotonin Reuptake Inhibitors (SSRIs) and Nonselective Reuptake Inhibitors (NRIs). These work only on the neurotransmitter serotonin. These medications have fewer side effects than the other available antidepressants and often are effective more quickly.

Tricyclic Antidepressants (TCAs). Have been used to treat depression for the past four decades. Patient education related to the time frame (up to four weeks) necessary before the individual may experience benefits from the medication needs to be reinforced.

Monoamine Oxidase Inhibitors (MAOIs). These medications were first prescribed for the treatment of tuberculosis. Patients did not experience a resolution of their bacterial infection; however, they did experience an improvement in mood. The discovery of the enzyme inhibition properties of the medication led to the belief that monoamines have a role in regulation of mood. Hypertensive crisis is a potential concern with this medication. Considered a medical emergency, hypertensive crisis symptoms will occur within two hours of consumption of tryamine. A pounding headache (in the occipital or temporal areas), feeling of choking, palpitations, and overall feeling of doom with a significant increase in systolic and diastolic readings are symptoms.

Dietary restrictions with MAOIs include the following:

- Aged cheese
- Raisins
- Fava beans
- Flat Italian beans
- Chinese pea pods
- Red wines
- Smoked and processed meats
- Caviar, pickled herring

NURSING DIAGNOSIS	NURSING INTERVENTIONS
Fatigue	1. Assess level, frequency, activities, and symptoms associated with increased fatigue, ability to perform ADL's, influence on socialization and everyday activities. 2. Assess individual's attention and concentration, mood and typical activity patterns. Use of appropriate fatigue rating scales as tolerated. 3. Evaluate adequacy of nutritional intake and sleep patterns 4. Patient teaching related to importance of appropriate sleep/wake schedule, promotion of periods of rest, and relaxation techniques to facilitate increasing self-calming effects 5. Encourage expression of feelings related to physical fatigue. 6. Administer medications as prescribed to promote sleep
Impaired verbal communication	1. Minimize the environmental stimuli and promote a quiet, nonthreatening environment to reduce anxiety/responsiveness 2. Introduce self and explain procedures in a calm manner with simple, brief terms 3. Encourage the patient to communicate needs in an unhurried and accepting manner 4. Provide reality orientation techniques 5. Use attentive listening behaviors, validate verbal and nonverbal communications 6. Assess appropriateness of touch
Disturbed thought process	1. Promote a nonjudgmental and trusting relationship with the patient through active listening and use of therapeutic communication techniques 2. Provide reality orientation; introduce self, call patient by name, provide relevant (brief) information 3. Orient the patient to the environment to facilitate awareness of self and surroundings 4. Do not argue, debate, or reason with a patient experiencing delusional thoughts as this will result in increased anxiety—provide comfort measures and support 5. Acknowledge realistic elements of the delusion, and when the dynamics are better understood, discourage expression of the delusions by focusing the 1:1 on the patient's underlying feelings 6. Administer neuroleptics, assessing for potential side effects 7. Provide patient education related to the signs and symptoms of the illness and the desired effects of the medications
Disturbed sensory perception	1. Establish a trusting therapeutic relationship with the patient, using therapeutic communication techniques and provide a safe and structured environment to decrease the patient's anxiety. 2. Encourage the patient to focus on you during experiences of hallucinations to decrease reaction intensity 3. Provide regular physical activity that requires concentration and energy as a distraction from internal stimuli 4. Assist the patient to identify situations that elicit hallucinations, teach to intervene in the experience to minimize intensity of the response. 5. Patient education related to the use of consensual validation of the experience as a reality test 6. Administer neuroleptic medication as prescribed, assess for potential side effects
Sexual dysfunction	1. Assist the patient in recognizing the potential negative implications of impulsive sexual acting out. 2. Encourage use of socially acceptable behaviors to express sexual needs 3. Engage the patient in discussions related to their hypersexuality and potential feelings to encourage an increase in insight 4. Provide a safe and nonjudgmental environment to ensure the individual's safety and that of other clients on the unit 5. Consider the use of a special monitoring status to prevent sexually inappropriate behaviors 6. Administer medications as prescribed to assist in decreasing impulsive behaviors, assess for potential side effects, and provide patient education related to the disease process and desired effects of the medications

Figure 11-2 Bipolar disorder care plan.

- Corned beef
- Chicken or beef livers
- Soy sauce
- Brewer's yeast
- MSG (meat tenderizer)

Medication restrictions with MAOIs include the following:

- Other antidepressants (tricyclic and SSRIs)
- Sympathomimetics (OTC cold remedies, epinephrine, dopamine, norepinephrine, ephedrine, pseudoephedrine, etc.)
- Stimulants (amphetamines, cocaine, diet medications)
- Antihypertensives
- Meperidine and other possible opioids, antiparkinsonian agents (levadopa)

See Figure 11-3 for a comparison of antidepressant medications.

CLASSIFICATION	NAME	ADULT DOSE RANGE	ADVERSE EFFECTS
Slow titration-therapeutic response can take up to a month, or longer			
Tricyclics	Amitriptyline (Elavil) Amoxapine (Asendin) Clomipramine (Anafranil) Despiramine (Norpramin) Doxepin (Sinequan) Imipramine (Tofranil) Nortriptyline (Pamelor)	50-300 mg 50-600 mg 25-250 mg 25-300 mg 25-300 mg 30-300 mg 30-100 mg	Dry mouth, drowsiness, blurred vision, urinary retention, constipation, lowered seizure threshold, arrhythmias, tachycardia, nausea and vomiting, blood dyscrasias, orthostatic hypotension, exacerbation of mania
Selective Serotonin Reuptake Inhibitors (SSRIs)	Citalopram (Celexa) Fluoxetine (Prozac) Fluvoxamine (Luvox) Escitalopram (Lexapro) Paroxetine (Paxil) Sertraline (Zoloft)	20-60 mg 20-80 mg 50-300 mg 10-20 mg 10-50 mg 50-200 mg	Headache, insomnia, nausea, diarrhea, constipation, sexual dysfunction, dry mouth, serotonin syndrome, somnolence
Monoamine Oxidase Inhibitors (MAOIs)	Isocarboxaid (Marplan) Phenelzine (Nardil) Tranylcypromine (Parnate)	20-60 mg 45-90 mg 30-60 mg	Dizziness, headache, orthostatic hypotension, constipation, tachycardia, palpitations, hypomania
Heterocyclics	Bupropion (Wellbutrin) Maprotiline (Ludiomil) Mirtazapine (Remeron) Trazedone (Desryl)	200-450 mg 50-225 mg 15-45 mg 150-600 mg	Dry mouth, sedation, dizziness, tachycardia, pripism (trazedone), seizures (Wellbutrin & Ludiomil)
Nonselective Reuptake Inhibitors (NRIs)	Nefazodone (Serzone) Venlafaxine (Effexor) Duloxetine (Cymbalta)	200-600 mg 75-375 mg 40-60 mg	Nausea, dry mouth, constipation, dizziness, somnolence, insomnia, sexual dysfunction, hepatic failure (Serzone warning)

Figure 11-3 Antidepressant medications.

Pharmacological Interventions for Bipolar Disorder (Mania)

Patients diagnosed with bipolar disorder may require multiple prescription medications for limited time frames to manage symptoms. Long-term medication management involves the use of mood-stabilizing prescriptions. The use of antianxiety medications assists in the reduction of feelings of agitation and anxiety, and antipsychotics reduce the influence of hallucinations and delusional thoughts while combating psychomotor agitation. Antidepressants are prescribed for the depression experienced in the bipolar spectrum.

Mood Stabilizers. These medications are also referred to as antimanic agents and are used to treat mood cycling. Except for lithium carbonate and Lamotrigine, mood stabilizers are not known to be effective in addressing symptoms of depression. The two first choice medications are Depakote (valproic acid) and lithium carbonate. See Figure 11-4 for comparison of various mood stabilizers.

NAME	INDICATIONS	DOSAGE	BLOOD LEVELS	THERAPEUTIC CONTRAINDICATIONS	SIDE EFFECTS
Lithium Carbonate	Acute treatment of mania, depressive episodes, prevent recurrence of episodes	900 - 2400 mg/day	0.4-1.3 mEq/L	Cardiovascular disease, brain damage, renal disease, thyroid disease, myasthenia gravis	Fine hand tremors, mild nausea, weight gain
				May be harmful to fetus, therefore not to be used during pregnancy, breastfeeding, use in children less than 12 years old	Early signs of toxicity (levels below 1.5 mEq/L), nausea and vomiting, thirst, polyuria, slurred speech, muscle weakness
Depakote (Valproic Acid)	Effective in Lithium nonresponders, acute mania, rapid cylcers, prevention of recurring mania	500 - 1500 mg/day	350-690 μmol/L (50-100 mg/L)	Patients with hepatic disease or significant hepatic dysfunction, as well as those known to be allergic to it	Drowsiness, sedation, dry mouth, blurred vision, weight gain, alopecia, hand tremor
Tegretol (Carbamazepine)	Patients experiencing treatment resistant bipolar, rapid cycling, patients with severe paranoia, anger, and mania, dysphoric mania	200 - 1200 mg/day	4 -12 μg/mL	Patients with a history of previous bone marrow depression, hypersensitivity to the medication or sensitivity to tricyclic compounds, use of MAOIs within 14 days	Drowsiness, dry mouth, blurred vision, sedation, rashes, orthostatic hypotension, Can cause aplastic anemia and agranulocytosis
Lamictal (Lamotrigine)	First-line treatment for bipolar depression, approved for acute and maintenance therapy	100 - 200 mg/day	1 - 5 mcg/ml	Hypersensitivity, impaired cardiac functioning	Ataxia, dizziness, headache, nausea, vomiting, photosensitivity, rash
Trileptal (Oxcarbazepine)	Similar to Tegretol. May be useful in difficult to treat bipolar disorder	600 - 1200 mg/day	15 - 35 μg/mL	History of allergies to Oxcarbazepine	Dizziness, somnolence, diplopia, fatigue, nasuea & vomiting, ataxia, tremor, dyspepsia, abnormal gait
Topomax (Topiramate)	Acute mania or mixed episodes in adults	50 - 400 mg/day	5 - 20 μg/mL	Allergies to topiramate, history of kidney stones, taking high-dose vitamin C or calcium supplementation (increase risk of kidney stones)	Paresthesia, somnolence, anorexia, dizziness, nausea, depression

Figure 11-4 Mood stabilizing medications.

11.4 Electroconvulsive Therapy

Electroconvulsive therapy (ECT) intervention is employed to treat depression for those patients who have not been responsive to antidepressants (or are unable to tolerate the side effects experienced at therapeutic levels), patients who are acutely suicidal, and for those individuals who are experiencing psychosis, severe psychomotor retardation, and neurovegetative symptoms. Evidence suggests that ECT is effective in decreasing acute suicidal ideations (see the section on the suicidal patient). Acute phases of mania have also been treated with ECT for those individuals who are unable to tolerate first-line medications or are exhibiting behaviors that are life-threatening (extreme impulsivity, exhaustion, etc.). ECT is safely used in pregnancy, with the only steadfast contraindication being increased intracranial pressure due to the side effect of a rise in cerebrospinal fluid pressure. Individuals considered high risk for complications related to ECT include those with cardiovascular problems, osteoporosis, and pulmonary disorders.

The procedure involves the delivery of an electrical impulse to the brain, resulting in seizure activity. Though there is no definitive implication of exactly how ECT works, it is believed that this electrical shock stimulates the brain chemistry and increases the presence of serotonin, norepinephrine, and dopamine, correcting the imbalance that causes depression. Treatment typically includes a series of 6 to 15 sessions, with maximum benefit achieved in 12 to 15 treatments. Adverse effects of ECT include temporary memory loss and confusion. Typically post treatment the patient experiences increased tiredness and often has a headache.

The role of the nurse in the care of the patient receiving ECT follows the steps of the nursing process. Priority interventions include the safety of the patient, facilitating appropriate management of fear and anxiety for the patient and significant others, providing patient education regarding the procedure and potential side effects, and documentation of care provided and response of the patient.

Evaluation

The fifth phase of the nursing process is evaluation. In this stage, a reassessment is done to determine if the nursing interventions selected were effective in assisting the patient to meet the objectives of care. Following are some of the outcomes that should be revisited:

- Has the patient been safe from injury to self and others?
- Has the patient demonstrated a decrease in psychomotor agitation?
- Has the patient exhibited a decrease in delusional thoughts or hallucinations?
- Is the patient able to maintain ADLs?
- Has the patient been able to sleep adequately? Is the nutritional intake sufficient?
- Does the patient express an understanding of the illness and treatment (medication, ECT, etc.)?

11.5 The Suicidal Patient

Individuals experiencing suicidal ideations and exhibiting suicidal behaviors can be encountered in various treatment settings. Suicide is the intentional killing of one's self. Suicidal ideations are thoughts centering on killing oneself, and while there may be a detailed plan involved, there is no action taken. There are three types of self-destructive actions that are categorized as suicidal behavior:

1. *Completed suicide*—An intentional act that results in death
2. *Attempted suicide*—An intentional act that is intended to result in death but does not.
3. *Suicidal gestures*—A self-harmful act that is unlikely to result in death

Prevalence

The World Health Organization reports that over one million people kill themselves each year, with an estimated 10 to 20 million unsuccessful attempts. It is the third leading cause of death for individuals 14 to 25 years of age. Those over the age of 65 are at highest risk for suicide.

Pathophysiology

There are many psychological, sociological, and biological implications in researching the causation of suicidality. Emotional responses including anger, hopelessness, worthlessness, guilt, shame, a history of aggressiveness and violence, and developmental stressors have all been connected as predisposing factors to suicide. Interactions of an individual and his or her environment, issues such as isolation, peer pressure, and stressors resulting from life events have all been identified as possible precipitants. Biologically, there is a genetic predisposition, as well as evidence supporting an imbalance of neurotransmitters, in particular serotonin.

Application of the Nursing Process

Assessment

- The nursing history data is collected from the individual, from family, from significant others, from prior treatment documentation, and from others involved in the care of the person.
- A mental status assessment (discussed in Chapter 4) is conducted, ensuring assessment related to suicidal ideations, suicidal plan/intent, and signs and symptoms of depression (discussed previously).
- Risk factors:
  - Marital status (married individuals are at lower risk)
  - Gender (7th cause of death for men, 16th for women)
  - Age (older individuals are more at risk)
  - Religion (activity can lower risk)
  - Ethnicity (highest rates are among Native Americans and non-Hispanic whites)
  - Presence of a mood disorder (presence of depression and other mental disorders or substance abuse increases risk)
  - Disturbance in sleep pattern (severe insomnia is associated with an increased risk)
  - Family or personal history (relationship of relative determines risk, the first two years for an individual after an attempt represent high-risk)
  - Presence of plan (lethality)
- Core symptoms:
  - Expressed feelings of hopelessness, worthlessness, helplessness, guilt
  - Impulsivity, aggressiveness, increased irritability
  - Expressed or observed anxiety (report of panic attack, anxious ruminations, increased psychomotor agitation)
  - Presence of command hallucinations
  - Expression of suicidal ideations
  - Anhedonia, sudden noticeable change in behavior, social isolation, interactions
  - Change in sleep or appetite habits
  - Substance abuse
  - In children and adolescents, potentially suicidal individuals may exhibit a dysphoric mood, aggression/hostility, frequent interpersonal problems and lack of friends/peer relations, marked loneliness, increased and exaggerated quietness, antisocial problems, prior suicidal behaviors, and substance abuse
- Cultural considerations:
  - As mentioned previously, ethnicity is a factor in assessing risk for suicide. Native Americans have the highest incidence of suicide.
  - Ethnic minorities with mental illness and mental disorders are less inclined to seek treatment from organized mental health systems.

- ○ Those financially disadvantaged have higher incidences of mood disorders, anxiety disorders, and alcohol and substance abuse problems.
- ○ Cultural and ethnic minorities face more stressors quantitatively and qualitatively than the rest of the population; there has been evidence that cognitive, emotional and social processes, perception of self, and motivation have been influenced by these factors.
- Assessment scales: Several suicide assessment tools are available in the screening of at-risk individuals. The questions typically address the presence of the risk factors addressed above.

Diagnosis

An analysis of the data will assist in determining the priority problems and help to formulate the plan of care. Common nursing diagnoses for the individual with suicidal behavior include the following:

- Risk for suicide
- Violence, risk for self-directed
- Self-mutilation, risk for
- Self-esteem, situation or chronic low
- Denial, ineffective
- Anxiety
- Hopelessness
- Ineffective individual coping

Planning/Implementation

Appropriate nursing interventions are to be selected to address specific problems identified for the patient experiencing suicidal behavior (see Figure 11-5). Priority interventions include the following:

- *Safety*—Implementation of suicide precautions to ensure a safe environment, minimize potential for suicidal behaviors in the hospital setting, and ensure the ability to continuously assess the patient.
- *Assessment and patient education*—Use of counseling skills (interviewing, crisis intervention, problem-solving techniques) to establish a trusting relationship with the patient.
- *Safety contract*—This can be a verbal or written contract where the patient agrees to refrain from self-harming behaviors by using adaptive alternative methods (expressing feelings to staff, journaling, etc.).
- *Administration of medication*—The use of prescribed medications can be effective in assisting the patient to regain and maintain self-control related to self-injurious behaviors. As discussed previously, antidepressant medications are used for those patients experiencing depressive or anxiety disorders. Use of lithium carbonate has shown evidence in decreasing suicidal thoughts. For those patients experiencing psychosis, antipsychotic medications (discussed previously) are prescribed, and anxiolytics are helpful with panic disorders and insomnia (frequently experienced in depressed patients).
- *Postvention*—This is required in the care of those family members and significant others of patients who successfully commit suicide, as well as the health professionals involved in their care. These individuals may need assistance in effectively managing the trauma experienced.

Evaluation

The fifth phase of the nursing process is evaluation. In this stage, a reassessment is done to determine if the nursing interventions selected were effective in assisting the patient to meet the objectives of care. Following are some of the outcomes that should be revisited:

- The patient has not acted on thoughts to harm self.
- Patient reports increased sense of safety and security with staff and is able to report presence of suicidal ideations.
- Patient will demonstrate increase in adaptive coping skills.
- Patient will be able to verbalize presence of hope, increased self-esteem.

NURSING DIAGNOSIS	NURSING INTERVENTIONS
Risk for Suicide Violence, (risk for self-directed)	1. Assess for suicidal ideation if patient has a history of depression, substance abuse, or other psychiatric disorders, family history of suicide, history of childhood physical or sexual abuse, chronic pain or illness, recent significant loss/stress. 2. Use of self-reporting assessment tools and/or screenings to determine presence of depressed mood or intent to die 3. Assess patient's willingness and ability to engage in no-suicide contract 4. Monitor for verbal expression of suicidality 5. Monitor nonverbal behaviors indicating mood and changes in mood 6. Establish a positive and therapeutic relationship via the use of therapeutic communication 7. Place patient on special monitoring status, assign bed placement in visible, close proximity to nurse's station 8. Provide a safe environment through diligent room and body searches for contraband or dangerous items 9. Patient education regarding suicide precaution, medications, and potential side effects 10. Explore with the patient precipitant's/motivation for suicidal behavior, encourage discussion of patient's view of consequences that may decrease probability of acting on suicidal thoughts (family response, cultural or religious implications, finality of actions). 11. Encourage patient to participate actively in care by formulating a plan to combat response to suicidal thoughts, identify supports and resources
Hopelessness	1. Assist the patient in identifying precipitants of current situation to allow clarification of patient's perception of stressors. 2. Assess patient's past coping skills with focus on patient's perception of effectiveness past and current to assist in identifying strengths, patient education to assist in the development and utilization of adaptive coping skills 3. Assess the implications of cultural beliefs, norms, and values on the patient's feelings of hopelessness 4. Using therapeutic techniques, provide support and hope about future to assist the patient in identifying positive aspects, assist in identifying sources of hope and hopelessness. Encourage expression of feelings and acknowledge acceptance of the feelings 5. Monitor and document potential for suicidal behaviors 6. Assist the patient with problem-solving and decision-making
Risk for Self-Mutilation	1. If the patient harms self, provide appropriate medical care in a nonjudgmental and calm manner. 2. Assess for risk of suicide or continuing self-injurious behaviors by asking the patient directly if suicide is a consideration and for presence of a plan. 3. Assess the patient for signs of depression, anxiety, and/or impulsive behaviors 4. Search the patient and room for dangerous items, remove as appropriate 5. As appropriate, place patient on special monitoring status. Room assignment to facilitate visibility. 6. In the presence of self-injurious behaviors, consider establishing a plan with the patient using behavior modification to decrease acting out behavior and increase self-control

Figure 11-5 Care plan for suicidal patient.

Reprinted from NANDA with permission.

Chapter 11 Questions

Multiple Choice

1. A patient diagnosed with bipolar disorder has been admitted to your unit. You are aware that bipolar is differentiated from unipolar disorder by this major factor:

    A. The presence of manic behavior.

    B. There is a higher incidence in women than men.

    C. The genetic etiology.

    D. The severity of the depression.

Scenario: Mrs. Smith is a 40-year-old, married woman who has been admitted to your unit after she attempted to kill herself in a drug overdose. During your assessment she tells you that she has been involved in outpatient treatment since her husband had told her he intended to file for a divorce. During a mediation session discussing the division of community property, Mrs. Smith and her husband had a verbal argument, and she subsequently took an overdose of her medication. Your initial assessment reveals that Mrs. Smith has dark circles under her eyes, frequently yawns, and has slow speech and responses. She is disheveled and slightly malodorous. During the interview she reveals to you that she believes a pimple she has on her right cheek is a cancer that has progressed and is "eating away my insides."

Questions 2 to 6 are based on the above scenario. Select the answer that is most appropriate.

2. Mrs. Smith is best classified as having:

   A. Major depression

   B. Depression with melancholia

   C. Dysthymic disorder

   D. Bipolar disorder

3. Analyzing your data regarding Mrs. Smith, what is a priority nursing diagnosis?

   A. Risk for suicide

   B. Alteration in thought process

   C. Disturbed family process

   D. Disturbed sleep pattern

4. What is an appropriate short-term goal for Mrs. Smith?

   A. Provide an environment conducive for sleep.

   B. Administer medications to promote rest and provide patient education regarding relaxation techniques.

   C. Mrs. Smith will sleep all night.

   D. Mrs. Smith will be able to rest comfortably for four to six hours within two nights.

5. Mrs. Smith is prescribed Lexapro (escitalopram) 10 mg q HS. What classification of antidepressants is this medication?

   A. Nonselective reuptake inhibitor

   B. Monoamine oxidase inhibitor

   C. Tricyclic

   D. Selective serotonin reuptake inhibitor

6. What unit activity would you initially encourage Mrs. Smith to participate in?

   A. Exercise and dance therapy

   B. Bingo

   C. None, she needs time alone to rest

   D. Brief 1:1 sessions with staff

7. The benefit of SSRIs over other antidepressants includes

   A. Fewer anticholenergic and cardiovascular side effects

   B. Need a lower dose of medication

   C. Result in an enzyme inhibition that decreases depressive symptoms

   D. Also address mania

8. As you are making rounds at 2 a.m. on the unit, you see that Jon Jones is making phone calls to his friends and family to discuss his new discovery to combat global warming. In his excitement, he is yelling and disturbing the unit. In reviewing his medical record, which of the following medications would you expect he is prescribed?

   A. Lithium carbonate

   B. An anxiolytic

   C. An SSRI

   D. A neuroleptic

9. The next evening you approach Jon to administer his evening dose of lithium carbonate. You note that he is experiencing ataxia, reporting "seeing double," informs you, "I have been having diarrhea all afternoon" and now "feels nauseous." What actions would you take?

   A. Tell him to go lie down after he takes his medication because he may be getting the flu.

   B. None. Manic patients frequently have somatic complaints.

   C. Tell Jon to go to his room and wait after you administer his evening dose of medication so you can talk to him some more.

   D. Do not administer to Jon his evening dose of medications and immediately contact the doctor on call.

10. The lab calls with a report of Jon's lithium level. It is 1.5 mEq/L. Based upon this information, you determine that

    A. Jon's symptoms are not associated with lithium toxicity.

    B. His therapeutic level of lithium is below therapeutic level.

    C. Jon's lithium level is high on the normal side.

    D. Interpreting lab values is not a nursing responsibility.

11. Supportive therapy for Jon may include all of the following except:

    A. Problem-solving therapy

    B. Cognitive therapy

    C. Interpersonal therapy

    D. Psychoanalysis

12. Which is an appropriate nursing diagnosis for a patient diagnosed with bipolar 1, single manic episode exhibiting poor boundaries, who is argumentative and hypercritical of peers?

    A. Defensive coping related to social learning patterns as evidenced by poor relations with peers.

    B. Social isolation related to dysfunctional interpersonal relationships as evidenced by projection of hostility in voice.

    C. Risk for injury related to increased psychomotor agitation, poor personal boundaries.

    D. Impaired social interaction related to altered thought processes as evidenced by use of dysfunctional social interaction skills.

Scenario: Debbie is a 77-year-old female brought into the emergency room by her niece who reports: "She told me today that she doesn't want to go on." She adds, "She hasn't been answering her phone, so today I went over to her house. She just sat in the chair saying how much she misses George [her husband] and how there is no reason for her to wake up every day. I am so worried about her." During your nursing assessment, you discover that Debbie's husband died eight months ago. They had been married for 58 years and did not have any children. Debbie's niece reports, "She looks much thinner than the last time I saw her. She is 5' 4" and weighs 95 lbs. When I looked in her refrigerator, there was only one stick of butter and a quart of milk." Debbie is wearing her nightgown, is disheveled, and is slightly malodorous. Throughout the interview, Debbie is tearful when asked about her husband.

Questions 13 to 15 pertain to this scenario.

13. Which of the following nursing impairments is a priority?

    A. Social isolation

    B. Imbalanced nutrition: less than body requirements

    C. Dysfunctional grieving

    D. Risk for suicide

14. The psychiatrist has decided that Debbie will be started on Celexa 20 mg BID. After the first week, during your one-on-one with Debbie, she states, "That medication doesn't work. I don't feel any differently." The best response would be

    A. "You should do other things than focus on how you feel. Why don't you go down to the recreation room and draw?"

    B. "The medication should be kicking in by now. I will tell the doctor that the medication isn't working for you. Perhaps she will change it."

    C. "You should be feeling good. You are here, your niece cares greatly for you, and maybe you can go home tomorrow."

    D. "Well, Debbie, the medication can take several weeks before you begin to notice the benefit."

15. Debbie asks you, "Why did this happen to me? How did I get depression?" The following theories all address the etiology of depression, except:

    A. Biological theory

    B. Contagion theory

    C. Psychosocial theory

    D. Transactional theory

Scenario: After two weeks of inpatient treatment, Debbie is discharged back to home and scheduled for outpatient treatment. Eight days after discharge, Debbie is brought into the ER by ambulance after her niece had gone to visit her and was not able to arouse her. Her empty medication bottle was found on the bedside table. After being medically cleared in the ER, Debbie was again admitted to your unit. The following day during multidisciplinary treatment rounds, the psychiatrist states that she feels Debbie is a good candidate for ECT. The required consents are obtained. Considering this updated treatment plan, answer the following questions:

Questions 16 to 20 pertain to this scenario.

16. ECT is used most commonly for which diagnosis?

    A. Paranoid schizophrenia

    B. Major depression

    C. Bipolar disorder

    D. Obsessive-compulsive disorder

17. Patient education related to the side effects of ECT would include

    A. Temporary memory loss, confusion, and headache

    B. Damage to bone or soft tissue

    C. Acute myocardial infarction

    D. Permanent brain damage

18. The following is the only absolute contraindication for the use of ECT:

    A. Recent myocardial infarction

    B. Severe hypertension

    C. Congestive heart failure

    D. Increased intracranial pressure

19. It is believed that electroconvulsive therapy works by
   A. Increasing neurotransmitters
   B. Causing intracellular chemical changes
   C. Modifying behavior
   D. Increasing stimulation of the central nervous system

20. After receiving her ECT treatment, Debbie enters the recovery room where you are assigned to provide her care. You expect
   A. Debbie will remain asleep for 45 minutes to one hour. You will monitor her vital signs every 5 minutes until stable.
   B. Debbie will awaken within 10 to 15 minutes and may be confused and disoriented. You will monitor vital signs every 15 minutes for the first hour and orient her to time and place.
   C. Debbie requires no special nursing care after ECT treatment; she will be immediately returned to her unit.
   D. Debbie will complain of paralytic ileus.

Matching

21. Melancholia

22. Dysthymia

23. Hypomania
24. Affect

25. Psychomotor retardation

26. Anergia

27. Hypersomnia

28. Vegetative signs of depression
29. Anhedonia

30. Mood

31. Rapid cycling

32. Cyclothymia

33. Lethality

A. Period in which mood is abnormally and persistently elevated, expansive, or irritable.

B. Period of abnormally and persistently elevated, expansive, or irritable mood lasting four days in which the patient's ability to function is not impaired and there are no psychotic features

C. Average affect and activity

D. The electrophysiological changes that occur in the brain as a result of repeated intermittent exposure to a subthreshold electrical or chemical stimulus (as one causing seizures) so that there develops a usually permanent decrease in the threshold of excitability)

E. Loss of sense of pleasure from activities formally enjoyed

F. Slowed body movement, cognitive processing, and verbal interactions

G. A severe form of major depressive episode in which symptoms are exaggerated, interest or pleasure in all activities is lost

H. Repeatedly going over the same thoughts

I. Chronic mood disorder involving numerous episodes of hypomania and depressed mood; not sufficient severity or duration to meet the criteria for bipolar disorder

J. A condition in which one sleeps for an excessively long time but is normal in the waking intervals

K. Nonfatal self-injury with a clear intent to cause bodily harm or death

L. Mild to moderate mood disturbance characterized by chronic depressive syndrome present for years; minimal social or occupational impairment

M. Thoughts an individual has to kill oneself

34. Suicidal ideations	N. Also referred to as a mixed episode, when an individual experiences both mania and depression every day
35. Mania	O. Lack of energy
36. Suicidal gesture	P. Any behavior or action that might be, or has been in the case of successful completion, interpreted as indicating a person's desire or intent to commit suicide
37. Parasuicide	Q. Effectiveness of, or related to, or causing death
38. Kindling	R. The behavioral expression of emotion
39. Ruminate	S. Changes in sleep patterns, eating habits, bowel movements
40. Euthymic	T. A pervasive and sustained emotion that significantly influences behavior, personality, and perception

Chapter 11 Answers

Multiple Choice

1. **A.** Unipolar and bipolar disorders both include episodes of depression. Bipolar disorder patients also experience episodes of mania.

2. **A.** This patient evidences psychomotor retardation, self-care deficit, disturbed sleep pattern, and a somatic delusion. These symptoms are consistent with the diagnosis of major depression.

3. **D.** Using Maslow's Hierarchy of Need as a guideline for selecting priority needs of a patient, the most appropriate response is related to physical needs of the patient. In this situation, the patient's insomnia is a priority nursing concern.

4. **D.** Responses A and B are nursing interventions. Response C is not a realistic short-term goal, and it does not have a time frame. It is essential that patient-centered goals include an expected time frame for achievement of the goal to allow for determining if the interventions selected are appropriate.

5. **D.** Lexapro is an SSRI.

6. **D.** Initially, Mrs. Smith may not be able to tolerate physical activities on the unit, and it could be expected that her attention and concentration may not support participation in an activity such as bingo. Social isolation is a relevant nursing problem; therefore, she should be encouraged to interact with staff and not remain by herself.

7. **A.** SSRIs have fewer anticholenergic and cardiovascular side effects than TCAs (tricyclic antidepressants) and work faster. It is MAOIs that have been demonstrated to inhibit the enzyme monoamine which has a part in mood regulation.

8. **A.** Lithium carbonate is a medication (antimanic) used in acute mania, maintenance of bipolar disorder, and prevention for future manic episodes.

9. **D.** Jon may be experiencing initial symptoms of lithium toxicity. Lithium toxicity is a life-threatening condition. You would hold his evening medication but would be required to promptly notify the doctor that the medication was not being administered and informed of the need for further assessment.

10. **C.** The therapeutic level for lithium carbonate is 1.0 to 1.5 mEq/L for acute mania. There is a narrow margin between therapeutic and toxic levels, and Jon is at the high end of normal and therefore is most probably experiencing initial symptoms of toxicity. Understanding lab values and their implications is most certainly a nursing responsibility.

11. **D.** Psychoanalysis is an in-depth, insight-oriented psychotherapy. This approach is not appropriate in the treatment of bipolar disorders.

12. **C.** This patient is at risk for injury by others as a result of his intrusiveness and provocativeness.

13. **B.** Nursing problems are determined according to Maslow's Hierarchy of Needs. Physical needs are a priority, followed by safety and security. Actions may occur simultaneously; however, physical needs take precedence.

14. **D.** While SSRIs often do work faster than TCAs, a subsiding of symptoms may not occur for up to four weeks after beginning antidepressant medication.

15. **B.** Biological, psychosocial, and transactional models all provide attempts to describe the etiology of depression. However, this disorder is not a contagious illness.

16. **B.** ECT is effective in the treatment of severe depression. It is also indicated in the treatment of acute mania but is rarely used due to use of antipsychotic medications and lithium. ECT can result in remission of acute schizophrenia if there is an affective component but has not proved useful in chronic schizophrenia.

17. **A.** The most common side effects of ECT are temporary memory loss, confusion, and headache.

18. **D.** The only absolute contraindication of ECT is increased intracranial pressure. ECT results in increased cerebrospinal fluid pressure during the treatment, which can lead to brain stem herniation.

19. **A.** Though the exact mechanism of ECT is an effective therapy is unknown; a biochemical theory most regarded is that the neurotransmitters serotonin; norepinephrine and dopamine are increased.

20. **B.** ECT is considered an operative procedure. However, paralytic ileus is not an expected result from this procedure. Most clients awaken within 10 to 15 minutes of the procedure and are often confused and disoriented. While some patients may sleep for 1 to 2 hours after the procedure, vital signs are monitored every 15 minutes for the first hour. Orientation to time and place, as well as providing a description of the events, will assist the patient with altered thought process following the therapy.

Matching

21. G
22. L
23. B
24. R
25. F
26. O
27. J
28. S
29. E
30. T

31. N
32. I
33. Q
34. M
35. A
36. P
37. K
38. D
39. H
40. C

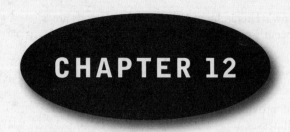

CHAPTER 12

Substance Abuse

12.1 Substance Abuse and Substance-Induced Disorders

In addressing substance-related disorders, this book's focus is centered on substance-use and substance-induced disorders. This book will review issues related to dependence, abuse, intoxication, and withdrawal. Substance use disorders address abuse and dependence (Box 12-1 and Box 12-2), while substance-induced disorders concentrate on intoxication (Box 12-3), delirium, withdrawal (Box 12-4), and alterations in mental states (amnesia, dementia, psychosis, mood, sleep and anxiety disorders, and sexual dysfunction).

Box 12-1: Diagnostic Criteria for Substance Abuse

Substance abuse is described as a maladaptive pattern of substance use leading to clinically significant impairment or distress, as manifested by one (or more) of the following, occurring within a 12-month period:

1. Recurrent substance use resulting in a failure to fulfill major role obligations at work, school, or home (e.g., repeated absences or poor work performance related to substance use; substance-related absences, suspensions, or expulsions from school; neglect of children or household).

2. Recurrent substance use in situations in which it is physically hazardous (e.g., while driving an automobile or operating a machine when impaired by substance use).

3. Recurrent substance-related legal problems (e.g., arrests for substance-related disorderly conduct).

4. Continued substance use despite having persistent or recurrent social or interpersonal problems caused or exacerbated by the effects of the substance (e.g., arguments with spouse about consequences of intoxication, physical fights).

Box 12-2: Diagnostic Criteria for Substance Dependence

At least three of the following characteristics must be present for a diagnosis of substance dependence:

1. Evidence of tolerance, as defined by either of the following:

   A. A need for markedly increased amounts of the substance to achieve intoxication or desired effects.

   B. Markedly diminished effect with continued use of the same amount of the substance.

2. Evidence of withdrawal symptoms, as manifested by either of the following:

   A. The characteristic withdrawal symptom for a substance.

   B. The same (or a closely related) substance is taken to relieve or avoid withdrawal symptoms.

3. The substance is often taken in larger amounts or over a longer period than was intended.

4. There is a persistent desire or unsuccessful effort to cut down or control substance use.

5. A great deal of time is spent in activities necessary to obtain the substance (e.g., visiting multiple doctors or driving long distances), use the substance (e.g., chain smoking), or recover from its effects.

6. Important social, occupational, or recreational activities are given up or reduced because of substance use.

7. The substance use is continued despite knowledge of having a persistent or recurrent physical or psychological problem that is likely to have been caused or exacerbated by the substance (e.g., current cocaine use despite recognition of cocaine-induced depression, or continued drinking despite recognition that an ulcer was made worse by alcohol consumption).

Box 12-3: Diagnostic Criteria for Substance Intoxication

1. The development of a reversible substance-specific syndrome caused by a recent ingestion of (or exposure to) a substance.

Note: Different substances may produce similar or identical syndromes.

2. Clinically significant maladaptive behavior or psychological changes that are due to the effect of the substance on the CNS (e.g., belligerence, mood lability, cognitive impairment, impaired judgment, impaired social or occupational functioning) and develop during or shortly after the use of the substance.

3. The symptoms are not due to a general medical condition and are not better accounted for by another mental disorder.

Box 12-4: Diagnostic Criteria for Substance Withdrawal

1. The development of a substance-specific syndrome caused by the cessation of (or reduction in) heavy and prolonged substance use.

2. The substance-specific syndrome causes clinically significant distress or impairment in social, occupational, or other important areas of functioning.

3. The symptoms are not due to a general medical condition and are not better accounted for by another mental illness.

The *DSM-IV-TR* lists disorders in the following categories:

- Alcohol-related disorders
- Amphetamine-related disorders
- Caffeine-related disorders
- Cannabis-related disorders

- Cocaine-related disorders
- Hallucinogen-related disorders
- Inhalant-related disorders
- Nicotine-related disorders
- Opinoid-related disorders
- Phencyclidine-related disorders
- Sedative-, hypnotic-, or anxiolytic-related disorders

Many drugs are used and abused; abuse of more than one substance at a time is referred to as polysubstance abuse. Certain substances are considered socially acceptable, such as alcohol, caffeine, and nicotine, despite information available indicating the health hazards associated with use or abuse of these substances. Prescriptive (amphetamines, depressants, anxiolytics, etc.) and over-the-counter substances (especially those items containing dextromethorphan, or DXM, are used to target symptoms experienced by individuals, and even some illegal substances have been able to gain acceptance for use (marijuana for glaucoma and pain management).

Prevalence

One of the leading health indicators (LHIs) established by Healthy People 2010 is substance abuse. Approximately two-thirds of the general adult population in the United States use alcohol, and surveys conducted by the National Institute for Mental Health evidence approximately 14 percent of adults in the United States of America meet criteria for an alcohol-related disorder and 6.2 percent meet criteria for a substance-related disorder other than alcohol or tobacco. Taking into consideration the course of illness or events leading to death in the United States, alcohol is ranked as the third leading cause of actual death, and illicit drug use is the ninth. Substance-related disorders and other psychiatric disorders are frequently comorbid, referred to as a "dual diagnosis." In comparison with the general population, patients with mood or anxiety disorders are twice as likely to have substance-related disorders. Assessment of an individual for the use of substances is essential, as the effects of substances results in alterations in mental status. Though there is no guarantee that discharged patients will not act out in a harmful way to self or others, those individuals under the influence of substances are more impulsive and therefore at high risk of such behaviors. These individuals should be appropriately monitored and reevaluated prior to release to a less restrictive environment.

Pathophysiology

Considerations addressing the etiology of this comorbidity include overlapping genetic vulnerabilities, overlapping environmental triggers, involvement of similar brain regions, and that both substance abuse and mental illness are developmental disorders. While a hereditary factor exists for most substance-related disorders, a family history is a significant risk factor for alcohol-related disorders. When alcohol is consumed, it affects various centers in the brain, directly related to the blood alcohol content (BAC). The BAC is the concentration of alcohol in an individual's blood, and is the measurement for an individual's level of intoxication for both medical and legal purposes. In most states the legal limit for alcohol is 0.08 percent. As an individual consumes alcohol, initially the cerebral cortex, then limbic system, cerebellum, hypothalamus and pituitary gland, and finally the medulla (brain stem) are affected.

Other drugs of abuse (such as marijuana and heroin) work by interfering with communication within the brain. Some mimic naturally occurring neurotransmitters and can activate neurons, and others (stimulants) result in a flooding of dopamine (regulates movement, emotion, cognition, motivation, feelings of pleasure) and subsequent euphoria.

There have been associations made between the experiences of low self-esteem and use/abuse of alcohol and other psychoactive substances. The use of such substances may serve to increase an individual's perception of self-worth and offer greater confidence. The temperaments of individuals diagnosed with depression and personality disorders and those experiencing esteem issues may demonstrate an inclination toward substance-related disorders.

Trends

The National Institute on Drug Abuse reports that overall the prevalence of underage alcohol and binge drinking has remained unchanged since 2002. Additionally, over 30 million people admitted that they had driven under the influence of alcohol at least one time within the past 12 months.

Use of nicotine has continued to drop and is now at its lowest rate. The use of illicit drugs continues to decline, specifically:

- Past-year marijuana use among 10th-graders dropped from a peak of 34.8 percent in 1997 to 24.6 percent in 2007.
- Among 12th-graders, use declined from a peak of 38.5 percent in 1997 to 31.7 percent in 2007.
- Annual prevalence of marijuana use by 8th graders is down to 10.3 percent in 2007, from a 1996 peak of 18.3 percent.
- In the five years between 2002 and 2006, the level of current marijuana use among persons aged 12 to 17 years declined from 8.2 percent in 2002 to 6.7 percent in 2006.
- The trend was also seen among older groups. From 2002 to 2006, the rate of current use of marijuana among 18- to 25-year-olds dropped from 17.3 to 16.3 percent.

Cocaine use has been stable since 2002, with a decline in the use of crack cocaine. A cause for concern, however, is the results that indicate that there is a drop in perception regarding the dangerousness of the drug Ecstasy among younger individuals. There has also been an increase in the abuse of prescription medications among young adults, aged 18 to 25 years (primarily Vicodin and Oxycontin).

Defense Mechanisms

While individuals who abuse substances employ various defense mechanisms (see Chapter 4), those primarily used are denial, rationalization, and projection.

Personality Traits of Substance Abusers

- Dominant and critical behavior toward others
- Personal insecurities
- Low self-esteem
- Rebelliousness
- Difficulty establishing interpersonal relationships

12.2   Substances Abused and Treatment Approaches

This chapter reviews alcohol, sedatives, hypnotics, anxiolytics, stimulants, cannabis, opioids, hallucinogens, and inhalants with regard to the effects of intoxication, overdose, withdrawal, and detoxification. After detoxification from these substances, the treatment approaches are quite similar.

Alcohol Abuse and Dependence

Intoxication. Alcohol (ethyl alcohol—ETOH) results from a reaction between fermenting sugar and yeast spores. It is rapidly absorbed into the bloodstream after ingestion and is a central nervous system depressant. It is rapidly dispersed throughout the body and immediate effects include the following:

- Slurred speech
- Lack of coordination
- Unsteady gait

- Impaired attention and memory
- Relaxation
- Disinhibition

Impairments in body movements, speech, vision, reaction time, judgment, and self-control begin to become affected when the BAC is approximately 0.07 to 0.090 percent. As the intoxication levels progress, an individual becomes increasingly impaired with significant coordination problems, euphoria reduces, and dysphoria increases. Physical symptoms begin, such as nausea, decreased gag reflex (leading to asphyxiation if vomiting occurs), and risk of serious injury related to falls. Stupor occurs at approximately 0.3 percent, coma at 0.35 percent, and possible death at 0.4 percent.

Withdrawal. Mild tremulousness can occur within 3 to 36 hours after cessation of or reduction in heavy and prolonged alcohol use. Characteristics of this include:

- Gross hand tremors
- Diaphoresis
- Elevated vital signs (pulse, blood pressure)
- Increased anxiety
- Nausea
- Vomiting

Left untreated, this withdrawal can advance to moderate withdrawal, characterized by:

- Intense anxiety
- Tremors
- Excessive adrenergic symptoms

Severe withdrawal typically occurs more than 48 hours after the cessation or reduction of alcohol use and presents with:

- A severe alteration in sensorium with hallucinations
- Disorientation
- Increased psychomotor agitation
- Severe autonomic hyperactivity (tremulousness, tachycardia, tachypnea, hyperthermia, and diaphoresis)

Withdrawal delirium. Acute withdrawal from alcohol is considered a medical emergency. Kindling is the term used where repeated alcohol detoxifications lead to an increase in the severity of symptoms of the withdrawal syndrome. Delirium tremens is an acute episode of delirium caused by withdrawal from alcohol in those individuals who have abused the substance for a long period of time. Usually peaking 2 to 3 days (48 to 72 hours) after cessation, or significant reduction, of alcohol intake, the delirium can last for 2 to 3 days.

Central Nervous System Depressants

Typically, CNS depressants (sedatives and tranquilizers) are prescribed to treat anxiety, muscular tension, sleep pattern disturbances, acute stress reactions, and pain. At high doses, these medications are used as general anesthetics. Examples of CNS depressants are barbiturates, benzodiazepines, alcohol (ETOH), and meprobamate. CNS depressants increase GABA activity, producing a calming effect to the brain. Many depressants have the potential to be both physically and psychologically addictive. As the body develops a tolerance for a depressant, larger doses are required to maintain the effect. Alcohol is the most frequently abused depressant.

Central Nervous System Stimulants

CNS stimulants are drugs that are used to increase activity in certain areas of the brain and work by releasing dopamine and noradrenaline to increase the rate of nerve impulses and/or block substances that would calm the nervous system. Disorders such as narcolepsy, ADHD, and other conditions with symptoms of impulsivity, inattention, and increased psychomotor activity are examples of indications for the prescription of stimulants.

Nonprescription examples of CNS stimulants include caffeine, nicotine, cocaine, and various amphetamines (e.g., levoamphetamine, dextroamphetamine, and methamphetamine).

Opiates

All opiates are derived either directly or in a synthetic form from the opium poppy. Opioids are medications (e.g., morphine, codeine, oxycodone, hydrocodone, dilaudid, fentanyl, methadone) that decrease the perception of pain, reaction to pain, and increase the tolerance to pain. They work by binding with opioid receptors (e.g., endorphin), causing a feeling of euphoria.

Hallucinogens

Hallucinogenic substances target specific areas of the brain that alter interpretations and result in alterations in sensory perceptions and reality disorientation. Some hallucinogens are synthetically manufactured (ketamine), while others occur naturally (peyote cactus). Following are the more common terms for these drugs:

Lysergic acid diethylamide (LSD)

- Acid
- Mellow yellow

Mescaline

- Cactus
- Peyote

Psilocybin/psilocin

- Boomers
- Shrooms
- Mexican/sacred mushrooms

Phencyclidine piperidine (PCP)

- Angel dust
- Hog
- Ozone

Inhalants

Inhalants are a diverse assortment of substances whose chemical vapors are inhaled to produce psychoactive effects. Typically abusers of these substances are those without access to other drugs or alcohol (i.e., young people, incarcerated and institutionalized individuals). Inhalants are breathed in through the nose or mouth by sniffing/snorting, spraying directly into the mouth or nose, saturating a cloth and placing it over the nose/mouth, inhaling fumes from a bag. This particular route of abuse displaces oxygen in the lungs, resulting in hypoxia in the brain. The term inhalant is generally used for those substances that are not used by any other route (e.g., cocaine, though it may be snorted, is not referred to as an inhalant). The following are inhalant categories:

- *Volatile solvents*—Liquids that vaporize at room temperature
  - Industrial or household products (paint thinners, gasoline)
  - Art or office supply (correction fluid, glue, markers)
- *Aerosols*—Sprays that contain propellants and solvents
  - Household (spray paint, hair and deodorant cans, aerosol cleaning products, vegetable oil sprays)
- *Gases*—Found in household or commercial products and medical anesthetics
  - Household or commercial products (butane lighters, propane tanks, whipped cream cans, refrigerant gases)
  - Medical anesthetics (ether, chloroform, nitrous oxide)

- *Nitrates*—Special class of inhalants used as sexual enhancers
  ○ Organic nitrates ("poppers"—cyclohexyl, butyl, amyl nitrates)

Marijuana

Marijuana is the most commonly abused drug in the United States. Derived from the Cannabis sativa hemp plant, the main active chemical is delta–9-tetrahydrocannabinol, or THC. Marijuana can be smoked as a joint/blunt, mixed with food (brownies, for example), brewed as a tea, or used as hashish (concentrated, resinous form). THC targets cannabinoid receptors (found in the basal ganglia and limbic system). There are no receptors in the medulla oblongata; therefore, marijuana is not a risk for respiratory or cardiovascular failure.

A number of studies correlates the chronic use of marijuana with increased occurrence of depression, anxiety, suicidal ideations, and even to schizophrenia (high doses can produce an acute psychotic reaction and may trigger the onset or relapse of schizophrenia in vulnerable individuals). Overdose and withdrawal from marijuana occur rarely.

- *Marinol*—A pharmaceutical product made with synthetic THC has been found to relieve nausea and vomiting to assist with anorexia associated with chemotherapy and AIDS patients, and it has been found to decrease intraocular eye pressure (glaucoma). It is available in pill form; there is no approved medical marijuana that is smoked. While it is legal to use marijuana in the smokeable form in some states for patients with terminal and/or painful illnesses, it remains a federal crime to buy or sell marijuana in the United States.

See Figure 12-1 for examples of pharmacological approaches to substance withdrawal and nursing considerations.

MEDICATION	INDICATION	NURSING CONSIDERATIONS
Benzodiazepines • lorazepam (Ativan) • chlordiazepoxide (librium) • diazepam (valium) • clonazepam (klonopin)	**CNS depressants** • alcohol • barbiturates • nonbarbiturate sedative/hypnotic • anxiolytics • opioids	• accepting and nonjudgmental attitude • monitor vital signs • monitor effectiveness of meds • assess for dizziness or drowsiness
Synthetic opioids • methadone • Subutex (antagonist) • Suboxone (antagonist) **Central-acting adrenergic stimulant** • clonidine	**Opioids**	• accepting and nonjudgmental attitude • monitor vital signs • monitor for nausea and vomiting • encourage fluid intake to minimize constipation • hold clonidine if hypotensive
Nutritional supplements • vitamin B$_1$ (thiamine) • folic acid (folate) • vitamin B$_{12}$ (cyanocobalamin) **Nonsteroidal anti-inflammatories** • ibuprofen • naproxen	**All substances**	• offer patient education related to proper nutrition • encourage nutrition and fluid intake
Antipsychotic • haloperidol (haldol) • phenothiazines (LSD only) **Anxiolytics** • diazepam (valium)	**Hallucinogens**	• accepting and nonjudgmental attitude • maintain low environmental stimuli • assign 1:1 to "talk down" individual (except for PCP) • speak clearly

Figure 12-1 Pharmacologic treatment.

12.3 Application of the Nursing Process

Assessment

Assessment of an individual experiencing substance abuse is complicated by the escalation in polysubstance abuse, and comorbidity with psychiatric and medical illnesses. Data is collected related to psychiatric issues, as well as substance abuse or dependence. Knowledge of risk factors will help to guide the clinical interview in assessing the individual's potential for substance abuse and facilitate a more in-depth discussion. See Figure 12-2 for an overview of signs and symptoms that may be assessed in the individual abusing substances.

- The nursing history data is collected from the individual, from family, from significant others, from prior treatment documentation, and from others involved in the care of the person.
- A mental status assessment (discussed in Chapter 4) is conducted, ensuring assessment-related general appearance, mood and affect, thought process and content, sensorium and intellectual processes, judgment and insight, self-perception, role performance and interpersonal relationships, and physiological concerns (nutritional status, system damage from substance abuse, etc.). Special consideration of the presence of suicidal ideations is emphasized, as well as any other self-destructive or injurious thoughts or behaviors.

Risk factors include the following:

- Biological factors
  - Genetics
  - Age (Illicit drug use has the highest rate among those 18 to 20 years old; alcohol use is highest among those ages.)
  - Race/ethnicity (Caucasians are more likely to use alcohol than other groups; binge drinking is relatively equal. Asians have the lowest use, including both binging and heavy alcohol use. Native Americans have the highest rate of alcohol use.)
  - Gender (The percentages are generally equal between male and female alcohol users; however, males are four times as likely as females to be heavy drinkers.)
  - Route of administration (inhalation, oral, injection, mucosa)
- Psychosocial factors
  - Family (family history is a significant risk factor, especially in alcohol abuse)
  - Education (in regard to alcohol use among adults 18 and older, the rate of use is increased as their education level is increased.)
  - Occupation (stress level, employment status, satisfaction)
  - Cultural/religious beliefs (attitudes, influencing patterns of use, learned coping skills)
- Environmental factors
  - Availability of substance
  - Peer pressure
  - Media
  - Substance abuse by family/significant others (children ages 8 to 17 cite parents as a primary influence in their decision to drink or not)
  - Community environment (poverty, unemployment, crime)
  - Geographic location (Illicit substance abuse is the highest in large metropolitan areas; alcohol use is lowest in the southern part of the United States.)
  - Legal ramifications (Illicit substance use is higher for those individuals involved on parole or other supervised release from incarceration.)
- Urine toxicology screening, breathalyzer, or blood alcohol calculator (BAC) will determine if substances are present in the individual's system,
- Substance abuse assessment tools determine the presence of a substance-related disorder. There are various screening tools available, such as CAGE (for "cut down/annoyed/guilty/eye-opener") questions:
  - Have you ever felt you ought to cut down on your drinking?
  - Have people annoyed you by criticizing your drinking?
  - Have you ever felt bad or guilty about your drinking?
  - Have you ever had to have a drink in the morning (eye-opener) to steady your nerves or get rid of a hangover?

A score of two to three "yes" answers indicate a possible problem with alcohol.

- If it is known, or discovered during the nursing history, that the individual has been using a substance, it is essential that assessment for signs of overdose, intoxication, and/or withdrawal be completed to determine need for immediate medical attention.

Central Nervous System Depressants

- *Physical symptoms*:
  - *Intoxication*—slurred speech, unbalanced gait, sedation, hypotension, uncoordinated motor skills, psychomotor retardation, bradycardia
  - *Withdrawal*—Nausea and vomiting, tachycardia, diaphoresis, increased irritability/anxiety, tremors, marked lethargy
- *Psychoemotional symptoms*:
  - *Intoxication:* Disinhibition, impaired judgment, impaired social and occupational functioning, impaired attention and memory, irritability
  - *Withdrawal:* Marked insomnia, hallucinations, and delirium tremens

Central Nervous System Stimulants

- *Physical symptoms*:
  - Intoxication—Hypertension, dilated pupils, tachycardia, nausea, and vomiting
  - *Withdrawal*—Psychomotor agitation/retardation, anxiety, lethargy, craving
- *Psychoemotional symptoms*:
  - *Intoxication*—Aggressiveness, grandiosity, impairments in social and occupational functioning, impaired judgment, hyperkinesia, euphoria
  - *Withdrawal*—Depression, vivid and disturbing dreams, insomnia/hypersomnia, paranoia

Hallucinogens

- *Physical symptoms*:
  - *Intoxication*—Dilated pupils, tachycardia, diaphoresis, palpitations, tremors, elevated vital signs (PCP additionally causes nystagmus, ataxia, muscle rigidity, chronic jerking, impulsivity).
  - *Withdrawal*—Hallucinogens are minimally addictive and have no physical withdrawal symptoms upon cessation of use.
  - *Overdose*—Unlikely to be life-threatening; however, overdoses are contributory to deaths due to behavioral responses to the drug (running from hallucinations, believing one has superhuman strength and can stop a car); can also result in permanent psychosis.
- *Psychoemotional symptoms*:
  - *Intoxication*—Alterations in sensory perceptions, disorientation, flashbacks, blissful calmness, impaired concentration and motivation
  - *Overdose*—Psychosis

Opiates

- *Physical symptoms:*
  - *Intoxication*—Constricted pupils, psychomotor retardation, nausea and vomiting, hypotension, sedation (nodding), euphoria, agitation
  - *Withdrawal*—Though the experience of withdrawal symptoms is uncomfortable, they are not life-threatening; nausea and vomiting, lacrimation, rhinorrhea, piloerection, diaphoresis, muscular cramping, muscle aches, yawning
  - *Overdose*—Medical emergency due to potential for respiratory arrest
- *Psychoemotional symptoms:*
  - *Intoxication*—Impaired attention and memory, apathy, dysphoria
  - *Withdrawal*—Irritability, panic, impulsivity

Inhalants:

- *Physical symptoms:*
  Intoxication—Dizziness, slurred speech, depressed reflexes, blurred vision, excitation followed by lethargy, ataxia, alterations in sensory perceptions; rapid and irregular heartbeat may result in sudden death (especially in prolonged single session).
  Withdrawal—Insomnia, headache, nausea, cravings, hallucinations, tremors, diaphoresis
- *Psychoemotional symptoms:*
  Intoxication—Similar to those individuals abusing depressants or anxiolytics; initial euphoria, a depressant effect on the CNS, feeling of floating, disinhibition
  Withdrawal—Sleep pattern disturbance, irritability, illusions

Assessment Data in Substance Abuse

- Family history of substance abuse
- Irritability of mood
- Use of minimization, projection, denial, rationalization, intellectualization as defense mechanisms
- Possible neurologic deficits from long-term abuse
- Poor judgment and insight
- Impulsivity
- Low self-esteem
- Ineffective coping skills
- Avoidant behaviors
- Impairment in occupation, social, and family roles
- Impaired nutritional status
- Report of sleep disturbances
- Medical complications from abuse (hepatitis, impaired skin integrity from injection sites, organ damage)
- Presents as intoxicated (see specific symptoms identified under the assessment section)
- Signs and symptoms of withdrawal from substance (see specific symptoms listed under the assessment section)

Diagnosis

An analysis of the data will assist in determining the priority problems and help to formulate the plan of care. See Figure 12-2 for common nursing diagnoses for the individual with substance abuse.

CHARACTERISTICS	NURSING IMPAIRMENT
Nausea & vomiting, diarrhea, abdominal cramping, anorexia, poor nutritional and fluid intake, body weight 20% less than ideal, review of lab values, reported or observed sleep changes, poor personal hygiene, inability to meet basic needs, poor skin turgor	Imbalanced nutrition: less than body requirement Deficient fluid volume Disturbed sleep pattern Self-care deficit
Neurologic deficits from acute or long-term abuse, unsteady gait, impaired judgment, report of suicidal ideations or behaviors, guilt, losses resulting from abuse (relationship, occupational, financial, etc.), impulsivity	Risk for injury Risk for self- or other-directed violence Risk for suicide Ineffective health maintenance
Increased family relationship issues and crises, parent-child and/or martial discord, presence of or increase in abusive behaviors towards others (verbal, emotional, physical, or sexual), inability to effectively communicate, irritability	Interrupted family process Impaired parenting Social isolation Anxiety
Expression of feelings of guilt, shame, hopelessness, helplessness, loss of motivation, sense of powerlessness over ability to manage without use of substance	Chronic low self-esteem Spiritual distress Hopelessness Powerlessness

Figure 12-2 Diagnosis of substance abuse.

Planning/Implementation

This phase of the nursing process is directed by the assessment data collected and diagnostic statement in the formulation of the patient-centered goal and selection of appropriate nursing actions focused on prevention, reduction, or elimination of the patient's health problems (nursing impairments). Identification of appropriate goals requires participation from both the patient and significant others. The focus of treatment is encouragement of the individual's responsibility and accountability in compliance, not specifically the compliance itself. Effective treatment results demand that the individual (not significant others) desire to address his or her substance abuse behaviors.

Treatment is available on an inpatient and outpatient basis. The decision of which is most appropriate will take consideration of ability of the individual (financial, occupational, social support systems, ability for self-care, etc.). Regardless of the treatment setting, the nurse's role is to select appropriate nursing interventions to address specific problems identified for the patient experiencing substance abuse. See Figure 12-3 for an example of a plan of care. Priority interventions include the following:

- Assess for signs and symptoms of detoxification or withdrawal from substances.
  - Monitor vital signs.
  - Administer scheduled and PRN medications for detoxification (see Figure 12-1).

Ineffective health maintenance	1. Assess individual's ability to maintain health status, support system(s) available, motivational level, and any dependency issues 2. Assist the individual and significant others to identify both strengths and weaknesses in health maintenance to assist with prioritizing 3. Assist improvement in communication to increase understanding of the disease process and allow for better acceptance by significant others, and facilitate discussions of concerns related to situation by the significant others and patient 4. Assist the individual and significant others to identify community resources and offer referrals
Risk for injury	1. Vital signs monitored for signs and symptoms of acute substance withdrawal, seizure precautions may by instituted 2. Decrease environmental stimuli to minimize impulsivity and effects of altered thought processes 3. Provide a safe and nonthreatening environment to convey security and safety to the individual 4. Reality orientation as required to help decrease anxiety 5. Monitor I&O, encouraging quality food & fluid as tolerated
Dysfunctional family process: alcoholism	1. Assessment of the family's behaviors related to alcohol abuse, denial, addiction to other substances, communication, impulsivity, and codependency issues 2. Encourage significant others to recognize the existence of substance abuse as a problem, and their personal responsibilities in relation to the process 3. Consider employing a contract to focus behavioral changes, encourage discussion of ramifications of abusive or violent behaviors (to self and others) 4. Patient education to encourage assertive expression of feelings and needs by significant others to the individual 5. Encourage involvement in supportive groups for significant others
Powerlessness	1. Assist the individual to identify realistic goals 2. Support review of life and recognition of aspects where control remains 3. Encourage the individual to participate as fully as possible in care options 4. Use of open-ended questions to encourage expression of opinions and feelings 5. Support attempts to regain control through education of the disease process and treatment options

Figure 12-3 Care plan for substance abuse.

  ○ Monitor intake and output, encouraging adequate and quality food and fluids.

  ○ Assess for deterioration of physical condition due to acute withdrawal (seizure, fall risk, etc.).

- Establish a therapeutic relationship employing nonjudgmental and accepting behaviors to facilitate communication of feelings and increase self-esteem.

- Provide health teaching for the individual and significant others.

  ○ Educate regarding signs and symptoms of withdrawal from substance.

  ○ Educate about the specific abused substance(s), including risk factors and physical affects (including impact on health status—HIV, hepatitis, etc.).

  ○ Educate regarding recovery and relapse.

  ○ Address family issues (codependence, communication impairment, caregiver strain, etc.).

  ○ Promote the development and utilization of effective coping skills (relaxation techniques, improving verbalization of feelings, etc.).

- Assess knowledge of support systems (self-help groups); assist with identification of accessibility and referrals.

- Assist the individual and significant others in identifying lifestyle changes to promote abstinence of substance use and sobriety.

Evaluation

As discussed in the previous chapter, in this phase of the nursing process, a reassessment is performed to determine the effectiveness of the selected nursing interventions in meeting the goals of care. This assessment determines if the nursing actions will be ended, continued, or revised. The evaluation of care is continuous and occurs at various times during the care period. Evaluation while intervening, or shortly afterward, allows for immediate adjustment in care during specific intervals during the patient's hospitalization (or other care setting) and enables assessment in progress towards goals. The evaluation of care is discontinued only when the patient had successfully achieved the goal established or is terminated from nursing care.

The fifth phase of the nursing process is evaluation. In this stage, a reassessment is done to determine if the nursing interventions selected were effective in assisting the patient to meet the objectives of care. Following are some of the outcomes discussed in previous chapters that should be revisited:

- The individual will not sustain injury.

- The individual and significant others will be able to effectively express feelings and concerns.

- The individual and significant others will be able to identify appropriate social and community resources.

- The individual will experience a safe withdrawal from the substance abused.

- The individual will be able to identify aspects that remain in personal control.

- The individual will express hopefulness for the future and participate fully in the planning of care.

Chapter 12 Questions

Multiple Choice

Scenario: Mr. Smith, a 59-year-old male, was brought into the emergency room by the police after they responded to a 911 call to his home. He states to you during the initial nursing assessment, "My wife started screaming about me drinking beer. I told her that if she didn't shut up, I was gonna punch her." The officer reports to you that the wife was scared to come to the ER but would be able to give information by phone. He added, "On the way here, Mr. Smith said that if he gets into any more trouble, he'll lose his job. Then he said, "If that happens, I might as well shoot myself in the head."

Questions 1 to 4 apply to this scenario.

1. During triage, Mr. Smith registers a 0.22 on the breathalyzer. You would expect his behaviors and thought processes to include all of the following except:

    A. Disinhibition

    B. Impaired reasoning

    C. Severe motor impairment

    D. Sense of well-being

2. Mr. Smith came into the ER at 10 p.m. When would you expect signs of alcohol withdrawal to begin?

    A. 11 p.m.

    B. 24 hours later

    C. In 3 to 5 days

    D. Between 2 a.m. and 10 a.m.

3. The data provided by the police officer and Mr. Smith's wife is considered to be

    A. Irrelevant

    B. Collateral

    C. Subjective

    D. Circumstantial

4. Which of the following are priority nursing interventions in the care of Mr. Smith?

    A. Monitor his vital signs; encourage food and fluids.

    B. Provide patient education related to alcohol withdrawal symptoms.

    C. Use firm limit-setting to decrease aggressive behaviors.

    D. Provide a community referral to Al-Anon for Mrs. Smith.

5. Symptoms of alcohol withdrawal include

    A. Disinhibition, mood lability, impaired social skills

    B. Coarse tremors, nausea and vomiting, elevated pulse and blood pressure, irritability

    C. Restlessness, nervousness, insomnia, GI disturbance

    D. Nystagmus, lethargy, psychomotor retardation, dizziness

6. You suspect that a colleague has a problem with substance abuse after noting alcohol on his breath a couple of times over the past month. What is the best way for you to handle this situation?

    A. Do nothing; you cannot be the only one who has noticed this.

    B. Confront him and tell him if it happens again that you will tell the supervisor.

    C. Ask around and see if anyone else has noticed it.

    D. Report your concerns to the unit nurse manager.

7. After discussing the desired effects of naltrexone with your patient, you determine that reinforcement is indicated when she responds

    A. "This medication can make withdrawal worse."

    B. "If I drink or use heroine taking this, I will get very sick."

    C. "I might have nausea and vomiting or stomach pains taking this medication, right?"

    D. "Taking this will not cure my substance abuse problems, but it will help me manage my addiction better."

8. During a one-on-one with your patient, she states, "I don't really have a problem with drinking. I just had a couple too many; it was a stressful day at work." She is exhibiting

   A. Suppression

   B. Denial

   C. Avoidance

   D. Displacement

9. Substance use disorders focus on which of the following characteristics?

   A. Intoxication, alterations in mental states, delirium, and withdrawal

   B. Abuse and dependence

   C. A and B

   D. None of the above

10. Acute withdrawal from which of these substances is considered a life-threatening emergency, requiring immediate medical care and treatment?

    A. Opioids

    B. Hallucinogens

    C. Alcohol

    D. Marijuana

11. Common methods used in the abuse of inhalants are called

    A. Sniffing and snuffing

    B. Gasping and snorting

    C. Huffing and bagging

    D. Infusing and imbuing

12. Marijuana, an illicit drug, is known to have medicinal qualities in the treatment of glaucoma and to combat nausea experienced during chemotherapy treatment. The pharmaceutical product made with synthetic THC, is called

    A. Marinol

    B. Sinsemilla

    C. Cannabella

    D. There is no marijuana-type medication available.

13. A priority intervention for the intoxicated patient is

    A. Allow sufficient time for the individual to sober up.

    B. Establish a trusting relationship by offering your own experiences with intoxication.

    C. Immediately engage the patient is establishing goals of care.

    D. Assess for other substance use.

14. During the evaluation phase of the nursing process, the following statement indicates that the patient has not achieved an expected goal and exhibits poor expectation of maintaining recovery:

    A. "I feel that I have the ability to not use drugs if I make sure I go to my program."

    B. "The best thing I learned, so far, is that there are people around who want to help me."

    C. "My husband came to visit me yesterday. We had a really good session with the doctor."

    D. "I got this thing beat. Now that the holidays are coming, I am sure I'll be able to control my drinking better."

15. Many substance abusers experience the following difficulties. The most common is

    A. Setting personal boundaries

    B. Dealing with work performance

    C. Dealing with social interactions

    D. Effectively managing life stressors and/or anxiety

16. Chronic abuse of alcohol can result in serious multisystem impairments, including:

    A. Peripheral neuropathy

    B. Wernicke's encephalopathy

    C. Korsakoff's psychosis

    D. Cirrhosis of the liver

    E. All of the above

17. It is important that the nurse ensures a self-assessment (examination of attitudes, feelings, beliefs) prior to participating in any patient care activities, but especially in the treatment of individuals experiencing problems with alcohol and other substances. Attending to this will assist the nurse in:

    A. Setting limits

    B. Participating in multidisciplinary meetings

    C. Establishing a trusting and therapeutic relationship with the individual

    D. Addressing the patient's poor coping strategies

18. While assigned to the emergency room, a 28-year-old male is brought in with constricted pupils, semiconscious. His roommate tells you, "I came home and found George with a needle in his arm; he was slumped over in a chair. I called 911 right away." What medication would you expect to be ordered for administration based upon this data?

    A. Naloxone

    B. Librium

    C. Clonidine

    D. Thorazine

19. Primary prevention is an essential intervention strategy because it

    A. Focuses on inhibiting development of substance abuse problems.

    B. Is aimed at detecting the presence of substance abuse to facilitate interventions to disrupt progression of symptoms.

    C. Reduces the negative impact of an established problem through restoration of functioning and reducing related complications.

    D. Teaches self-responsibility and accountability.

20. In your role as the school nurse at the middle school, you are providing a class about substance abuse. In your discussion of inhalant abuse, you would offer the following information about the potential dangers of huffing:

    A. Acquiring of infectious diseases

    B. Experiencing flashbacks

    C. Physical and psychological dependency

    D. Possibility of death due to cardiac or respiratory depression

Matching

21. Addiction

22. Antagonistic effect

23. Tolerance

24. Withdrawal

25. Enabling

26. Tolerance

27. Flashback

28. Detoxification

29. Abuse

30. Intoxication

31. Ascites

32. Delirium

33. Blackout

34. Flushing

35. Codependence

36. Polysubstance abuse

37. Tapering

38. Dual diagnosis

39. Tremor

40. Overdose

A. The administration of decreasing dosages of a medication

B. The state of being beholden to a substance or behavior that is psychologically or physically habit-forming

C. To make able or give means, power to someone to pursue an activity

D. Accumulation of serous fluid in the peritoneal cavity, symptom of severe alcoholic hepatitis

E. Need for higher doses of a substance to achieve desired effect

F. Transitory recurrences of perceptual disturbance as a result of hallucinogenic use occurring in a drug-free state

G. Use of a drug to weaken or inhibit the effect of another drug

H. An unhealthy relationship where one person is psychologically dependent on an addicted individual

I. An excessive dosage

J. State of mental confusion characterized by anxiety, disorientation, hallucinations, delusions, and incoherent speech

K. Reddening of the face and neck resulting from increased blood flow—involved with enzymes associated in the metabolism of alcohol

L. An episode where an individual continues to function but will have no conscious awareness nor be able to recall the events

M. Use wrongly or incorrectly

N. Discontinuation of an addictive substance

O. Behavioral and physiological changes resulting from excessive use of a substance

P. Combination of both substance abuse and another psychiatric illness

Q. Ability to endure or resist the action of a drug

R. Treatment that assists one to overcome physical and psychological dependence on a substance

S. Involuntary shaking of the body or an extremity, trembling or quivering movement

T. Abuse of more than one substance at a time

Chapter 12 Answers

Multiple Choice

1. **D.** Patients with a BAC of 0.03 to 0.05 may exhibit a general sense of well-being; however, as the effects of alcohol progress, they experience growing difficulties in both motor functioning and thought processes. The level of 0.22 would include stupor, loss of understanding, impaired sensations, impaired gross motor skills, and decreased reaction times.

2. **D.** Alcohol withdrawal typically begins within 4 to 12 hours of cessation or reduction of heavy use of alcohol.

3. **B.** Collateral sources of information include others involved with the individual and provide objective data. Subjective data is information provided by the patient (individual); objective data is provided by others.

4. **A.** Physical needs always take precedence in patient care (refer to Maslow's Hierarchy of Needs). While each of the identified nursing interventions is appropriate, it is important to understand the concept of how to prioritize care.

5. **B.** Answer A is characteristics of alcohol intoxication. C is symptoms of caffeine intoxication, and D is signs of inhalant intoxication.

6. **D.** The best response is to inform the nurse manager. Once you have notified the appropriate supervisor, your legal and ethical responsibilities for facility reporting are met. If no action is taken, you should report up to the next level of supervision.

7. **B.** Naltrexone blocks the response of the brain to the "pleasure" of alcohol and narcotics, encouraging less use. It does not "cure" addiction, but it allows for better management of urges. Unlike disulfiram (Antabuse), naltrexone does not make you ill if you drink alcohol while using it. Nausea is the most common side effect of this medication. The others listed are included as well.

8. **B.** Denial is the failure to recognize the reality of a given situation. Suppression is a conscious exclusion of unacceptable thoughts and feelings from conscious awareness. Avoidance is the refusal to encounter situations, objects, or activities because of the representation of sexual or aggressive impulses and/or punishment of those impulses. Displacement is the ventilation of intense feelings toward individuals less threatening than the one who is the cause of the feelings.

9. **B.** Substance use disorders address issues of abuse and dependence, while substance-induced disorders focus on intoxication, delirium, withdrawal, and changes in mental states.

10. **C.** Acute withdrawal from alcohol is considered a medical emergency that requires close monitoring and prompt treatment. Withdrawal from marijuana or hallucinogens rarely occurs. Opioid withdrawal is physically uncomfortable but not life-threatening.

11. **C.** Methods of use for inhalants include huffing (the use of a substance-soaked rag over the mouth/nose to breath in) and bagging (the substance is put into a plastic or paper bag and inhaled).

12. **A.** Marinol is a Schedule III drug that is a synthetic version of delta–9-THC. Sinsemilla is marijuana from the seedless female hemp plant that has high THC levels.

13. **D.** The assessment of chemical impairment is an increasingly complex intervention due to the increase of polysubstance use. It is essential that the nursing assessment include exploring the use of the obvious substance (alcohol) and possible other substances.

14. **D.** In the last statement, the patient demonstrates knowledge deficit related to the common approach to substance treatment—abstinence (total avoidance of an activity)—by verbalizing her opinion that alcohol/drugs may be used if "self-control" is exhibited. While for some individuals controlled drinking is successful, those who are dependent on substances rarely experience success using this approach.

15. **D.** Ineffective coping skills are an underlying impairment for each of the characteristics identified.

16. **E.** A, B, and C are conditions that all result from deficiencies in the B vitamins, particularly thiamine. Peripheral neuropathy results in pain, burning, tingling, or prickly sensations of the extremities; Wernicke's encephalopathy includes paralysis of the ocular muscles, double vision, ataxia, somnolence, and stupor; and Korsakoff's psychosis is a syndrome of confusion, loss of recent memory, and confabulation. Cirrhosis of the liver results in widespread destruction of liver cells, replaced by fibrous tissue.

17. **C.** Trust is a basic component of the therapeutic relationship. Conveyance of an attitude of acceptance promotes dignity and self-worth and allows for the delivery of appropriate patient-centered care.

18. **A.** Naloxone (Narcan) is an opioid antagonist that reverses opioid toxicity. Chlordiazepoxide (Librium) is used in the treatment of alcohol withdrawal. Clonidine (Catapres) is used to suppress effects of withdrawal (nausea, vomiting, diarrhea). Chlorpromazine (Thorazine) is an antipsychotic.

19. **A.** Primary prevention targets avoidance of a disease, secondary prevention focuses on early detection to allow for halting progress, and tertiary prevention aims to improve the quality of life through reduction of complications. Unlike primary and secondary prevention, this level involves actual treatment of the disease.

20. **D.** As a CNS depressant, inhalants can result in respiratory or cardiac failure. Flashbacks are possible in the use of hallucinogens, infectious disease is associated more so with IV drug abuse, and while psychological dependence is a possibility with most substance abuse, physical dependency has not been associated with inhalants.

Matching

21.	B	31.	D
22.	G	32.	J
23.	Q	33.	M
24.	N	34.	K
25.	C	35.	H
26.	E	36.	T
27.	F	37.	A
28.	R	38.	P
29.	M	39.	S
30.	O	40.	I

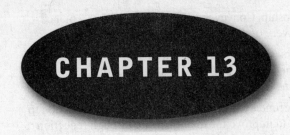

CHAPTER 13

Eating Disorders

13.1 Eating Disorders

Consumption of food serves many purposes. On a basic level, it provides the nutrients required for survival. It is also an integral component of socialization and is involved in various cultural activities. Though experiences with food can be joyful and celebratory, food consumption also provides those individuals experiencing lack of control in their lives a venue to manipulate a level of authority. Eating disorders are characterized by asymmetry in eating behaviors. The incidence of this health issue is increasing, with females more commonly identified as experiencing difficulties. The APA (2000) reports that there is an identified comorbidity with eating disorders and other psychiatric illnesses, especially major depressive disorder and dysthymia. Additionally, the report states that females of industrialized countries are at greatest risk due to accessibility of foods and perception that thinness is associated with beauty. For this review, this chapter will examine anorexia nervosa, bulimia nervosa, and binge-eating disorder.

Anorexia (see Box 13-1) and bulimia (see Box 13-2) are eating disorders occurring primarily in highly developed cultures, such as the United States, where there is great focus on beauty and youth. Obesity is the term used for those individuals who have a body mass index (BMI) of 30 or higher. Though obesity is not a classified psychiatric disorder in the *DSM-IV-TR*, it is a factor of the recently considered research criteria of binge-eating disorder (BED, see Box 13-3), where the individual eats copious amounts of food but does not engage in behaviors to dispose of the excess calories. See Figure 13-4 for data and statistics related to obesity in the United States.

Sociocultural Factors	Geographical location: Southeast, Appalachia, tribal lands in the West and Northern Plains; In relation to the occurrence of obesity in Caucasians (23% of population); African Americans 51% higher prevalence; Hispanic 21% higher prevalence
Psychosocial Factors	From a psychoanalytical perspective, obese individuals experience unresolved dependency/needs and remain in the oral stage of development.
Risk Factors	Genetics (amount and distribution of body fat storage), family history, age (physical changes, activity tolerance), cessation of addictive behaviors, social and economic issues (lack of access to exercise, knowledge deficit regarding food, lack of access to healthy foods, influence of social network)

Figure 13-1 Obesity statistics.

The BMI is a number that is calculated based upon an individual's height and weight used to determine a body's fatness and screen for weight categories identifying potential health problems. See Figure 13-2.

$$BMI = \frac{Weight\ (lbs.)}{Height\ (Inches)^2}$$

BMI	WEIGHT STATUS
Below 18.5	Underweight
18.5-24.9	Normal
25.0-29.9	Overweight
30.0-39.9	Obese
40 & Above	Morbidly Obese

Figure 13-2 BMI.

Obese individuals experience the following:

- Cardiovascular problems (CAD, hypertension, dyslipidemia)
- Osteoarthritis, cancer (endometrial, breast, and colon)
- Sleep disturbances
- Type 2 diabetes
- Liver and gallbladder disease
- Females only: greater incidence of gynecological problems (infertility, irregular menses)

13.2 Anorexia Nervosa

This disorder is characterized by an individual's refusal to maintain minimally normal body weight, a fear of gaining weight or becoming fat, a significantly disturbed perception of one's body shape or size, and a continuous inability or refusal to acknowledge the existence and seriousness of the problem. Though the actual definition of anorexia is the loss of appetite, individuals experiencing anorexia nervosa do experience physical symptoms of hunger. Individuals experiencing anorexia nervosa are characterized by restricting or binge-eating/purging types.

Those diagnosed with anorexia nervosa are centrally focused on weight loss and typically present with a body weight that is within 15 percent of the expected weight for their age and height. There is frequently a preoccupation with food-related activities, and many individuals participate in ritualistic approaches in their eating behaviors. Many individuals report anxiety and dislike/discomfort with their perception of self.

Some consequences of behaviors related to anorexia nervosa include the following:

- Amenorrhea
- Depressive symptoms
- Gastrointestinal issues (constipation)
- Hypothermia
- Lanugo
- Emaciation
- Cardiovascular effects (hypotension, bradycardia)
- Electrolyte imbalances

Prevalence

This disorder generally occurs pre- or post-puberty, though it can be experienced at any point throughout the lifespan. Occurrence is more common in adolescent and young adult females, regarded as due to societal pressure to achieve the "perfect" figure. Individuals experiencing eating disorders often relate to the sense of control offered through regulation of food consumption in relation to feelings of being out of control in other life aspects. It is estimated that 0.5 percent to 1 percent of females in the United States develop anorexia nervosa.

Etiology

Precise etiological considerations for this disorder are unknown, though there is evidence that both genetic and environmental factors are involved. The neurotransmitters norepinephrine, dopamine, and serotonin are thought to contribute in the etiology of this disorder. The obsessive dieting behaviors associated with this disorder support temperaments of perfectionism, neuroticism, esteem issues, and socialization impairments.

Box 13-1: Diagnostic Criteria for Anorexia Nervosa

A. Refusal to maintain body weight at or above a minimally normal weight for age and height (e.g., weight loss leading to maintenance of body weight less than 85 percent of that expected; or failure to make expected weight gain during a period of growth, leading to body weight less than 85 percent of that expected).

B. Intense fear of gaining weight or becoming fat, even though underweight.

C. Disturbance in the way in which one's body weight or shape is experienced, undue influence of body weight or shape on self-evaluation, or denial of the seriousness of the current low body weight.

D. In post-menarchal females, amenorrhea, or the absence of at least three consecutive menstrual cycles (a woman is considered to have amenorrhea if her periods occur only following hormone treatment, e.g., estrogen administration).

Specify type:

Restricting Type: During the current episode of anorexia nervosa, the person has not regularly engaged in binge-eating or purging behavior (e.g., self-induced vomiting or the misuse of laxatives, diuretics, or enemas).

Binge-Eating/Purging Type: During the current episode of anorexia nervosa, the person has regularly engaged in binge eating or purging behavior (e.g., self-induced vomiting or the misuse of laxatives, diuretics, or enemas).

American Psychiatric Association, with permission.

13.3 Bulimia Nervosa

This disorder occurs more frequently than anorexia nervosa and is typically referred to simply as bulimia. Food amounts consumed by those individuals experiencing this disorder are generally much larger than normally ingested and occur in a shorter than usual time period (binge eating). Bulimia is a behavior that the person strives to perform secretly, and the frequency is at least twice a week for three months. The behavior of binging is a coping response to emotional stress and typically results in feelings of guilt, remorse, and shame with subsequent behavior to negate the consumption through purging, fasting, or excessive exercise.

The majority of individuals experiencing bulimia nervosa present within the normal range of weight. Many individuals report anxiety and dislike/discomfort with their perception of self. Following are some consequences of purging behaviors:

- Dental complications (perimyolysis, caries, broken teeth)
- Electrolyte abnormalities (hypokalemia, hypomagnesemia)
- Metabolic acidosis
- Elevated uric acid
- Gastrointestinal difficulties (peptic ulcers, pancreatitis, constipation)

Prevalence

Bulimia nervosa typically occurs in either late adolescence or early adulthood (5 percent develop the disorder at an age older than 25). There is a higher incidence of affective illness in individuals experiencing bulimia nervosa (it is aligned with personality disorders—especially those characterized by rigid thinking and impulsivity). Recent research indicates that the occurrence is higher in Caucasians.

Etiology

As discussed in the review of anorexia nervosa, etiological indications are unspecified in eating disorders. There are many suppositions, including biologic (serotonin imbalance, genetics) and environmental (interpersonal and family relationships, sociocultural considerations, and self-perceptual implications) effects.

Box 13-2: Diagnostic Criteria for Bulimia Nervosa

A. Recurrent episodes of binge eating. An episode of binge eating is characterized by both of the following:

    1. Eating, in a discrete period of time, (e.g., within any 2-hour period) an amount of food that is definitely larger than most people would eat during a similar period of time and under similar circumstances.

    2. A sense of lack of control over eating during the episode (e.g., a feeling that one cannot stop eating or control what or how much one is eating).

B. Recurrent inappropriate compensatory behavior in order to prevent weight gain, such as self-induced vomiting, misuse of laxatives, diuretics, enemas, or other medications, fasting, or excessive exercise.

C. The binge eating and inappropriate compensatory behaviors both occur, on average, at least twice a week for 3 months.

D. Self-evaluation is unduly influenced by body shape and weight.

E. The disturbance does not occur exclusively during periods of anorexia nervosa.

Specify type:

Purging Type: During the current episode of bulimia nervosa, the person has regularly engaged in self-induced vomiting or the misuse of laxatives, diuretics, or enemas.

Nonpurging Type: During the current episode of bulimia nervosa, the person has used other inappropriate compensatory behaviors, such as fasting and excessive exercise, but has not regularly engaged in self-induced vomiting or the misuse of laxatives, diuretics, or enemas.

American Psychiatric Association, with permission.

13.4 Binge-Eating Disorder

Binge-eating disorder (see Box 13-3) is a recently identified eating problem where individuals consume significantly larger quantities of food (up to 20,000 calories in an episode). The frequency of these eating episodes is at least two per week, on average, for six months. It differs from bulimia nervosa as individuals who binge-eat do not participate in purging behaviors. Physical consequences of this disorder include the following:

- Hypertension
- Hyperlipidemia
- Osteoarthritis
- Type 2 diabetes
- Gallbladder and liver disease
- Cardiovascular disease

Prevalence

Binge-eating disorder affects about 2 percent of adult Americans (1 to 2 million persons). While dieting has been identified as a risk factor in both anorexia nervosa and bulimia nervosa, it does not have a clear correlation in binge-eating disorder. There is a connection with impulsivity, depression, and substance abuse, and the occurrence of sexual abuse has been reported by some individuals.

Etiology

As discussed previously, there is no specified etiology for eating disorders. While research continues to uncover the causation of eating disorders, there are some probable relations and risk factors. As discussed in Chapter 2, the hypothalamus controls the appetite. There is some evidence that the correct hunger messages are not being transmitted. Decreased levels of the neurotransmitter serotonin has been evidenced to have a part in compulsive eating—a characteristic in eating disorders. The presence of a depressive disorder, along with self-esteem issues and disturbed self-image, also contribute to possible causes of eating disorders. Societal pressures related to appearance and perception of beauty, along with peer relations, play a significant role in the development of an eating disorder.

Box 13-3: Research Criteria for Binge-Eating Disorder

A. Recurrent episodes of being eating. An episode of binge eating is characterized by both of the following:

    1. Eating, in a discrete period of time (e.g., within any 2-hour period), an amount of food that is definitely larger than most people would eat in a similar period of time under similar circumstances.

    2. A sense of lack of control over eating during the episode (e.g., a feeling that one cannot stop eating or control what or how much one is eating).

B. The binge-eating episodes are associated with three (or more) of the following:

    1. Eating much more rapidly than normal

    2. Eating until feeling uncomfortably full

    3. Eating large amounts of food when not feeling physically hungry

    4. Eating alone because of being embarrassed by how much one is eating

    5. Feeling disgusted with oneself, depressed, or very guilty after overeating

C. Marked distress regarding binge eating is present.

D. The binge eating occurs, on average, at last 2 days a week for 6 months.

Note: The method of determining frequency differs from that used for bulimia nervosa; future research should address whether the preferred method of setting a frequency threshold is counting the number of days on which binges occur or counting the number of episodes of binge eating.

E. The binge eating is not associated with the regular use of inappropriate compensatory behaviors (e.g., purging, fasting, excessive exercise) and does not occur exclusively during the course of anorexia nervosa or bulimia nervosa.

American Psychiatric Association, with permission.

13.5   Application of the Nursing Process

As with any of the other psychiatric illnesses discussed, it is essential that a nurse evaluate his or her own response to the diagnosis of an eating disorder. Nurses communicate more through nonverbal behaviors than verbal words, emphasizing the importance of ensuring the messages relayed to patients are supportive, objective, and therapeutic.

Assessment

Data is collected related to psychiatric issues, as well as substance abuse or dependence. Knowledge of risk factors will help to guide the clinical interview in assessing the individual's potential for eating disorders and facilitate a more in depth discussion. See Box 13-4 for an overview of signs and symptoms that may be assessed in the individual experiencing an eating disorder.

Box 13-4: Characteristics Assessed in Eating Disorders

Weight loss not explained by any other condition
Increased or decreased sleep
Irregularity of menses
Pallor
Discoloration of nails and skin (brittleness of nails)
Alopecia
Increased frequency and ease of bruising
Poor healing
Report of dizziness, fatigue
Fluid and electrolyte imbalance
Hypoglycemia
Lanugo, dry skin
Constipation
Difficulty chewing and swallowing
Dental caries
Expressed fear of weight gain
Distortion of body image
Report or presence of affective illness
History of sexual abuse
Loss of muscle mass

- The nursing history data is collected from the individual, from family, from significant others, from prior treatment documentation, and from others involved in the care of the person.
- A mental status assessment (discussed in Chapter 4) is conducted, ensuring assessment related to general appearance and motor behavior, mood and affect, thought process and content, sensorium and intellectual processes, judgment and insight, self-perception, role performance and interpersonal relationships, physiological concerns (nutritional status, system damage from eating disorder, etc.). Special consideration of the individual's eating habits, history and methodology of dieting, self-perception, values and beliefs associated with appearance and weight, interpersonal functioning, and socialization is recommended.
- Risk factors include the following:
  - Biological factors
    - Genetics
    - Age race/ethnicity
    - Gender
  - Psychosocial factors
    - Family relationships and influences
    - Occupation (athlete, gymnast, actor, model)
    - Cultural/religious beliefs
    - History of sexual abuse (focus on body image, dietary habits, etc.)
    - Life transitions

- ○ Environmental factors
  - – Peer pressure
  - – Media
  - – Community environment (peer pressure)
  - – Geographic location
- Physical assessment
  - ○ Laboratory values (hypokalemia, hypocalcemia, hypoglycemia, elevated BUN, hypothyroidism)
  - ○ Cardiovascular (hypotension, bradycardia, hypothermia)
  - ○ Skin, hair, teeth, bone, voice (dry, cool to touch, pallor, discoloration, lanugo, alopecia, hoarseness of voice, dental caries, difficulty chewing, Russell's sign)
  - ○ Gastrointestinal (constipation, esophagitis, esophageal tears, abdominal pain, increased gas, diarrhea)
  - ○ Reproductive (amenorrhea, decreased luteinizing and follicle-stimulating hormones)
  - ○ Musculoskeletal (loss of muscle mass, loss of subcutaneous fat, osteoporosis, osteoarthritis)
  - ○ Calculation of BMI
- Assessment tools—If it is suspected that an individual is experiencing an eating disorder, there are several assessment tools available to assist in gathering specific information related to the person's values, beliefs, and practices with regard to dietary habits.
  - ○ EAT: Eating Attitudes Test is one tool that helps to discern anorexia nervosa. This tool assesses concerns and beliefs commonly found in individuals with an eating disorder. While not diagnostic (diagnosis of an eating disorder is determined by an evaluation by a qualified clinician), as a learning tool it does highlight concerning behaviors/beliefs.
  - ○ Self-assessments that individuals can complete that assess thinking patterns and behavioral characteristics of individuals with an eating disorder.
  - ○ Body image assessments assess body image disturbances, a significant predictor in the development of eating disorders.

Diagnosis

An analysis of the data will assist in determining the priority problems and help to formulate the plan of care. See Figure 13-3 for common nursing diagnoses for the individual with an eating disorder.

CHARACTERISTICS	NURSING IMPAIRMENT
Presents under- or overweight, BMI <18,> 30, use of laxatives, severe calorie restriction, excessive exercising, fluid & electrolyte imbalance, difficulty with chewing r/t dental problems	Imbalanced nutrition: Less than/More than Body requirement Deficient fluid volume (risk for or actual) Risk for infection
Presents slow, lethargic, delayed response, decisional conflicts, occupational or school failure, withdrawal from peers, secretive eating, sleep disturbances, abdominal discomfort, esophageal tears, compulsive behaviors	Fatigue Pain Ineffective individual coping Social isolation
Expressed feelings of helplessness, hopelessness. Feelings of worthlessness, inability to control impulses mood lability, dislike of self	Anxiety (moderate to severe) Chronic low self-esteem
Envisions self as obese, obsessed with food and weight loss, unrealistic fear of weight gain, limited insight and poor judgment about health status, feel that others are sabotaging weight loss efforts, not receptive to patient education regarding health status affects of eating disorder	Ineffective denial Disturbed body image Knowledge deficit
Family enmeshment, unclear familiar boundaries, inattention to illness, exacerbation of individual's symptoms due to family stress, changes in availability of support, roles	Ineffective family coping Disturbed family process Knowledge deficit

Figure 13-3 Nursing diagnoses in eating disorders.

Planning/Implementation

This phase of the nursing process is directed by the assessment data collected and diagnostic statement in the formulation of the patient-centered goal and selection of appropriate nursing actions focused on prevention, reduction, or elimination of the patient's health problems (nursing impairments). The level of care provided is determined by the presentation of the individual at the time of the assessment. Inpatient hospitalization is required in the following cases:

- If the eating disorder has resulted in acute physical/medical problems that may be life threatening (weight loss over 30 percent in six months, inability to gain weight in outpatient treatment, cardiovascular complications, acute electrolyte imbalances, etc.)
- If the individual has reached an acute level of psychiatric crisis (severe depression, suicidal tendencies, self-mutilation/injurious behaviors, extreme abuse of laxatives, diuretics, etc.).
- If the family has reached the stage of crisis and inability to manage the situation. Treatment is provided on an inpatient and outpatient basis due to the chronicity of the disorders.

Identification of appropriate goals requires participation from both the patient and significant others. The focus of inpatient treatment is to restore body weight and address acute complications (electrolyte imbalances, cardiac irregularities, etc.). Once the individual is medically stabilized, the treatment centers on addressing the causes of the eating disorder, typically occurring on an outpatient basis. Regardless of the treatment setting, the nurse's role is to select appropriate nursing interventions to address specific problems identified for the patient experiencing substance abuse. See Figure 13-4 for an example of a plan of care. Priority interventions include the following:

- Establish therapeutic relationship (building trust is an essential component to care).
- Address physiologic needs of the patient.
- Address safety needs (initiation of observational status for suicidal tendencies /self-injurious behaviors).
- Establish nutritional eating patterns (work collaboratively with all disciplines involved in the care of the patient).
- Monitor eating habits (I&O); observation afterward to reduce purging.
- Monitor weights (patient should be weighed in fewest possible clothes to prevent secreting extra weight—no pockets, etc.)
- Encourage verbalization related to fear of weight gain and loss of control; assist in identifying correlation of feelings of self and eating behaviors.
- Teach adaptive coping skills to increase feelings of control and reduce anxiety.
- Encourage and allow active participation in treatment planning to increase self-esteem.
- Pharmacological interventions may include the use of antidepressants (see Chapter 11) in anorexia nervosa.

Evaluation

The fifth phase of the nursing process is evaluation. In this stage, a reassessment is done to determine if the nursing interventions selected were effective in assisting the patient to meet the objectives of care. It is during this phase of care that a determination will be made for nursing actions to end, continue, or be revised. The evaluation of care is continuous and occurs at various times during the care period. Evaluation while intervening, or shortly afterward, allows for immediate adjustment in care during specific intervals during the patient's hospitalization (or other care setting). This enables assessment in progress toward goals. The evaluation of care is discontinued only when the patient had successfully achieved the goal established or is terminated from nursing care.

Following are some of the outcomes that should be revisited:

- Has the patient been able to establish an adequate nutritional eating pattern?
- Is the patient free from signs and symptoms of malnutrition and dehydration?

NURSING IMPAIRMENT	NURSING INTERVENTION
Imbalanced nutrition: less than body requirements	1. If patient is severely malnourished, or refusing nutrition it may be required that tube feedings be instituted. At each feeding, offer opportunity to take nutrients by mouth, if tube feeding is necessary-approach in a nonjudgmental and nonpunitive manner 2. After feedings, monitor to reduce purging 3. Monitor vital signs until stable, repeat EKG and laboratory tests (electrolytes, acid-base balance, liver enzymes, albumin, etc.) until stable 4. Weigh weekly or biweekly—same time of the day. Best practice is before meals, after voiding, in minimal clothing (decreases ability to manipulate weight) 5. Establish a contract addressing treatment goals 6. Once tube feedings are no longer required, encourage meals to be eaten in the community area, monitor to ensure food is not thrown away or hidden, observe after meals to prevent purging. 7. Monitor elimination patterns 8. Use of privilege system to encourage compliance and weight gain.
Disturbed body image	1. Establish therapeutic relationship, conveying a positive, caring attitude 2. Provide facts regarding patient's weight and the impact on health status in a nonjudgmental and nonconfrontative manner 3. Acknowledge the perception of self of the patient. 4. Encourage expression of feelings through use of therapeutic communication techniques. 5. Encourage expression of self, eating, exercise to correct misconceptions and help clarify and reinforce a more realistic self-appraisal 6. Encourage identification of positive physical attributes 7. Use behavior modification strategies 8. Encourage participation in groups to foster insight and group support

Figure 13-4 Nursing plan for eating disorders.

- Has the patient been able to gain 2 to 3 lbs. per week during hospitalization?
- Has the patient been able to eliminate the use of compensatory behaviors (laxative, diuretics, excessive exercise, caloric limitation)?
- Has the patient been able to identify a positive physical attribute?
- Is the patient able to report a more realistic perception of and increased feeling of comfort with body image?
- Is the patient able to engage in discussion how maladaptive eating behaviors were used to exercise control in life events?

Chapter 13 Questions

Multiple Choice

Scenario: Allison is an 18-year-old female admitted to your unit with a diagnosis of anorexia nervosa. She is 67 inches tall and weighs 115 lbs. Her vital signs are BP: 98/60, P: 58, T: 97.2, R: 14. She reports that she has not had her period in over six months, and complains of feeling fatigued. Laboratory results indicate the following: K+: 3.0. She does admit to inducing vomiting after eating to "keep my weight down."

Questions 1 to 4 apply to the above scenario. Select the answer that is most appropriate.

1. What is your priority nursing action?

   A. Complete the nursing assessment and assign Allison to her room.

   B. Notify the doctor of the laboratory results.

    C. Place Allison on a strict observational status.

    D. Assess Allison for suicidal ideations.

2. What is Allison's BMI?

    A. 18

    B. 19.5

    C. 2.0

    D. 25

3. You are assigned to observe Allison during her evening meal. She states, "I don't know why you have to stare at me while I eat. Don't you trust me?" Your best response would be

    A. "If you could be trusted to eat properly, you wouldn't need to be admitted to the hospital."

    B. "It is not a matter of trust; it's my assignment."

    C. "I understand that it is uncomfortable for you to have someone watching you eat. The reason that I am watching you to monitor what you eat is because we recognize that your behaviors are difficult to stop and we want to offer you support."

    D. "You're right. I'll wait until you do something that warrants such close observation."

4. An appropriate actual nursing diagnosis for Allison is

    A. Altered thought process as evidenced by disturbed perception of self

    B. Anorexia nervosa related to fear of being overweight

    C. Electrolyte imbalance as evidenced by hypokalemia

    D. Imbalanced nutrition: less than body requirements related to self-induced vomiting as evidenced by patient stating, "I vomit to keep my weight down."

5. With the diagnosis of anorexia nervosa, you would expect to see these symptoms:

    A. Normal body weight, recurrent episodes of binge-eating, expressed feeling of loss of control over eating pattern

    B. Refusal to maintain body weight, expressed fear of weight gain, amenorrhea, bradycardia

    C. Loss of dental arch, dental caries and erosions, consuming large quantities of food in a short period of time and then purging

    D. Above-average body weight, BMI of 29, hyperlipidemia, osteoarthritis

6. In providing care for your patient diagnosed with bulimia nervosa, you acknowledge an understanding that the patient experiences feelings of shame and guilt over the loss of control related to bingeing and purging. This type of disorder is referred to as:

    A. Ego syntonic

    B. Ego dystonic

    C. Ego distorting

    D. Ego enhancing

7. An initial treatment priority in hospitalization of an individual experiencing anorexia nervosa is to

    A. Assist in identifying self-image.

    B. Identify implication of family processes.

    C. Promote autonomy and independence in eating patterns.

    D. Initiate a refeeding program.

8. Within four days of instituting a refeeding program, your patient experiences fluid and electrolyte disorder, with neurologic, pulmonary, cardiac, neuromuscular, and hematologic complications. This phenomenon is referred to as:

    A. Refueling syndrome

    B. Refeeding syndrome

    C. Silage syndrome

    D. Pasturage syndrome

9. Which of the following patients with an eating disorder is most likely to develop hypokalemia?

    A. A patient with nonpurging bulimia nervosa

    B. A patient with anorexia nervosa: restricting type

    C. A patient with anorexia nervosa: binge-eating/purging type

    D. A patient diagnosed with an eating disorder at risk for hyponatremia

10. A 15-year-old, diagnosed with anorexia nervosa, is admitted to your unit. During the admission procedure, you discover a bottle of pills she describes as "Tums." She reports that she has been experiencing stomach pains. The best response would be

    A. "No one can use their own medication on the unit without the pharmacy's approval."

    B. "Tell me more about the stomach problem you have been having."

    C. "Some people take pills to help them lose weight."

    D. "What other drugs do you use?"

11. Behavior modification is a nursing intervention used in the care of a patient experiencing an eating disorder. Which of the following is an example of behavior modification?

    A. Ensuring the patient gets balanced, high-protein, high-calorie meals and snacks each day

    B. Encouraging participation in unit groups to facilitate expression of feelings

    C. Encouraging expression of anger through music and exercise

    D. Not allowing off-ward privileges until the patient gains 3 lbs.

12. Which of the following statements is true?

    A. Eating disorders were first diagnosed in the Middle Ages.

    B. The occurrence of eating disorders is equal in men and women.

    C. Eating disorders are major health problems in only the United States and Canada.

    D. Cultures where beauty is linked to thinness have an increased risk for eating disorders.

13. The following goals are all appropriate for the patient diagnosed with anorexia nervosa. Which is not a priority?

    A. The patient will gain no more than 1 to 2 lbs. in the first week of refeeding.

    B. The patient will have a correction of electrolytes.

    C. The patient will develop a nurse–patient contract supporting collaboration and demonstrating personal responsibility toward treatment.

    D. The patient will be able to verbalize two positive attributes of self.

14. During your shift in the emergency room, a teenage girl is brought in to be evaluated for an eating disorder. Which of the following would suggest bulimia nervosa?

    A. Unrealistic view of her physical self

    B. Refusal to maintain body weight over a minimum normal for age and height

C. Amenorrhea

D. Recurrent inappropriate compensatory behavior to prevent weight gain

15. Your patient has been diagnosed with bulimia nervosa. Together you established a goal that she would be able to employ the technique of self-monitoring. Which of the following nursing actions would be the most advantageous for this patient?

A. Encourage the patient to use distraction to minimize feelings and impulsivity surrounding food.

B. Provide patient education related to the nutritional composition of favorite foods.

C. Encourage the use of a journal to record awareness of responses and experiences related to food.

D. Assist the patient in identifying the best foods to eat.

16. Which of the following medications would you expect the nurse practitioner to prescribe for your patient diagnosed with anorexia nervosa?

A. Phenelzine (Nardil)

B. Ativan (Lorazepam)

C. Orlistat (Xenical)

D. Fluoxetine (Prozac)

17. Which of the following statements is true?

A. Obesity is not classified as a psychiatric disorder in the *DSM-IV-TR*.

B. Obesity is classified in the *DMS-IV-TR* as of 2008.

C. Obesity is not considered a psychiatric disorder; it is considered a life choice.

D. Individuals who are obese have a BMI between 25 to 29.

18. An appropriate nursing intervention for the patient with a nursing diagnosis of ineffective denial is

A. Assist the patient in developing a more realistic perception of body image.

B. Avoid arguing or bargaining with the patient if the patient is resistant to treatment.

C. Discuss with the patient feelings and emotions related to food.

D. Practice and role play with the patient alternative responses to stressors.

19. The milieu of an inpatient eating disorder unit has as primary goals:

A. Reduce overwhelming environmental stimuli and prevent destruction of property.

B. Supervised environment for medication stabilization and protection from suicidal behaviors.

C. Interruption of binge-eating cycle and prevention of disordered eating behaviors.

D. Safety, resources for resolving conflicts, and opportunities to learn social and vocational skills.

20. Health teaching for an individual diagnosed with an eating disorder should include

A. Relaxation techniques

B. Physical and emotional ramifications of binge-eating and purging

C. The disease process and meal planning

D. All of the above

E. B and C

Matching

21. Amenorrhea	**A.** A less than normal amount of hair on the head or body
22. Binging	**B.** A bluish discoloration of the extremities resulting from inadequate oxygenation
23. Emaciated	**C.** How an individual perceives his or her body
24. Alexithymia	**D.** To entangle, involve
25. Satiety	**E.** Satisfaction of hunger
26. Body image	**F.** Consumption of a large amount of food in a relatively short period of time
27. Enmeshment	**G.** A covering of fine, soft hair
28. Lanugo	**H.** Actuated or swayed by emotions
29. Body mass index	**I.** Presence of abrasions, scars, or calluses on the back of the hand resulting from self-induced vomiting
30. Russell's sign	**J.** Cavity formation in teeth, complication of purging behaviors
31. Anorexia	**K.** Difficulty in experiencing, expressing, and describing emotional responses
32. Pallor	**L.** Low potassium
33. Alopecia	**M.** Actions taken to correct binge eating (excessive exercise, use of laxatives, purging, fasting, etc.)
34. Dental caries	**N.** Absences of menses
35. Hypotrichosis	**O.** Heart rate lower than 60 bpm
36. Bradycardia	**P.** Unusual or extreme paleness
37. Hypokalemia	**Q.** Measure of body fat that is the ratio of body weight to height squared.
38. Impulsivity	**R.** Loss of hair
39. Acrocyanosis	**S.** Presenting as abnormally thin or lean
40. Compensatory behavior	**T.** Loss of appetite, inability to eat

Chapter 13 Answers

1. **B.** Normal value for potassium is 3.5 to 5.0 mEq/L. Fatigue can be a symptom of hypokalemia. Treatment can be oral supplements, but this must be addressed to prevent complications. While each of the other responses may be appropriate, correction of Allison's potassium level is a priority.

2. **A.** The formula to assess an individual's BMI is weight divided by height (squared).

3. **C.** It is important to acknowledge feelings experienced by the patient and offer rationale for the nursing intervention. Uncomfortable feelings associated with others watching eating habits as well as the inability to discard food may cause an increase in anxiety for the patient.

4. **D.** The diagnostic statement for an actual nursing diagnosis is composed of three components: impairment, etiology, and current signs and symptoms (A is wrong format). The nursing problem/impairment must be derived from the NANDA approved list (B is not an approved NANDA impairment). Medical diagnoses are not included in the nursing diagnosis (C contains a medical diagnosis).

5. **B.** The response under A and C depicts symptoms of bulimia nervosa, and D evidences obesity.

6. **B.** Ego dystonic disorders are ones in which the patient feels that his or her symptoms or behaviors are not aligned with self-image and subsequently experiences distress. Ego distorting and ego enhancing are strategies that do not apply to this situation. An ego syntonic disorder evidences congruency between symptoms/behaviors and self-image.

7. **D.** A priority goal is to reestablish near normal body weight to prevent physiologic complications of anorexia nervosa. While the other interventions may be appropriate, the priority intervention is to assist the patient in weight gaining.

8. **B.** Refeeding syndrome occurs when aggressive support measures are taken with significantly malnourished individuals. It can occur with either enteral or parenteral feedings, typically within four days of initiating the refeeding program. Patients experience fluid and electrolyte disturbances, along with neurologic, pulmonary, cardiac, neuromuscular, and hematologic complications. To reduce the chance of occurrence, nutrition support should be introduced slowly in conjunction with vitamins and minerals. Monitoring of organ functioning and fluid and electrolyte balance should be done daily initially and then less often as the patient evidences stabilization.

9. **C.** Hypokalemia is not commonly caused by poor dietary intake; rather, it is a result of excessive loss (vomiting, laxative use). Neither patient A nor B participate in purging. Risk for hyponatremia is not an indication in hypokalemia.

10. **B.** The primary focus should be the pain experienced by the patient. More information is required to determine if an acute medical condition exists. While it may be prudent to assess use of substances, that is not the priority.

11. **D.** Behavior modification strategies involve using positive and negative rewards for behaviors. The goal is weight gain. Therefore, when the patient achieves the desired goal, a privilege is awarded.

12. **D.** It was the 1960s when anorexia nervosa was established as an eating disorder. More than 90 percent of cases of anorexia nervosa and bulimia occur in females. Though more common in the industrialized countries, as access to technology becomes more available, less developed countries are demonstrating the occurrence of eating disorders, and the perception of beauty in relation to body shape/thinness in conjunction with the temperament (sensitive to perceptions of others, in need of approval, perception of self-worth in relation to physical appearance) of an individual at risk for eating disorders are ingredients in the formula for the etiology of the disorder.

13. **D.** Priority is determined using Maslow's Hierarchy of Needs. Physical needs take precedence, though addressing the individual's perception of physical self is an appropriate objective.

14. **D.** Answers A, B, and C are characteristics of anorexia nervosa.

15. **C.** Self-monitoring is a cognitive-behavioral approach that serves to increase awareness about one's behavior and offers a means to regain control other than through foods. Many times it is easier for the individual to write feelings instead of verbalizing them, and it allows identification of the association between emotional responses and eating behaviors.

16. **D.** SSRI antidepressants (Prozac) have been successful in the treatment of patients diagnosed with anorexia nervosa. MAOI antidepressants (Nardil), antianxiety (Ativan), and medication to treat obesity (Xenical) would not be indicated for anorexia nervosa.

17. **A.** Obesity is not classified in the *DSM-IV-TR*. Etiological implications of obesity include genetics, physiological factors, and lifestyle factors. Obesity is defined as a BMI of 30 or greater.

18. **B.** An individual who uses denial and has a weakened ego uses manipulation to try to gain control of situations. Arguing, bargaining, or defending your position will result in a greater defensive response by the patient. Response A is appropriate for a patient with disturbed body image, C is appropriate for the patient diagnosed with imbalanced nutrition: more/less than body requirement, and D for the patient diagnosed with ineffective coping.

19. **C.** Milieu varies dependent upon the patient population of the unit. Answer A depicts the purpose of the milieu for patients placed in seclusion, B for those diagnosed with major depression, and C for those individuals diagnosed with schizophrenia.

20. **D.** Health teaching would include all of the components identified. Provision of this information provides the groundwork for the patient to build upon the information as treatment progresses.

Matching

21. N
22. F
23. S
24. K
25. E
26. C
27. D
28. G
29. Q
30. I

31. T
32. P
33. R
34. J
35. A
36. O
37. L
38. H
39. B
40. M

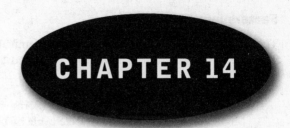

CHAPTER 14

Sleeping Disorders

14.1   Sleep

Sleep is defined as an unconscious state that allows for rest of voluntary bodily functions. It is an essential need for maintaining health, especially with regard to learning and memory, metabolism and weight, safety, mood, cardiovascular health, and disease prevention. Sleep deprivation (insufficient amount of sleep) results in impairments in attention and concentration, lowering of body temperature, decrease in the immune system (WBC lowers), decrease in the release of HGH (human growth hormone), and lethargy, to name just a few effects. Understanding the basic principles of sleep requires review of the stages of sleep:

- *Stage I*—Transitional period between wakefulness and sleep, light sleep. Initial muscle relaxation, occurs just as one falls asleep and intermittently throughout the sleep cycle; person is easily aroused. Accounts for 10 percent of sleep time.

- *Stage II*—Cessation of eye movement, slowing of brainwaves. Accounts for 40 to 50 percent of sleep time.

- *Stages III and IV*—Referred to as deep sleep, no eye or muscle movement occurs. Delta waves appear with interspersed faster brain waves; stage IV is primarily delta waves. The differentiation between these two stages is the amount of delta activity. Difficult to arouse the individual; upon awakening, he or she experiences disorientation. Accounts for 20 percent of sleep time.

- *Rapid Eye Movement Sleep (REM)*—This level of sleep follows non-REM sleep. There is significant eye movement, heart rate and breathing increase and may be irregular, and increase in blood pressure occurs. Brain activity is increased, muscles are essentially paralyzed. Infants can spend up to 50% of their sleep in the REM stage of sleep, and adults spend only about 20% in REM.

Sleep requirements by age:

- Infants (birth to 1 year): 14 to 16 hours per day
- Children (1 year to 12 years): 10 to 14 hours per day
- Adolescent (13 years to 18 years): 8 to 9 hours per day
- Adults (18 years and older): 8 to 10 hours per day
  Special note:
  - Geriatric population: Though appearance is increased time in bed, there is more light sleep occurring and for shorter periods of time as one ages.

Factors Influencing Sleep

The circadian rhythm is the cycle in the biochemical, physiological, or behavioral processes of a living entity. The sleep and wakefulness rhythm is regulated by the hypothalamus but can be influenced by external stimulus:

- *Cycle of light and dark*—Melatonin (hormone produced by the body mostly at night, in response to light that regulates the sleep/wake cycle by causing drowsiness and lowering the body temperature).
- *Body temperature*—Increases during wakefulness, decreases during sleep.
- *Daily routines*—Shift work, meal times, travel (crossing time zones).
- *Substances*—Caffeine consumption, stimulants, nicotine, alcohol, other drugs.

The National Sleep Foundation's Sleep in America Polls

Per the National Sleep Foundation's 2008 (2009) Sleep in America Poll, shift workers are more likely to

- Spend in bed/sleep less than six hours on workdays.
- Have been told they have sleep apnea.
- Have driven while drowsy at least once a month for the past year.
- Take 30 minutes or more to fall asleep; use a sleep aid at least three times/week.
- Experience daytime drowsiness that interferes in daily activities

  Types of sleep aids used:

  - Alcohol, beer, or wine
  - Over-the-counter medications
  - Prescription sleep medications
  - Alternative therapies or herbal supplements

The National Sleep Foundation's 2005 poll evidenced that

- 75 percent of adults in the United States report sleep disturbances a few nights or more per week over the past year.
- Two-thirds of children experience sleep disturbances at least a few times a week.
- Prevalence increases up until age 64 of sleep disturbances, then begins to decrease.
- Indirect costs of insomnia to the national health care bill are at least $28 billion dollars.

Two major types of *DSM-IV-TR* sleep disorders are *dyssomnias* (trouble getting enough sleep, timing of sleep, and impairments in the quality of sleep) and *parasomnias* (abnormal behavioral and physiological events occurring during sleep). Common sleep disturbance disorders are *insomnia, hypersomnia, parasomnias,* and *circadian rhythm sleep disorders.*

14.2   Insomnia

Insomnia is a sleep disturbance characterized by difficulty falling asleep or staying asleep. The level of sleep disturbance (mild to severe) is determined by the frequency and duration of symptoms.

- *Chronic insomnia*—Three times per week, more than one month
- *Acute insomnia*—Occurrence less than one month

Insomnia can result from medical conditions, medications, sleep disorders, and use of substances. The most common type of insomnia is referred to as secondary, or comorbid insomnia. Primary insomnia occurs independent of precipitants. Certain life stressors may result in the occurrence of acute insomnia. Individuals experiencing insomnia typically report excessive daytime lethargy, feelings of anxiety, depression, or irritability. They also identify decreased attention and concentration abilities; memory difficulties; and subsequent impairments in social, occupational, and school functioning.

Prevalence

Primary insomnia affects more women than men and begins in middle adulthood, increasing in occurrence with age.

14.3 Hypersomnia

Also referred to as somnolence, hypersomnia is characterized by an individual who experiences abnormal increases in sleepiness. Primary hypersomnia is considered when the individual has no other cause for the excessive sleepiness (sleep disorder narcolepsy, sleep apnea, sleep deprivation, being overweight, substance abuse, neurological injury or disease, prescription medication).

Prevalence

Usually begins later in adolescence to early adulthood; occurrence is more common in men than women.

14.4 Narcolepsy

This disorder, similar to hypersomnia, is a neurological disorder that affects the control of an individual's sleep and wakefulness. Individuals experience an increase in daytime sleepiness and experience intermittent, uncontrollable episodes of falling asleep. Symptoms of narcolepsy include the following:

- Excessive daytime sleepiness (EDS)
- Cataplexy
- Hallucinations
- Sleep paralysis

Prevalence

Onset of narcolepsy is adolescence to early adulthood, and occurrence is similar in males and females.

14.5 Parasomnias

These disruptive sleep disorders occur during arousal from REM sleep or partial arousals from non-REM sleep.

- *Nightmares*—Frightening dreams that lead to awakenings from sleep. A nightmare disorder is diagnosed when there is a repeated occurrence, and a subsequent impairment in social or occupational functioning. Occurs during REM sleep.
- *Sleep terror*—Also referred to as "night terrors," the individual abruptly awakens from sleep in a terrified state. Though appearing awake, there is confusion and inability to communicate. The individual is difficult to awaken and is nonresponsive to verbal commands. Typically, upon waking in the morning, the individual has amnesia regarding the incident. There is a danger of injury related to movement with this disorder, and it is closely associated with sleepwalking.

Prevalence

From 1 to 6 percent of children will experience sleep terror. It is more common in boys, and it will usually resolve spontaneously in adolescence.

- *Sleepwalking*—Employment of physical activities when the individual is asleep (walking, dressing, using the bathroom, talking, etc.). Often occurs during non-REM sleep (stages III and IV) early in the night, and during REM sleep early in the morning. Most commonly occurs between the ages of 8 and 12, but it is not limited to those ages. Length of occurrence can be up to 30 or so minutes.

Prevalence

From 1 to 5 percent of children will experience sleep walking. It resolves during adolescence with no treatment.

14.6 Circadian Rhythm Disorders

Extrinsic Type:

- Shift work
- Jet lag

Intrinsic Type:

- *Delayed sleep phase syndrome*—Later-than-normal timing of sleep, alertness during the middle of the night.
- *Advanced sleep phase syndrome*—Difficulty with wakefulness in the evening, later sleep in the morning.
- *Non–24-hour sleep-wake syndrome*—Occurrence of sleep is later each day; peak alertness moves around the clock as well.
- *Irregular sleep pattern*—Sleeping occurs irregularly (more than once per 24-hour period); frequent night waking occurs and daytime naps are taken.

Prevalence

The prevalence of circadian rhythm sleep disorders is not known.

14.7 Influencing Factors in Diagnosis of Sleep Disorders

There are multiple precipitating factors influencing the occurrence of sleep disorders. Considerations include the following:

- The normal aging process
- Presence of medical conditions
- Familiar patterns of sleep disorders
- Presence of psychiatric disorders
- Environmental changes

14.8 Application of the Nursing Process

Assessment

Data is collected related to the presence of medical and/or psychiatric issues, as well as substance abuse or dependence. Knowledge of risk factors will help to guide the clinician during the interview in assessing the individual's potential for sleep disorders and facilitate a more in-depth discussion. See Box 14-1 for an overview of signs and symptoms that may be assessed in the individual experiencing an sleep disorder.

Box 14-1: Characteristics Assessed in Sleep Disorders

General Symptoms:

- Increased irritability
- Difficulty staying awake when sitting still and engaging in sedentary activities
- Feel excessively tired or falling asleep while driving
- Impaired concentration
- Impaired attention
- Decreased reaction time
- Appearance of tiredness
- Increased emotionality
- Need for a nap during the day
- Use of caffeinated beverages for a "boost" most every day
- Frequent yawning

- The nursing history data is collected from the individual, from family, from significant others, from prior treatment documentation, and from others involved in the care of the person.
- A mental status assessment (discussed in Chapter 4) is conducted, ensuring assessment-related general appearance and motor behavior, mood and affect, thought process and content, sensorium and intellectual processes, judgment and insight, self-perception, role performance and interpersonal relationships, and physiological concerns from sleep disturbance. Special consideration of the individual's sleep hygiene, history and methodology of facilitating sleep, and interpersonal functioning and socialization is recommended with a focus on assessing for anxiety, depression, and so on.
- Risk factors include the following:
  - Biological factors
    - Genetics
    - Age, race/ethnicity—Insomnia increases with age; parasomnias occur most frequently in late adolescence and early adulthood.
    - Gender—Insomnia is more common in women, and hypersomnia in men.
  - Psychosocial factors
    - Occupation—Shift work can result in disturbed sleep pattern.
    - Cultural/religious beliefs—Cultural beliefs and practices related to sleep behaviors should be considered in the assessment.
    - Life transitions—Ensure assessment of recent life stressors.
  - Environmental factors
    - Change in time zones
    - Conduciveness for rest (temperature, noise, darkness, etc.)
- Physical assessment
  - Electroencephalograph (EEG)—Monitors leg movements and brain activity
  - Electrooculograph (EOG)—Monitors eye movement
  - Electromyography (EMG)—Monitors muscle movement
  - Assess for the presence of pain, sleep apnea syndrome, restless leg syndrome
  - Assess for abuse of/withdrawal from substances
  - Presence of metabolic or endocrine disorders, any other medical illness

- Assessment tools—If you suspect that an individual is experiencing a sleep disorder, there are several assessment tools available to assist you in gathering specific information related to the person's values, beliefs, and practices with regard to sleep hygiene.

Diagnosis

As discussed previously, the nursing diagnosis is formulated by analysis of the data (subjective and objective) collected during the assessment phase. In conjunction with knowledge of factors influencing the occurrence of sleep disorders, the nurse will be able to determine appropriate problems or impairments. Priority nursing diagnoses for the individual experiencing sleep disorders include the following:

- Disturbed sleep pattern
- Risk for injury
- Fatigue
- Sleep deprivation

Planning/Implementation

In the planning and implementation phase, the assessment data and diagnostic statements direct the formulation of the patient-centered goals and the designing of appropriate nursing actions to prevent, reduce, or eliminate the individual's health problem (nursing impairment). See Figure 14-1 for an example of a nursing care plan for a patient experiencing a sleep disorder. Priority interventions include the following:

- Establish a therapeutic relationship (building trust is an essential component to care).
- Address the physiologic needs of the patient.

NURSING DIAGNOSIS	NURSING INTERVENTION
Disturbed sleep pattern	1. Active listening to encourage verbalization of concerns preventing sleep 2. Nursing care is planned to prevent interruption of sleep 3. Provide sleep inducing measures (warm shower or bath before sleep, comfortable sleeping area and supports (pillows), encouragement of milk and/or high-protein snack (L-tryptophan is a sleep promoter) 4. Provide an environment conducive for sleep (quiet, comfort, darkness, safety) 5. Administration of prescribed medication 6. Assess and encourage appropriate sleep-wake pattern (awake during the day, sleep at night, etc.) 7. Assess the patient's perception of quality of sleep 8. Patient education r/t relation techniques, avoidance of stimulants, decreasing hydration prior to sleep, etc.
Risk for injury	1. Use of side rails to prevent fall of patient from bed due to night terrors, nightmares) 2. Maintain bed in a low position for those individuals who sleepwalk 3. Use of monitoring equipment that will alert caretaker/staff that individual has exited the bed to provide closer supervision 4. Patient education to ensure use of a night light and consideration in furniture positioning to promote safety for the patient who awakens at night 5. Administration of prescribed medications 6. Encourage verbalization of frightening episodes, provide validation of fearfulness, and emphasize safety
Sleep deprivation	1. Assess sleep-wake history (consider work and activity schedules; history of sleeping problems, medications used, etc.) 2. Encourage patient to keep sleep-wake journal (bedtime, waking time, night awakenings, daytime sleep, recognized disturbance factors) 3. Assess presence of and level of anxiety 4. Patient education r/t relaxation techiques, avoidance of stimulants (caffeine, nicotine, etc.), sleep hygiene 5. Assess for presence of psychiatric or medical conditions 6. Encourage environment conducive for sleep (quiet, dark, comfortable)

Figure 14-1 Nursing care for sleep disorders.

- Address safety needs (side rails, night lights, closer observation to prevent risk for falls, etc.).
- Establish nutritional eating patterns (work collaboratively with all disciplines involved in the care of the patient); discuss effect of caffeine and alcohol on sleep.
- Encourage verbalization related to current life stressors.
- Teach adaptive coping skills to increase feelings of control and reduce anxiety related to disturbed sleep pattern.
- Encourage and allow active participation in treatment planning to increase compliance.
- Pharmacological interventions may include the use of sleep agents (see Chapter 11 for side effects of TCAs and MAOIs) in sleep disorders.

Medications are effective in the treatment of sleep disorders. The type of medication prescribed is dependent upon the specific type of disorder the individual is experiencing. When medications are used to assist the patient in meeting goals of care, it is essential that you incorporate standard nursing actions related to the administration of medications (assessment of knowledge, education as indicated, etc.). Refer to Figure 14-2 for an overview of medications commonly prescribed for sleep disorders and potential side effects.

Evaluation

In this phase of the nursing process, a reassessment is performed to determine the effectiveness of the selected nursing interventions in meeting the goals of care. This important aspect of nursing care determines if the nursing actions will be ended, continued, or revised. The evaluation of care is continuous and occurs at various times

CONDITION	MEDICATION	COMMON SIDE EFFECTS
Insomnia	CNS Depressants	headache
		dizziness
	Benzodiazepines	confusion
	1. flurazepam (Dalmane)	lethargy
	2. temazepam (Restoril)	unsteadiness in gait
	3. triazolam (Halcion)	
	Nonbenzodiazepines	
	1. zolpidem (Ambien)	
	2. zaleplon (Sonata)	
	3. eszopiclone (Lunesta)	

- sleep-driving, along with other less dangerous "complex sleep-related behaviors" (making phone calls, fixing and eating food, and having sex while still asleep) have been reported with use of sleep agents
- gradual discontinuation and tapering is recommended with long-term users to reduce risk of withdrawal symptoms and possible rebound insomnia

Hypersomnolence	CNS Stimulants	
	1. amphetamine	restlessness
	2. methamphetamine	irregular heart rhythms
	3. dextroamphetamine	tremors
	4. methylphenidate	headaches
	5. selegiline	loss of appetite
		psychosis and slowed growth rates
	Tricyclic Antidepressants (TCAs)	See Chapter 11: Mood Disorders
	Monoamine Oxidase Inhibitors (MAOIs)	
		nausea & vomiting
	Dopamine Agonists	dizziness/fainting
	1. Clonidine	orthosatitc hypotension
	2. Levadopa	confusion
	3. Bromocriptine	dyskinesias
	4. Amantadine	irregular heart rate

Figure 14-2 Pharmacological approaches.

during the care period. Evaluation while intervening, or shortly afterward, allows for immediate adjustment in care during specific intervals of the patient's hospitalization (or other care setting) to enable assessment in progress toward goals. The evaluation of care is discontinued only when the patient had successfully achieved the goal established or is terminated from nursing care. The evaluation of the selected nursing interventions employed with the individual experiencing a sleep disorder may include the following data:

- Has the individual remained free from injury?
- Is the individual able to engage in a discussion related to his or her experience with sleep disturbance and to identify possible precipitants?
- Is the individual able to incorporate appropriate sleep hygiene behaviors to promote sleep?
- Does the individual report an improvement in sleep quantity/quality?
- Is the individual observed to sleep the specified number of hours per night?
- Does the individual exhibit complications related to sleep deprivation (sleep apnea, nocturnal hypoxic episodes, etc.)?
- Is the individual able to return demonstration of relaxation techniques taught?
- Has the individual been able to make adjustments to daily activities to promote sleep (dietary changes, activity regulation, etc.)?

Chapter 14 Questions

Multiple Choice

1. Which of the following statements is true?

   A. When you sleep, both your body and brain shut down to rest and recover.

   B. Sleep is a state of unconsciousness, but the brain and body remain active and functioning.

   C. Older adults require less sleep than younger adults.

   D. Sleep deprivation does not result in any problems.

Scenario: A patient is admitted to your unit with the diagnosis of a sleep disorder. (The following questions are related to your understanding of sleep disorders and care that is required)

Questions 2 to 5 apply to the above scenario. Select the answer that is most appropriate.

2. You are aware that the reticular activating system (RAS) is

   A. An area of the brain responsible for regulating arousal and sleep-wake transition

   B. An area of the eye that is responsible to light regulation

   C. A network of neurotransmitters that induce sleep

   D. A complex hormonal system of the body

3. The RAS is located in the

   A. Cerebral cortex

   B. Hypothalamus

   C. Cerebellum

   D. Brain stem

4. This patient is diagnosed with insomnia. Which of the following is not a true statement about insomnia?

   A. Insomnia is a common sleep complaint.

   B. When insomnia lasts for longer than a month, it is referred to as "chronic."

   C. Two risk factors of insomnia may be age and gender.

   D. There is no treatment for insomnia.

5. During your nursing assessment, the patient informs you that she has been using Dalmane every night for the past seven months to get to sleep. She states that she wants to stop using the medication. The best response you could offer is

   A. "You couldn't possibly stop taking the medication after all this time. You will never get to sleep without it."

   B. "When you decide to stop, just don't take any more pills."

   C. "Keep taking the pill until you are ready to go on vacation. That way you'll be able to make up for any lost sleep."

   D. "I can understand that you want to not rely on medication for sleep. You should continue taking the medication, as directed by your doctor, but discuss with her your wish to stop and arrange a plan to taper the dose."

6. Upon graduation, you have accepted a position working at night at the local hospital. Which of the following actions will assist you the best in facilitating sleep during the day?

   A. Exercise immediately after work to make sure you are physically tired.

   B. Have a glass of wine to relax when you get home.

   C. Wear sleep mask and get room-darkening shades for your bedroom.

   D. Eat a big breakfast.

7. Your patient tells you that "I am a light sleeper. Once I wake up, I have a hard time getting back to sleep." Which of the following actions is appropriate?

   A. Encourage the patient to ask her family to bring in a white noise machine.

   B. Enforce the hospital's policy to decrease noise at night to minimize disturbance to the patients.

   C. Plan the patient's care between the hours of 10 p.m. and 6 a.m., as able.

   D. All of the above.

8. Your patient is prescribed zolpidem (Ambien) as a PRN for insomnia. It differs from benzodiazepine sedative-hypnotics because

   A. It does not reduce REM sleep durations or cause rebound insomnia when discontinued.

   B. It does reduce REM sleep durations and may cause rebound insomnia when discontinued.

   C. It is not considered a narcotic.

   D. It is the same as a benzodiazepine sedative-hypnotic.

Scenario: During your nursing assessment, Mr. Smith reports, "I have been having a hard time getting to sleep at night." As he speaks, he suppresses a yawn. He adds, "I recently applied for a promotion at work, I could really use the money. I find out next week if I get the position."

Considering the above information, answer questions 9 to 11. Select the answer that is most appropriate.

9. An appropriate actual nursing diagnosis for Mr. Smith would be

   A. Tiredness related to lack of sleep.

   B. Disturbed sleep pattern related to anxiety, as evidenced by the patient stating, "I have been having a hard time getting to sleep at night."

   C. Insomnia related to increased stress, as evidenced by the patient stating, "I recently applied for a promotion at work."

   D. Fatigue due to complaint of difficulty sleeping.

10. An appropriate nursing action for Mr. Smith would be

    A. Mr. Smith will be able to sleep, uninterrupted, for 5 to 8 hours per night within one week.

    B. Provide patient education related to reducing or eliminating use of caffeine, limiting fluid intake, increasing physical exercise during the day, and establishing a regular sleep time.

    C. Mr. Smith is able to return demonstration of deep breathing and relaxation techniques.

    D. Mr. Smith reports, "I have a hard time getting to sleep at night."

11. Which of the following medications would you expect to be prescribed for Mr. Smith?

    A. Chlorpromazine (Thorazine)

    B. Benzotropine (Cogentin)

    C. Zolpidem (Ambien)

    D. Provigil (Modafinil)

12. The average number of sleep cycles experienced by an adult is

    A. 8 to 10

    B. 4 to 6

    C. 1

    D. 2 to 3

13. Which of the following is the third stage of sleep?

    A. Light sleep where the body processes continue to slow down, eyes are still, heart and respiratory rates decrease slightly, and body temperature falls.

    B. Very light sleep, person feels drowsy and relaxed, his eyes roll from side to side, and he is easy to arouse.

    C. Deep sleep begins; brain begins to generate slow delta waves.

    D. Very deep sleep with rhythmic breathing, limited muscular movement; delta waves are produced by the brain.

14. During sleep, REM occurs

    A. Every 90 minutes

    B. Twice a night

    C. Every 30 minutes

    D. Every 10 minutes

15. Which of the following statements is true about the function of sleep?

    A. The effects of sleep on the body are not completely understood.

    B. Sleep restores the balance within the nervous system and is necessary for protein synthesis.

    C. Inadequate sleep will result in a deterioration of mental functioning.

    D. All of the above.

16. The most common sleep disorder is

    A. Hypersomnia

    B. Narcolepsy

    C. Insomnia

    D. Parasomnia

17. A main focus in the care of an individual experiencing a sleep disturbance would be

    A. Enhance the person's feeling of well-being.

    B. Improve the quality of sleep.

   C. Improve the quantity of sleep.

   D. Develop or maintain a sleeping pattern that will allow for sufficient energy for ADLs.

18. Sleep hygiene is defined as:

   A. Ensuring that one is clean before going to bed.

   B. Interventions used to promote sleep.

   C. Health teaching about sleep habits, support of bedtime rituals, providing a restful environment, promotion of comfort and relaxation, and use of sleep medications.

   D. B and C.

19. Most sleep medications affect which phase of sleep the most?

   A. Stage II

   B. Stages III and IV

   C. REM

   D. NREM

20. You are asked to provide an information presentation on sleep at the monthly PTA meeting. During the question-and-answer phase, a woman makes the comment, "My 10-year-old daughter sleeps eight hours a night. I have a terrible time getting her up in the morning." The most appropriate response you could offer is:

   A. "At her age, she needs to be responsible to awaken without help."

   B. "Children your daughter's age need 10 to 11 hours of sleep each night, but many don't get that much because of the demands on them and free-time activities."

   C. "During the school week you should not allow her to watch TV in the evening."

   D. "If she is tired, you should encourage her to take a nap after school."

Matching

21. Biological rhythms	**A.** The inability to fall asleep or remain asleep
22. Electro-oculogram	**B.** The study of sleep
23. Sleep	**C.** A cyclical, repeated variation in a biological function that exists in plants, animals, and humans controlled from within the body and synchronized with environmental factors
24. Somnology	**D.** Rest with suspension of voluntary bodily functions and consciousness
25. REM sleep	**E.** A condition characterized by sudden, brief attacks of muscle weakness, causing the body to fall helplessly (is usually associated with narcolepsy)
26. RAS	**F.** Recurrent period of sleep, typically totaling two hours a night, during which most dreaming occurs
27. Electroencephalogram	**G.** Of or pertaining to the night
28. Sleep hygiene	**H.** Transient immobility experienced when falling asleep or waking up
29. Sleep apnea	**I.** Visual, auditory, or tactile sensory impairments experienced at sleep onset or when waking up

30. Circadian

31. Delta sleep

32. Tryptophan

33. Hypnotic

34. Insomnia

J. Characterized by frequent short breathing pauses during sleep

K. A condition where an individual gets sufficient sleep at night, but is unable to remain awake during the day

L. An amino acid that can promote sleep

M. Also referred to as an EEG, used to monitor brain waves

N. Part of the reticular formation that extends from the brain stem to the midbrain and thalamus with connections distributed through the cerebral cortex that controls the activity of the CNS (sleep, wake)

O. A term used to describe actions used to promote sleep

P. Occurs during stages III or IV of sleep where it is difficult to awaken, represented by slower brain waves

Q. A disorder of excessive daytime sleepiness caused by lack of hypocretin in the area of the CNS that regulates sleep

R. Also known as EOG, monitors eye movement

S. Category of medication that induces sleep

T. Rhythmic biological cycle recurring at approximately 24-hour intervals

Chapter 14 Answers

Multiple Choice

1. B. Sleep is a time when the body rests and restores itself; however, it is an active state. The sleep requirement does not change as an individual ages. Cognitive functioning deteriorates with sleep deprivation.

2. A. The reticular activating system is a network of ascending nerve fibers involved with the sleep-wake cycle (bodily and behavioral alertness).

3. D. The reticular activating system (RAS) is located in the brain stem.

4. D. Insomnia is treated by assisting the individual to learn new behavior patterns (creating an optimal sleep environment, developing a more positive approach to sleep, developing appropriate sleep patterns) and medications effectively. The other statements are true about insomnia.

5. D. Sudden cessation of barbiturate medication can result in withdrawal problems. These medications must be tapered under supervision of the prescribing clinician. This response incorporates that knowledge and validates the individual's wishes.

6. C. Night-shift workers typically experience difficulty falling asleep during the daylight hours and experience less sleep than other workers. Minimizing the exposure to light will assist you in facilitating sleep. Melatonin, a hormone produced by the pineal gland, helps to control the wake-sleep cycle. Light affects how much melatonin your body produces (typically levels are higher at night than during the morning/day). Exercise can result in stimulating the body, thereby increasing the difficulty to fall asleep.

Alcohol disrupts REM sleep, although it may well hasten sleep itself. Foods containing tryptophan may be helpful in inducing sleep; however, it is not recommended that a large meal be ingested for various reasons (proper weight management, increased work to digest large quantities of food, etc.).

7. **D.** Staff communication is a significant interruption of sleep, particularly at the shift change report. Awareness of this should be reinforced, as well as planning care to interrupt, as minimally as possible, the patient's night sleep. The use of white noise to block or decrease the negative affect of environmental stimulus is recommended, if available.

8. **A.** Zolpidem (Ambien) is used for short-term management of insomnia, reduces sleep latency and awakenings, and lengthens sleep duration. It does not reduce REM sleep durations or cause rebound insomnia when discontinued.

9. **B.** An actual nursing diagnosis is a problem present at the time of the nursing assessment and is based upon the presence of associated signs and symptoms. An actual nursing diagnosis has three components: the NANDA-approved nursing impairment, the factors contributing (or probable causes of the response), and defining characteristics manifested by the patient. In the formulation of the diagnostic statement, the nursing problem and etiology are joined by the words "related to" rather than "due to." The focus is to identify a relationship between the two. The phrase "due to" specifies that one causes the other. The other responses are incorrect because they do not contain NANDA-approved impairments or are formatted incorrectly.

10. **B.** The nursing action (intervention) is the fourth phase of the nursing process. It is the action phase where the nurse performs the nursing interventions. A is an example of a goal, C is an example of the evaluation phase, and D demonstrates an assessment.

11. **C.** A is an antipsychotic, B is an anticholinergic, and D is a CNS stimulant (used to promote wakefulness for those diagnosed with narcolepsy, shift work sleep disorder, etc.).

12. **B.** During a normal night of sleep, an adult experiences four to six sleep cycles, each with NREM (quiet sleep) and REM (rapid-eye-movement) sleep.

13. **C.** The third stage of sleep is a transitional period between the second and fourth stage, where delta waves begin to emerge. Response A indicates the second stage of sleep, B is the first stage, and D is the fourth stage.

14. **A.** REM sleep recurs about every 90 minutes and lasts for 5 to 30 minutes.

15. **D.** While the functions of sleep are not fully understood, it is accepted knowledge that sleep is essential and exerts physiologic effects on the nervous system and other body structures. Individuals who experience inadequate levels of sleep experience increased emotionality, irritability, and impairments in concentration and decision making.

16. **C.** Insomnia is the most common sleep complaint.

17. **D.** While each of the goals offered are relevant, the major goal would be for the individual to establish/maintain an adequate sleep pattern to provide energy required to attend to ADLs.

18. **D.** Sleep hygiene is used to describe actions used to promote sleep, and includes nursing interventions employed to enhance the quantity and quality of an individual's sleep. It is typically focused on nonpharmacologic actions.

19. **C.** Sleep medications affect REM sleep more than NREM (stages I to IV) sleep. Patient education for those individuals receiving medications should include the information that they may experience increased dreaming (REM rebound) after the medication is discontinued.

20. **B.** The best response is to provide information about the sleep requirements for the age range and assist in formulating a plan to investigate options. A child of 10 would not be expected to be responsible to wake for school independently. Response C assumes that television watching is the cause, and naps during the day can result in sleep disturbances at night.

Matching

21. C
22. R
23. D
24. B
25. F
26. N
27. M
28. O
29. J
30. T

31. P
32. L
33. S
34. A
35. Q
36. K
37. H
38. E
39. I
40. G